Short Implants

Boyd J. Tomasetti • Rolf Ewers
Editors

Short Implants

Springer

Editors
Boyd J. Tomasetti
Department of Oral and Maxillofacial Surgery
Denver Health and Hospitals
Denver, CO
USA

Tomasetti and McLain Oral and
Maxillofacial Surgery
Littleton, CO
USA

Rolf Ewers
CMF Institute Vienna
Vienna, Austria

ISBN 978-3-030-44198-2 ISBN 978-3-030-44199-9 (eBook)
https://doi.org/10.1007/978-3-030-44199-9

This Springer imprint is published by the registered company Springer Nature Switzerland AG
The registered company address is: Gewerbestrasse 11, 6330 Cham, Switzerland

This book is dedicated to all of those who have been instrumental in our training and committed to advances in Dental Implantology. Of particular note are the following:

Professor Dr. Per Ingvar Branemark—the father of modern osseointegration. Without him, none of us would be involved in dental implants.

Professor Dr. Wilfried Schilli—he was the consummate teacher, training many of the present chiefs of Oral and Maxillofacial Surgery in Europe and sharing his knowledge around the world.

Dr. Axel Kirsch—one of the many who expanded upon Professor Branemark's original premise. He was always a willing sounding board for our thoughts and ideas.

Dr. Vincent Morgan—among the first to realize that short implants may actually work and then had the courage to continually push the envelope with short and ultrashort implants.

Dr. Stephen Quarcoo—the consummate mentor who spent his career training future Oral and Maxillofacial Surgeons. He always had a smile and willingness to help no matter the situation.

Finally, all of those practitioners who were willing to use short implants despite extremely harsh critics who berated them both in the literature and from the podium.

There are a multitude of other surgeons, restorative dentists, and organizations who supported us along the long path to making short and ultrashort implants a standard of care. Among them are the AAOMS—they were willing to give us a forum for short implants, Dr. Shadi Daher—always willing to share his knowledge, Dr. Rainier Urdaneta—a prodigious researcher, and Dr. John K Schulte, one of the first prosthodontists to recognize that short implants had a place in modern restorative dentistry.

We would be remiss without thanking Ms. Rosanna Jenkins and Dr. Hildegund Ewers for their encouragement and support.

Vail/Denver, CO Boyd J. Tomasetti DMD

Vienna, Austria Rolf Ewers DMD, MD, PhD

Foreword

You are at peace
when you don't need more or less.

—Rumi

Titanium orthopedic bone screws adapted by Branemark more than 50 years ago for use in the oral cavity were found to heal intimately to alveolar bone with biomechanical capacity to support a dental prosthesis [1]. The healed titanium bone interface, once stressed by dental occlusal function, led to significant bone strain increasing peri-implant bone density via the mechanostat termed "osseointegration." Remarkably, once osseointegrated, implant stability actually increased over time. But the dental restorative question remained: How much titanium surface area, that is, *how long*, did a titanium screw need to be?

Worldwide, the introduction of dental implants in the 1980s subsequently led to a *quantitative* bone classification in 1989 [2]. This first site classification used as a starting intuition *10 mm of osseointegration*, a somewhat arbitrary standard based on clinical expert opinion at the time for what became known as an optimal implant site. This implied that 10 mm of bone would osseointegrate upon a 10 mm titanium screw surface. When less bone was available, such as 7 mm, the site was described as less optimal and so on. This intuitive and seemingly self-evident classification became engrained in treatment planning bedrock. Basically, the surgeons of the time and since have looked for a 10 mm site as an ideal implant site without substantial scientific demarcation for doing so.

The schismatic idea of using shorter implants such as 7 or 8 mm length implants, and now 5 or 6 mm length implants, was considered biomechanically improbable if not impossible.

But recently, there have been symposia, even consensus conferences, on the use of short implants as an alternative for augmentation bone grafting to gain vertical height. Remarkably, short implants of approximately 6 mm in length were determined to be a clinically effective treatment suggesting a lack of necessity for bone grafting [3].

If the field of implant dentistry is undergoing a change in orthodoxy, a revision of the implant site classification is warranted as the net effect of short implant disruptive innovation is to decrease the amount of vertical bone height needed for optimal implant restoration.

Therefore, an updated classification describes a new "optimal" implant site as 8 mm in which no grafting is required (Class A) and a second category of 4–7 mm, where grafting may *also* not be required (Class B). This is a rather extraordinary change in thinking and is basically the subject of this book—a paradigm shattering exposition regarding *what is needed and what is not needed* in order to accomplish acceptable implant dentistry. Shockingly, what the classification advocates is that alveolar bone grafting may not be necessary except in markedly deficient states such as 3 mm or less in height (Class C)! [4].

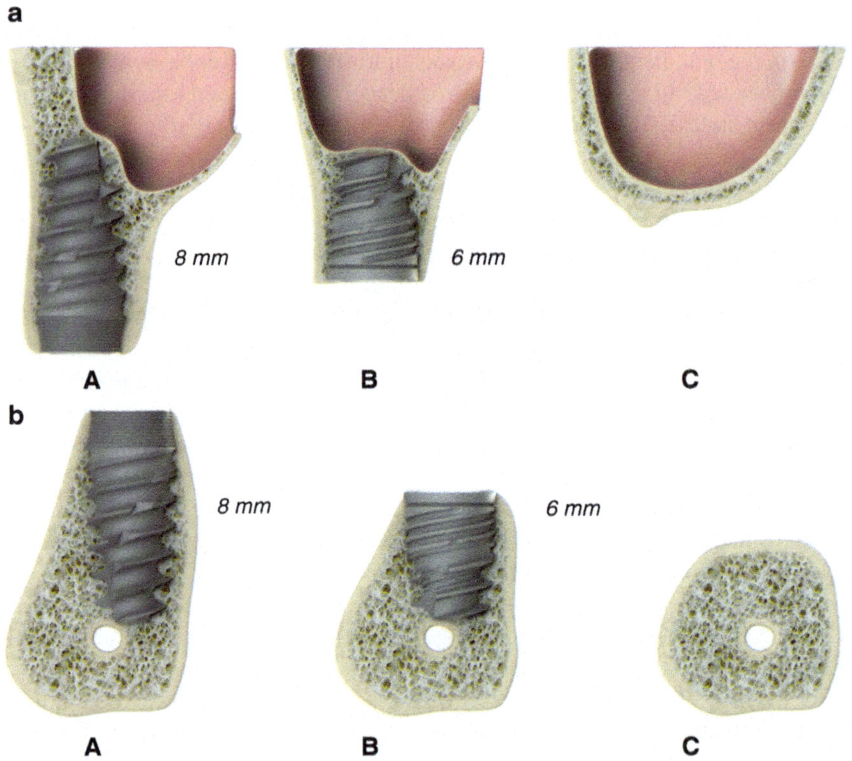

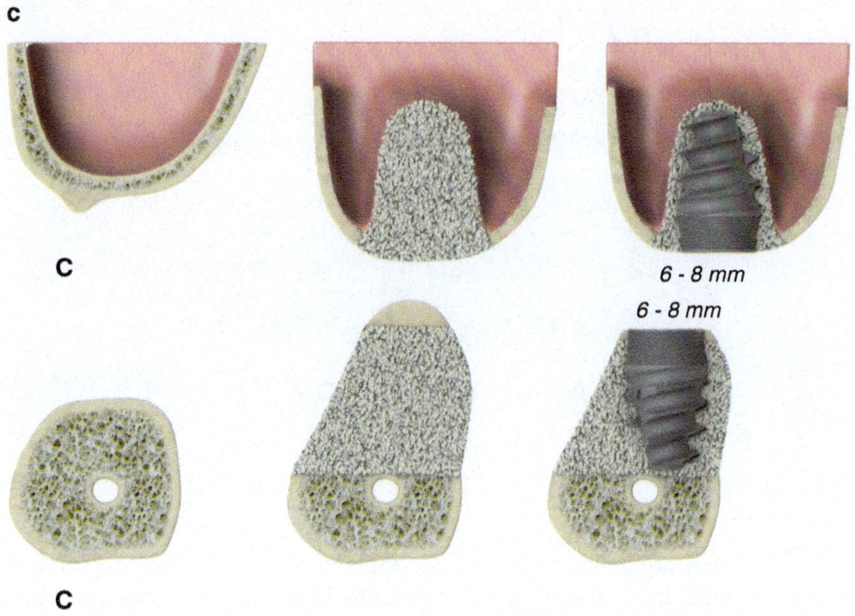

The diagram shown below was used to classify the sinus bone graft as it related to available bone in a study published in 1991 [5]. The way this might look today with shorter implants is shown in the second image where 8 mm of bone does not require sinus penetration, a 4–7 mm height requires minimal if any sinus membrane elevation with simultaneous implant placement; and only for the 1–3 mm sinus floor setting is a bone graft prescribed, done prior to implant placement—a much different practice than was recommended 30 years ago [4].

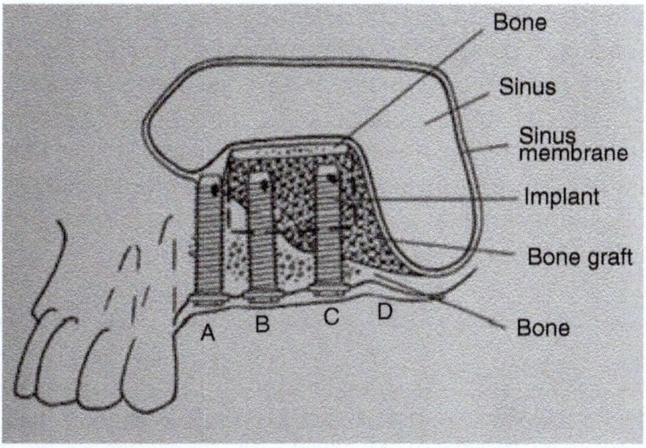

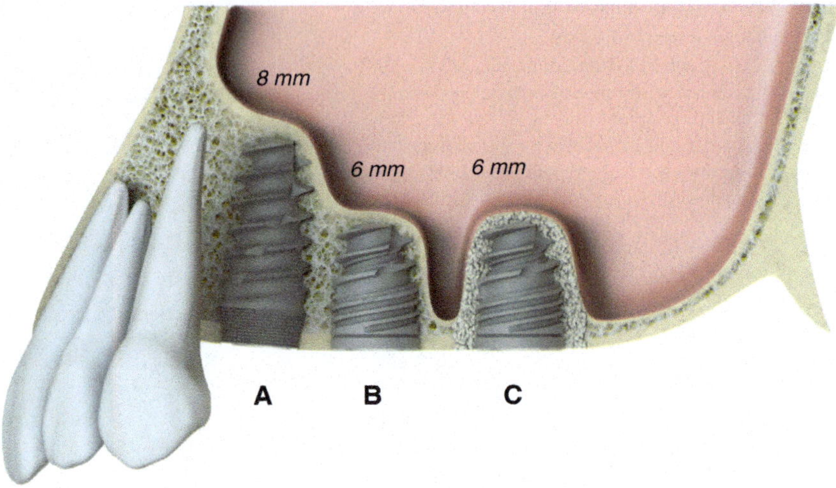

One common argument against short implants is prospective peri-implantitis leading to bone loss. Precision-fit abutments have lessened bacterial leakage decreasing the risk for peri-implant bone loss, but biofilm remains a problem whatever the connection or surface treatment. This then becomes the last problem to solve to demarcate implant length. If the risk of peri-implant bone loss is negligible, then one may surmise that the need for "fail-safe" length can be reduced proportionately such that perhaps only 5 or 6 mm of a well-osseointegrated implant height might be sufficient long term in the vast majority of settings.

Various antimicrobial technologies will likely be incorporated onto implant surfaces in the future which will serve to solidify a preference for shorter implants even more [6]. Thus, the recalcitrant need within the dental profession for treatment strategies using longer implants will likely subside.

Hopefully, this book and its many scientific chapters will lead the skeptical to cognitive dissonance, a sense of dis-ease so profound that the reader will soon find him or herself in a place of conciliation where one does not want for more or less than is needed. An adjustment from heuristic thinking is long overdue. This text then asks each practitioner to pause and reflect a moment, to consider recent clinical research findings for the use of shorter implants and take advantage of the technological development of implant macro- and micro-design in order to provide less invasive but still highly acceptable treatment for patients.

References

1. Branemark PI, Adell R, Breine U, Hansson BO, Lindstrom J, Ohlsson A. Intra-osseous anchorage of dental prostheses. I. Experimental studies. Scan J Plast Reconstr Surg. 1969;3(2):81–100.
2. Jensen O. Site classification for the osseointegrated implant. J Prosthet Dent. 1989;61(2):228–34.
3. Jung RE, et al. Group 1 ITI consensus report: the influence of implant length and design and medications on clinical and patient-reported outcomes. Clin Oral Implants Res. 2018; 29 Suppl 16:66–77.

4. Jensen OT, Evers R. Glick P. Site classification of the osseointegrated implant: update 2020. J Prosthet Dent. (In submission).
5. Jensen OT, Greer RO. Immediate placement of osseointegrating implants into the maxillary sinus augmented with mineralized cancellous allograft and Gore-tex membrane: second stage surgical and histological findings. In: Laney WR, Tolman DE, editors. Tissue integration in oral, orthopedic and maxillofacial reconstruction. Chicago: Quintessence; 1991. p. 321–33.
6. Zaltsman N. Ionescu AC, Weiss E, Brambilla E, Beyth S, Beyth N. Surface modified nanoparticles as anti-biofilm filler for dental polymers. PLoS One. 2017;12(12):e189397.

Ole T. Jensen
Department of Oral and Maxillofacial Surgery
University of Utah
Salt Lake City
UT, USA

Contents

1 **A Short History of Dental Implants** 1
Boyd J. Tomasetti

2 **Short Implants: Indications and Contraindications** 9
Boyd J. Tomasetti and Rolf Ewers

3 **Short Implants and Early Brånemark Team Developments: Heritage Established at the Outset** 25
Oded Bahat, Yvan Fortin, Martin L. Kolinski, Franck Renouard, and Richard M. Sullivan

4 **The Short Implant Heritage Continues: The Possibility of Reduced Grafting Without Restorative Compromise** 33
Oded Bahat, Yvan Fortin, Martin L. Kolinski, Franck Renouard, and Richard M. Sullivan

5 **The Straumann Short Implants** 47
Waldemar D. Polido and Dean Morton

6 **Short Implants: Historical Perspectives** 59
Clarence Lindquist

7 **Significance of Bone–Implant Contact in Short Implants and Clinical Impact** 81
Reha S. Kisnisci and Ismail Doruk Kocyigit

8 **The Survival of Short and Ultrashort Plateau Root Form Implants** 95
Rainier A. Urdaneta and Sung-Kiang Chuang

9 **Short Implant in Cleft Cases** 125
Dusan Poruban, Rastislav Slavik, and Adam Stebel

10 **Rehabilitation of Tumour Patients with Ultra-Short Implants and TRINIA Bridges** 143
Rolf Ewers and Rudolf Seemann

11 Minimally Invasive Sinus Lift Using Short Implants 161
Mauro Marincola, Rolf Ewers, and Boyd J. Tomasetti

12 The Use of Short and Ultrashort Implants in Atrophic Jaws 177
Rolf Ewers, Boyd J. Tomasetti, Vincent J. Morgan, and Angelo Perpetuini

13 Restorative Techniques for Bicon Short® Implants 205
Kristina Pisarik, Angelo Perpetuini, Laura Murcko, Katherine Morgan, Drauseo Speratti, Muneki Hirayama, and Jordyn Hollingsworth

14 Grow Your Practice Utilizing the Short Implant 315
Rosanna Jenkins

Contributors

Oded Bahat, BDS, MSD, FACD Private Practice Periodontology, Beverly Hills, CA, USA

Sung-Kiang Chuang Department of Oral Health Policy and Epidemiology, Harvard School of Dental Medicine, Boston, MA, USA

Rolf Ewers CMF Institute Vienna, Vienna, Austria

Yvan Fortin, DMD Private Practice-Retired, Levis, QC, Canada

Muneki Hirayama Implant Dentistry Centre, Boston, MA, USA

Bicon, Tokyo, Japan

Jordyn Hollingsworth Midwestern University College of Dental Medicine, Downers Grove, IL, USA

Rosanna Jenkins Founder of "the new face of 60", CEO Rx Marketing, Denver, CO, USA

Reha S. Kisnisci Professor, Department of Oral and Maxillofacial Surgery, School of Dentistry, Ankara University, Ankara, Turkey

Ismail Doruk Kocyigit Department of Oral and Maxillofacial Surgery, Former Resident in Ankara University, Currently Assoc. Prof, School of Dentistry, Kirikkale University, Kirikkale, Turkey

Martin L. Kolinski, DDS Midwest Dental Implantology, St. Charles, IL, USA

Clarence Lindquist Chevy Chase Oral and Implant Surgery, Chevy Chase, MD, USA

Mauro Marincola, DDS, MDS Clinical Director Implant Dentistry, University of Cartagena, School of Dentistry, Bolívar, Colombia

Katherine Morgan Implant Dentistry Centre, Boston, MA, USA

Vincent J. Morgan Bicon, Boston, MA, USA

Dean Morton Indiana University School of Dentistry, Indianapolis, IN, USA

Laura Murcko Implant Dentistry Centre, Boston, MA, USA

Angelo Perpetuini Dental Laboratory, Rome, Italy

Master Dental Technician, Bicon, Rome, Italy

Kristina Pisarik Bicon, Boston, MA, USA

Implant Dentistry Centre, Boston, MA, USA

Waldemar D. Polido Indiana University School of Dentistry, Indianapolis, IN, USA

Dusan Poruban Department of Maxillofacial Surgery, F.D. Roosevelt University Hospital, Banska Bystrica, Slovakia

Dental and Oro-Maxillofacial Surgery Office StomEst, Bratislava, Slovakia

Franck Renouard, DDS Private Practice Oral and Maxillofacial Surgery, Paris, France

Rudolf Seemann, PhD, MSc, MD, DMD, MBA Department of Otorhinolaryngology, Institute of Head and Neck Diseases, Evangelical Hospital, Vienna, Austria

Rastislav Slavik Department of Maxillofacial Surgery, F.D. Roosevelt University Hospital, Banska Bystrica, Slovakia

Medical Faculty of Comenius' University, Bratislava, Slovakia

Drauseo Speratti Bicon, Boston, MA, USA

Midwestern University College of Dental Medicine, Glendale, AZ, USA

Midwestern University College of Dental Medicine, Downers Grove, IL, USA

Adam Stebel Department of Maxillofacial Surgery, F.D. Roosevelt University Hospital, Banska Bystrica, Slovakia

Medical Faculty of Comenius' University, Bratislava, Slovakia

Richard M. Sullivan, DDS Vice President, Clinical Technologies, Nobel Biocare (Retired), Yorba Linda, CA, USA

Boyd J. Tomasetti Department of Oral and Maxillofacial Surgery, Denver Health and Hospitals, Denver, CO, USA

Tomasetti and McLain Oral and Maxillofacial Surgery, Littleton, CO, USA

Rainier A. Urdaneta Private Practice, Shrewsbury, MA, USA

A Short History of Dental Implants

1

Boyd J. Tomasetti

Contents

References.. 6

We like to think that dental implants have been around for only the last hundred or so years. Archaeologists, however, have found evidence of dental implants in both ancient Mayan and Egyptian civilizations [1, 2]. The Mayan find appears to have been a successful implant of a shell which osseointegrated. The ancient Egyptian findings were most likely placed postmortem. Fast forward to Renaissance times and there is evidence that implant placement was somewhat common, at least among the Nobility [3]. These implants were usually from a human donor (probably unwilling live donors or fresh corpses) or animals.

The use of donor implants from both live and dead persons seems to have fallen from favor by the mid-1600s. Perhaps, substantial failures were seen or there were significant life-threatening infections secondary to the implants—we certainly did not see sterile or even clean procedures being performed! Implants are seen again in the early nineteenth century when Maggiolo makes a tooth root replica from gold. Maggiolo, in his treatise in 1807 [4], mentions an aseptic technique which certainly had to help with implant survival. By the late 1800s there were a variety of implant shapes and materials in use.

B. J. Tomasetti (✉)
Department of Oral and Maxillofacial Surgery, Denver Health and Hospitals, Denver, CO, USA

Tomasetti and McLain Oral and Maxillofacial Surgery, Littleton, CO, USA
e-mail: bjtrmoms@aol.com

B. J. Tomasetti, R. Ewers (eds.), *Short Implants*,
https://doi.org/10.1007/978-3-030-44199-9_1

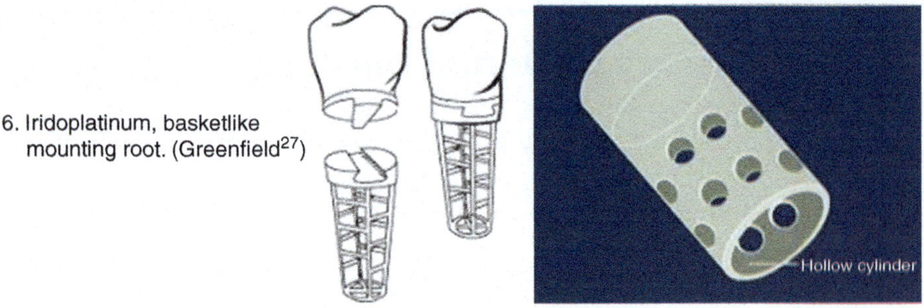

Fig. 1.1 The Greenfield basket implant and an early cylindrical implant

The beginning of the twentieth century heralded the early forays into the modern era of dental implants. In 1913, Greenfield [5] described an implant/prosthetic combination that can be considered the forerunner of implants as we know them. Greenfield was one of the first practitioners to give reports on long-term survival of his implants. He postulated on the mechanism of the implant to bone interface actually theorizing on what we now know as osseointegration. Some aspects of his designs were still being used in the late 1980s—compare his basket design to one of the early basket-type implants (Fig. 1.1).

Unfortunately, like many great pioneers, Greenfield's advancements were met with great skepticism, criticism, and mistruths. Within a few years, the Greenfield basket implant was abandoned.

One of Greenfield's mistakes was in the choice of materials used in his implants. He used an iridium/platinum alloy that was not as compatible with the soft tissue and bone as other materials. In the 1930s, there was a push by researchers to find a material that would meet the requirements of compatibility with both tissue and bone, resistance to oral fluids and the strength needed to withstand occlusal forces. In 1937, Venable [6] and his fellow researchers published a paper extolling the properties found in vitallium, an alloy of chrome cobalt and molybdenum. Bothe et al. [7], experimented with both vitallium and titanium. With respect to their findings with titanium, they reported that "… the bone had a tendency to grow into contact with it." Their results were published in 1940—a time when titanium was expensive and World War II was about to start, thus putting a damper on further research.

The 1950s and 1960s marked the beginning of the modern dental implant era. Foremost among the early pioneers was Leonard Linkow [8] who developed a blade implant and early screw implant. Per Ingvar Branemark [9] began his early research with titanium and started his landmark studies resulting in the establishment of osseointegration as the standard by which we measure all implants (Figs. 1.2 and 1.3).

In 1978, the NIH and Harvard held a Consensus Conference [10] that looked at blade, subperiosteal, staple, vitreous carbon, and transosteal implants. It is interesting that among the findings with respect to transosteal implants was the notation that there was insufficient data and that further research was needed.

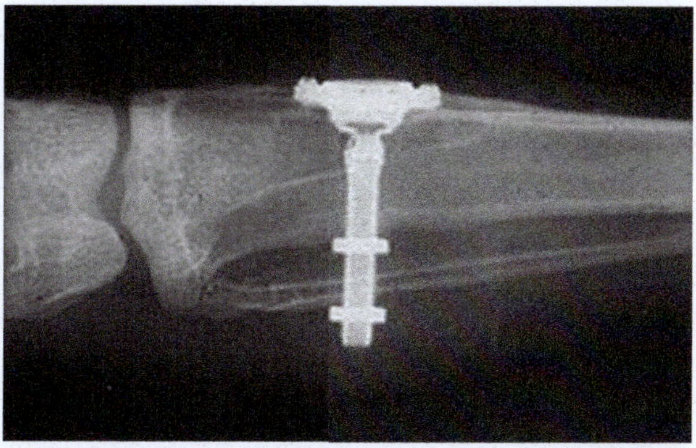

Fig. 1.2 Branemark's original rabbit study

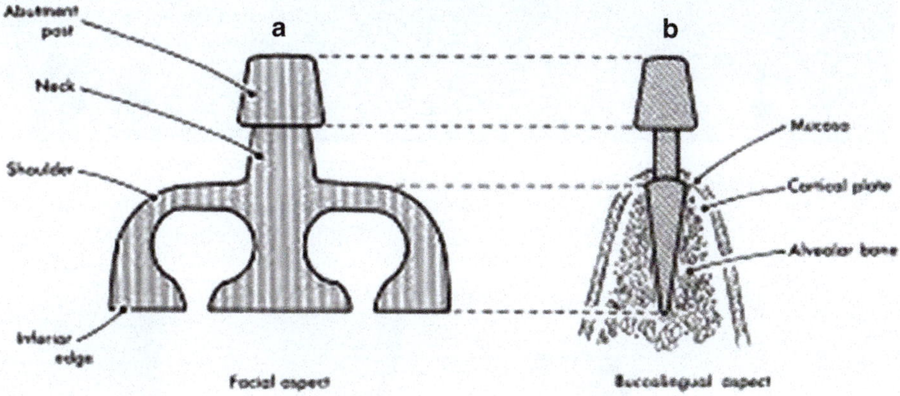

Fig. 1.3 The Linkow blade implant

One recommendation was that "… a minimum of 25 mm of available bone (measured) from alveolar ridge crest to inferior border" was needed for successful placement [10].

The dental implant world was dramatically changed in 1982 when Branemark presented his research and long-term findings at an invitational conference in Toronto [11, 12]. Shortly after, the Branemark implant system was brought to the US market and the whole implant world exploded! (Fig. 1.4).

Initially, osseointegrated implants were used for the treatment of edentulous patients only and, per the original Branemark protocol, were placed in the anterior mandible. It wasn't long before Branemark had competition and implants were being used in the maxilla and as single tooth replacements. At this time, implants were still fairly long (13–16 mm) but many companies were beginning to produce shorter ones. By the mid- to late-1980s 10–11 mm implants were bring used and research was beginning on even shorter implants (Fig. 1.5).

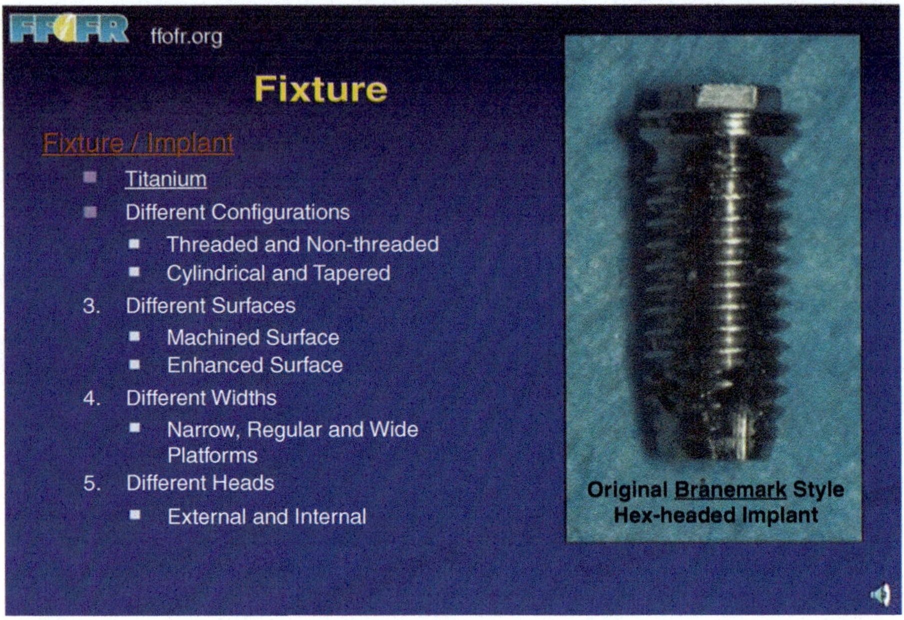

Fig. 1.4 The original Branemark threaded implant

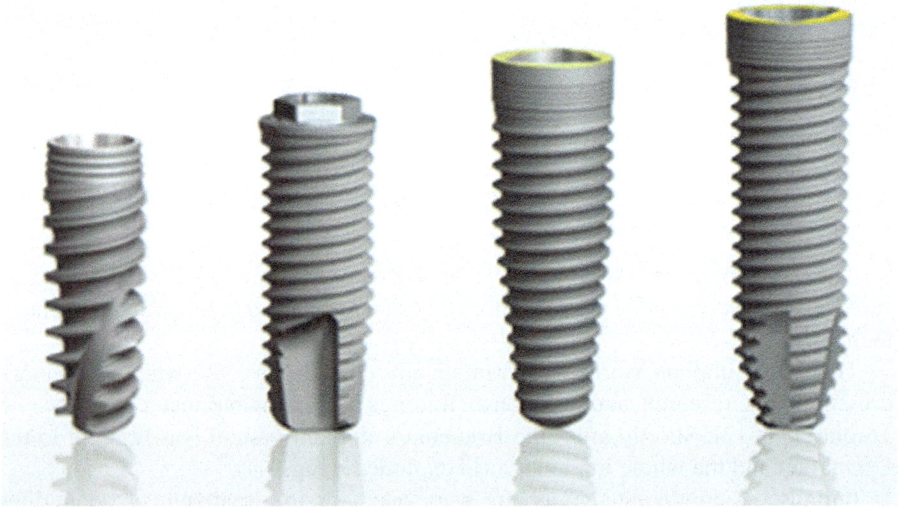

Fig. 1.5 Early coated threaded implants

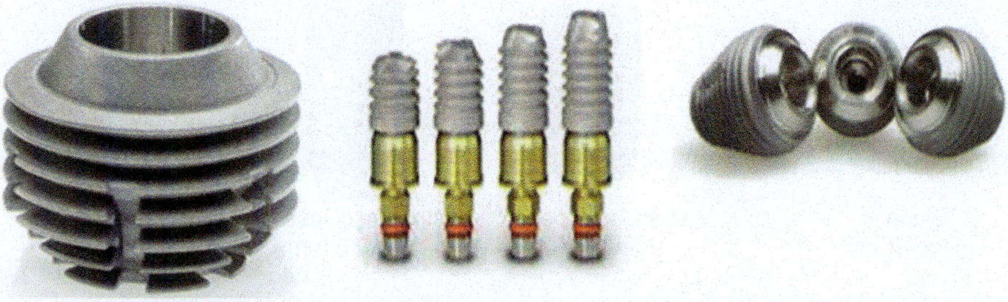

Fig. 1.6 Early short implants

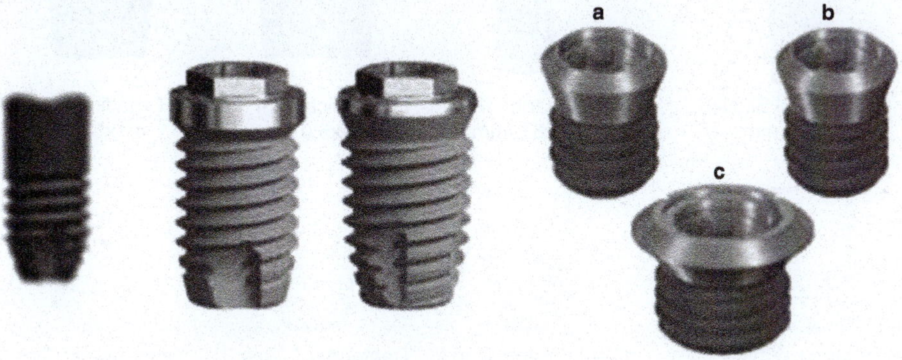

Fig. 1.7 Early Nobel, Astra, and Straumann short implants

Short implants, those that were 8–10 mm, initially were the purview of the smaller implant companies. 7br, MegaGen, Bicon, Jeneric, and BTI among others began to develop these 8–10 mm implants (Fig. 1.6).

It was not long before the larger implant companies—Nobel, Astra, and Straumann—released their research and development of short implants (Fig. 1.7).

The next obvious question for the R&D people was how short can we make an implant and still have long-term success? The result was the development of the ultrashort osseointegrated implant (Fig. 1.8).

Implants are now produced with 5–6 mm lengths, obviating the need for extensive grafting. Short and narrow implants allow the practitioner to place implants in locations that would have been impossible 10–15 years ago. Many practitioners are still skeptical of the ultrashort implant but recent research has shown success similar to short (8–10 mm) and traditional (above 10 mm) length implants. In many cases the use of short and ultrashort implants has obviated the need for grafting.

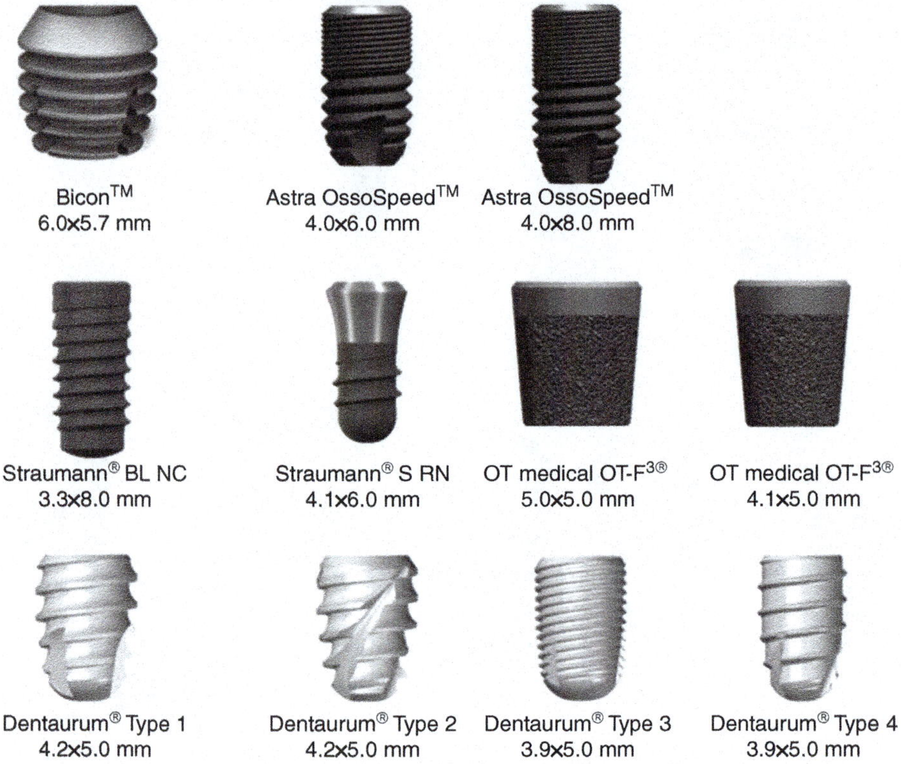

Fig. 1.8 Short and ultrashort implants 5–8 mm with and without collars

References

1. Bobbio A. The first endosseous alloplastic implant in the history of man. Bull Hist Dent. 1972;20:1–6.
2. Forshaw R. The practice of dentistry in ancient Egypt. Br Dent J. 2009;206:481–6.
3. Noble H. Tooth transplantation: a controversial story. History of Dentistry Research Group Newsletter. 2002.
4. Maggiolo J. Le Manuel De L'Art Du Dentiste. 1807.
5. Greenfield E. Implantation of artificial crown and bridge abutments. Dent Cosmos. 1913;55:364–9.
6. Venable C, et al. The effects on bone of the presence of metals based upon electrolysis: an experimental study. Ann Surg. 1937;105:917–38.
7. Bothe R, et al. Reaction of bone to multiple metallic implants. Surg Gynecol Obstet. 1940;71:598–602.
8. Linkow L. Clinical evaluation of the various designed endosseous implants. J Oral Implant Transplant Surg. 1966;12:35–46.
9. Branemark P, et al. Intra osseous anchorage of dental prostheses, experimental studies. Scand J Plast Reconstr Surg. 1969;3:81–100.

10. National Institutes of Health Dental Implants Benefits and Risks Consensus Development Conference Statement June 13–14 1978.
11. Branemark P. Osseointegration and its experimental background. J Prosthet Dent. 1983;50:399–410.
12. Branemark P, et al. Osseointegrated implants in the treatment of the edentulous jaw: experience from a 10 year period. Scand J Plast Reconstruct Surg Suppl. 1977;16:1–132.

Short Implants: Indications and Contraindications

2

Boyd J. Tomasetti and Rolf Ewers

Contents

References 22

For the most part, the indications and contraindications for short and ultrashort implants are not significantly different than those for traditional length implants. A review of the literature shows considerable indications for implant usage—both traditional lengths, short and ultrashort implants. It is well documented that the initial indication for osseointegrated traditional length implants was to assist in mandibular denture retention [1, 2]. It was not long before the indications expanded and at the present time there is a plethora of clinical uses for both traditional and short osseointegrated implants. Among these indications are the following:

- Edentulous mandibular and maxillary arches.
- Single tooth replacement.
- Multiple tooth replacements to include implant supported prostheses.
- Inability to tolerate the material, coverage, bulk, etc. of a traditional prosthesis.
- The patient's desire to not have a removable prosthesis.
- Patient inability to tolerate a removable prosthesis.

B. J. Tomasetti (✉)
Department of Oral and Maxillofacial Surgery, Denver Health and Hospitals, Denver, CO, USA

Tomasetti and McLain Oral and Maxillofacial Surgery, Littleton, CO, USA
e-mail: bjtrmoms@aol.com

R. Ewers
CMF Institute Vienna, Vienna, Austria
e-mail: rolf@cmf-vienna.com

B. J. Tomasetti, R. Ewers (eds.), *Short Implants*,
https://doi.org/10.1007/978-3-030-44199-9_2

With respect to contraindications for dental implants, one needs to look at both absolute and relative contraindications. Over the past 40–50 years, there has been a significant change in both absolute and relative types of contraindications. What was once considered an absolute contraindication has now become mainstream. For example, at one time smoking (or any tobacco use) was thought to be an absolute contraindication. Studies in the past 10–15 years have shown that there is no to very little change in implant success rate when nonsmokers and smokers are compared. In 2005, Ewers reported on a 95.6% implant success rate of implants placed in grafted sinuses—this included smokers [3].

When dental implants were first introduced, many of the initial contraindications revolved around the amount of bone available for implant placement. Initial Branemark training recommended bicortical placement of the implants in the edentulous mandible. The general thinking was that a minimum of a 10 mm length was needed in the mandible and 13 mm in the maxilla. A 1991 report by Friberg et al. [4] looked at 4641 consecutively placed Branemark implants. They found a failure rate of 7.1% of 7 mm implants in the fully edentulous maxilla and 3.1% in fully edentulous mandibles. Interestingly, they found no difference between the 7 mm implants and traditional length implants in partially edentulous jaws. With the advent of extensive grafting procedures along with the continuing success of short and ultrashort implants, implant length no longer plays a role in implant success. A 2017 European Consensus Conference on short, angulated and diameter reduced implants found that short implants were a reliable treatment option [5].

Presently, it appears that absolute contraindications to dental implant placement are primarily related to advanced medical problems

- Significantly medically compromised patients including those patients that are unable to withstand the anesthetic—local or sedation—necessary for the procedure.
- Uncontrolled diabetic patients. Once controlled, these patients have either a relative or no contraindication.
- Patients who have undergone treatment with bisphosphonate-related medications and have documented evidence of bisphosphonate-related bone necrosis. The mere usage of, or exposure to, bisphosphonates is a relative contraindication to dental implant placement.
- Placement of implants in bone that has had heavy radiation exposure to both the bone and surrounding soft tissue.
- Uncontrolled immuno-suppressive disease.

When we begin to discuss relative contraindications for dental implants, there are factors that may apply to traditional length implants but not to short and ultrashort implants. Some relative contraindications may include:

- A variety of systemic diseases. Consultation and coordination with the relevant Medical personnel will go a long way to alleviating any potential problems.
- Heavy smoking. Patients should be counseled on the potential detrimental effects on implant longevity as well as general health problems.
- Poor oral hygiene. Those patients who have lost their teeth through dental neglect or periodontal problems secondary to poor oral hygiene should be counseled about the need for good home care and regular preventive dental care.
- Lack of adequate alveolar bone. All implants—traditional, short and ultrashort—require a certain amount of alveolar bone height and width.

The lack of alveolar bone is where we find a divergence between the traditional, short, and ultrashort implants. For example, an alveolar bone height of less than 8 mm may be a contraindication to placement of traditional length implants if the patient elects not to have a graft procedure. This same patient may be able to have an ultrashort 5–6 mm implant placed. Along the same vein, posterior maxillary alveolar bone height of 4–6 mm may require grafting with all implants. However, with short or ultrashort implants, this grafting may only require an internal minimally invasive sinus graft versus a full lateral approach sinus graft [6].

An additional relative contraindication for implant placement has been in adolescents. It has been long been held that implants should not be placed until growth has ceased [7]. Recent reports have shown that short implants can be successfully placed in adolescents as young as 8–9 years of age. Ewers and Seeman [8] followed 54 adolescents who had short implants placed over a 1-, 5- and 10-year period. They reported a cumulative success rate of 94.6% (Figs. 2.1, 2.2, 2.3, 2.4, 2.5, 2.6, and 2.7).

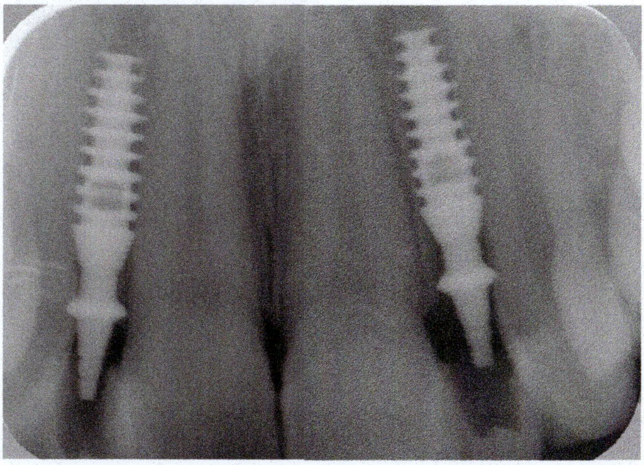

Fig. 2.1 Adolescent Male Case #1: implants placed at age 16

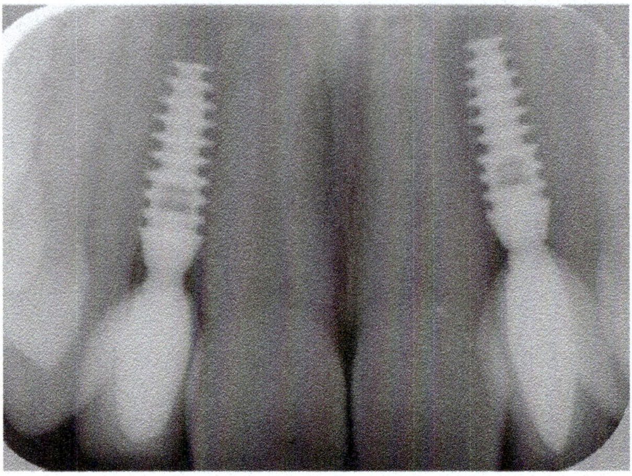

Fig. 2.2 Implants restored at age 16 in 2003

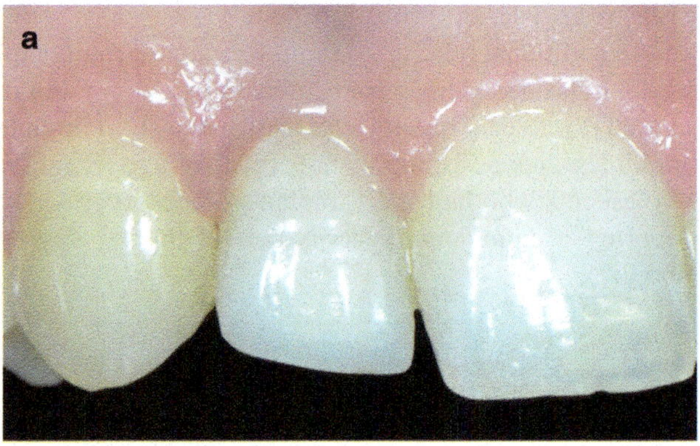

Fig. 2.3 (**a**, **b**) Restored implants at age 28 (right side)

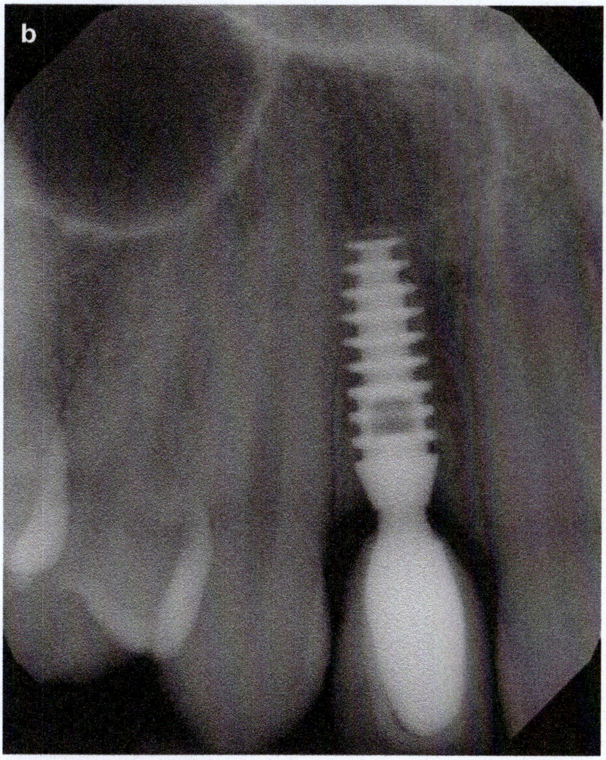

Fig. 2.3 (continued)

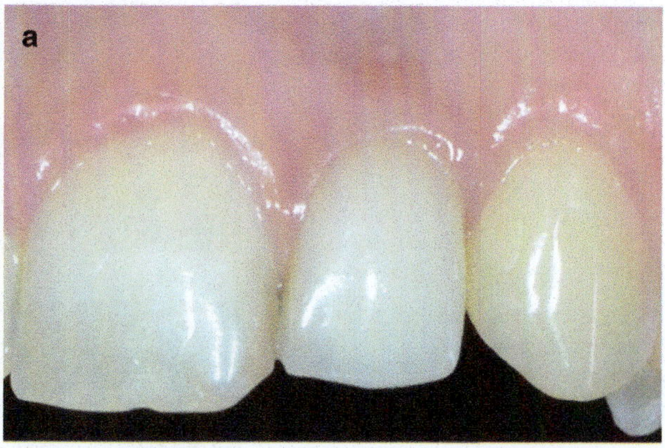

Fig. 2.4 (**a**, **b**) Restored implants at age 28 in 2015 (left side)

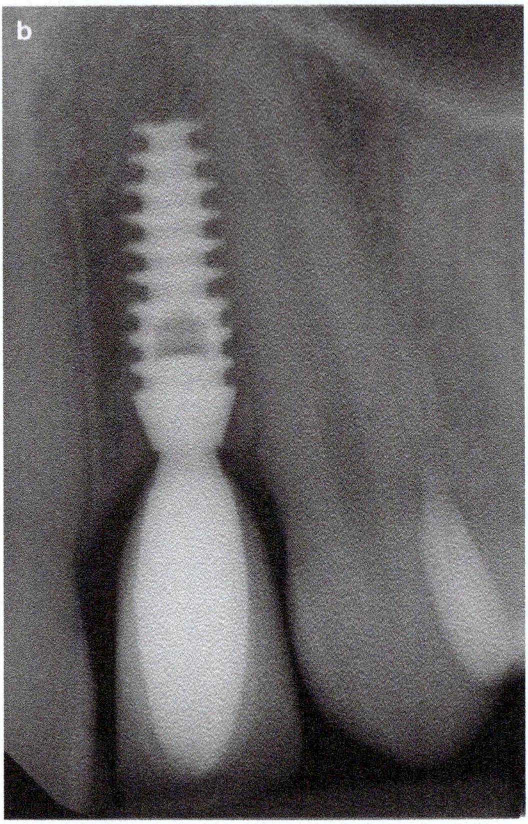

Fig. 2.4 (continued)

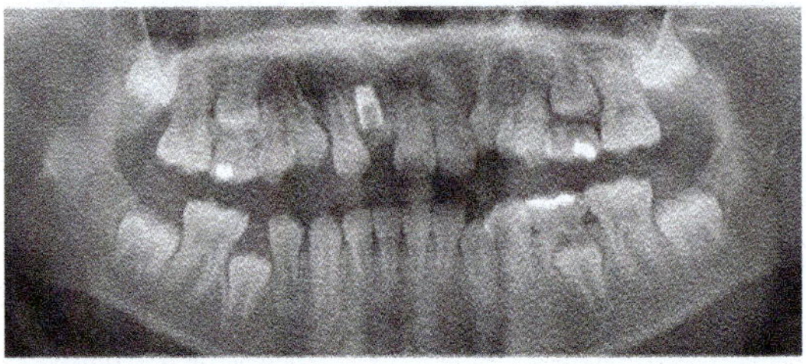

Fig. 2.5 Adolescent Case #2: implant placed in 2007 female age 8

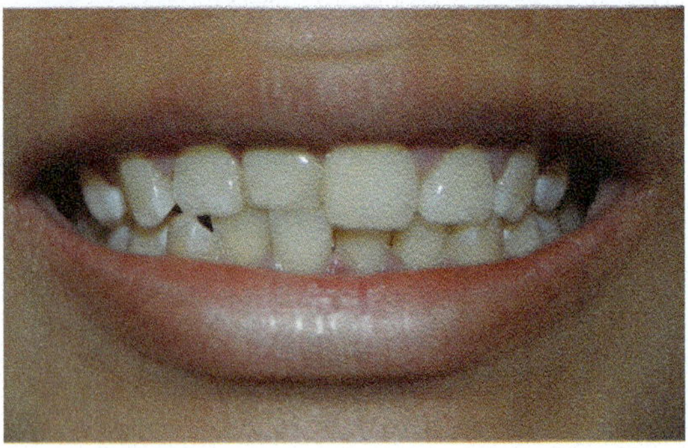

Fig. 2.6 Patient at age 15 showing obvious size difference in teeth

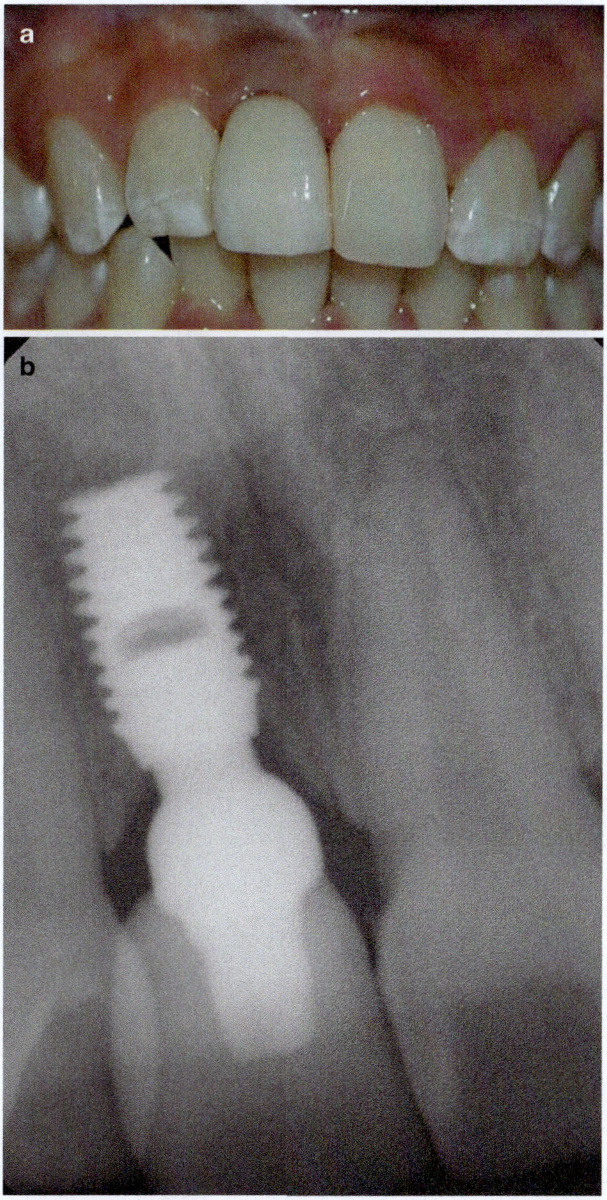

Fig. 2.7 (**a**, **b**) The unique aspects of the implant system allow the crown to be remade at age 16

A number of factors played a part in allowing these implants to be placed in adolescents. These include the ability to place the implants about 2–3 mm subcrestally. This appears to be one of the major factors in placing these short implants. The subcrestal placement allows for future growth. Deeper implant placement is better that an implant placed at the ridge crest. The other factor concerns the restorative aspect—the implant design allows for periodic restorative adjustments for esthetic concerns.

There are also clinical situations in which a narrow—less than 4.0 mm diameter—implant is needed. In some cases, a narrow traditional length implant may encroach on adjacent teeth or structures. In these instances, a short or ultrashort narrow implant may solve this often difficult problem. The use of a 3.0–3.5 mm × 6.0–8.0 mm implant will often allow an implant to be placed in areas where a more traditional size implant could not be used. The short and ultrashort narrow implant is ideal in clinical situations with congenitally missing lateral incisors and angled cuspid roots. It is also useful in replacing missing mandibular incisor teeth (Figs. 2.8 and 2.9).

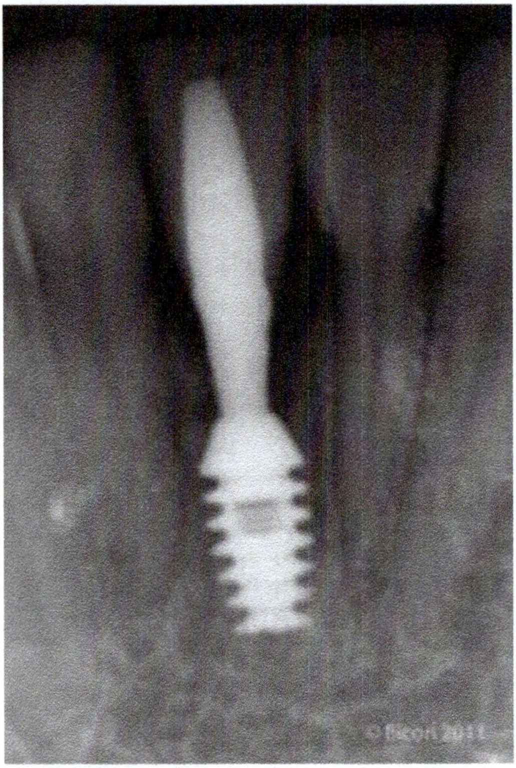

Fig. 2.8 Short and narrow implant replacing a mandibular incisor

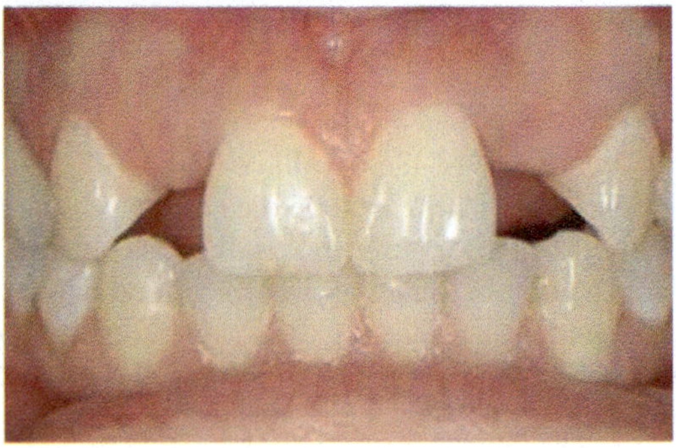

Fig. 2.9 Congenitally missing maxillary lateral incisors

The position of adjacent tooth roots makes cases such as these difficult to restore with traditional length implants [9]. With traditional length implants, the long held rule was that a minimum of 2 mm was needed between implants and natural tooth roots. Long-term studies appear to show that some short and ultrashort implants can actually come in contact with adjacent tooth roots (Figs. 2.10 and 2.11).

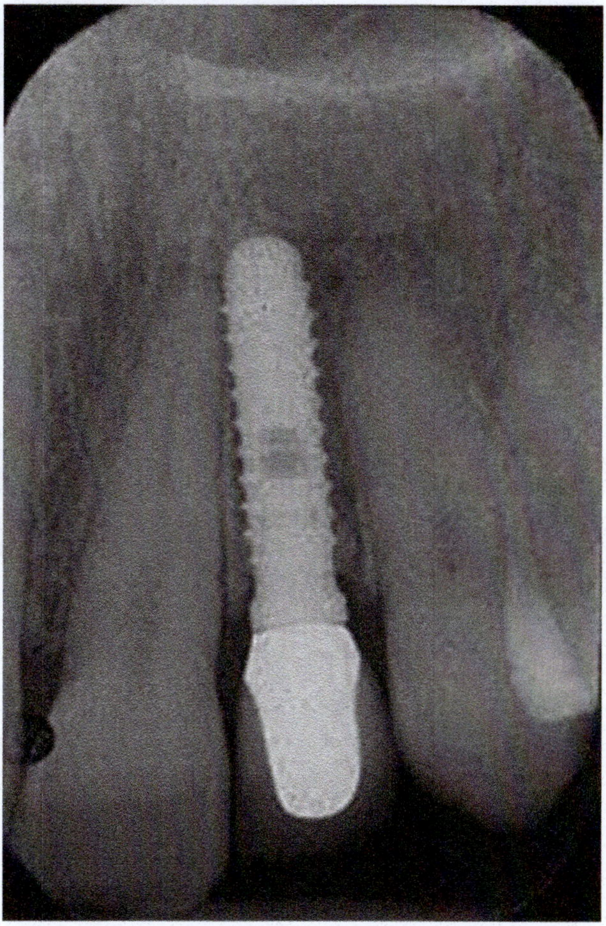

Fig. 2.10 Congenitally missing maxillary lateral incisor replaced with a traditional implant

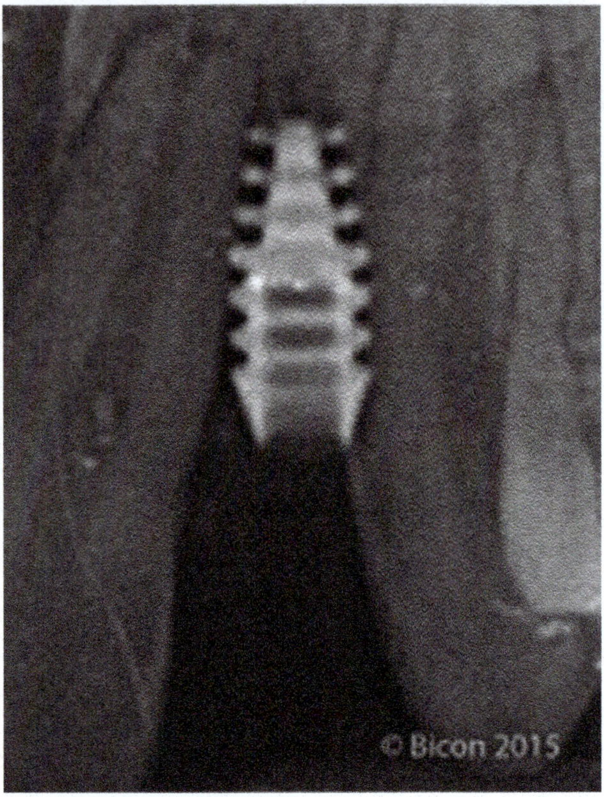

Fig. 2.11 Congenitally missing maxillary lateral incisor replaced with a narrow short implant

The short and ultrashort implants in both standard width (4.0–6.0 mm) diameter and narrow width (3.0–3.5 mm) diameter gives the clinician another option to use when treating those patients who would not otherwise be a good implant candidate. The use of the incisive canal as an implant site is an additional indication for short and ultrashort implant usage. In very complex cases, the options for augmentation reconstructions and implant placement in the anterior maxilla are very limited due to the lack of alveolar ridge height and width.

In order to decide whether it is possible to insert an implant in the area of the incisal foramen, a preoperative CBCT is essential [10]. The middle implant is inserted into the incisal foramen and the nasopalatine canal. The incisal foramen provides the thickest and highest bone structure in the atrophic maxilla for implant placement. In the usually one-chambered incisal foramen, there are often two incisal nerves [11] (Fig. 2.12).

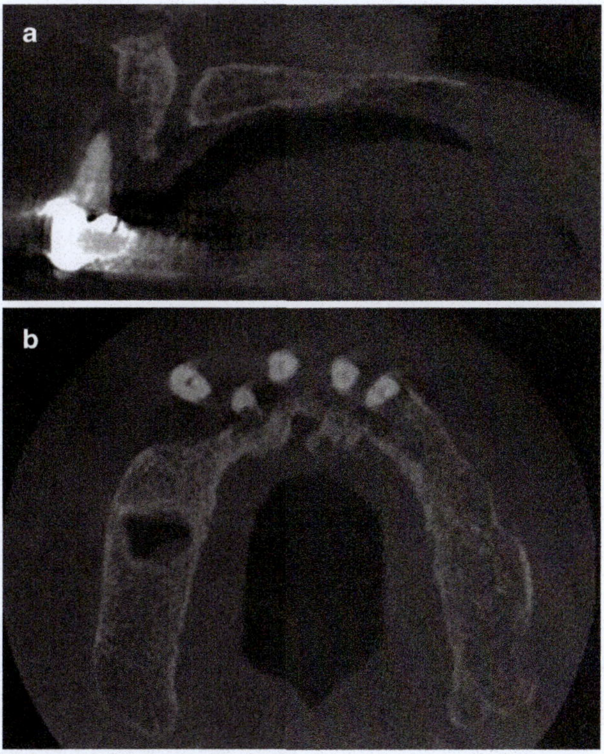

Fig. 2.12 (**a**, **b**) CBCT through the incisive foramen

One concern has been that damage to the incisal nerve may occur with implant placement. As surgeons we understand that nerve and vascular structures usually need to be severed in a Le Fort I osteotomy and horseshoe Le Fort I osteotomy. In a large-scale systematic review and meta-analysis, de Mello et al. [12] filtered 10 out of 238 articles and found a success rate of 84.6–100% for a total of 91 implants placed in the incisal foramen. Regarding permanent nerve disorders, all 10 articles reported only one permanent nerve disorder.

Case Study

A 65-year-old patient with periodontally involved non-restorable anterior maxillary teeth was seen for implant placement and a fixed prosthesis. Eight weeks after the teeth were removed a CBCT image was taken. After consultation with the patient and restoring dentist, it was decided to place three implants using the incisal foramen for the anterior implant. Images taken 8 weeks after removal of the teeth showed pronounced bone loss in the anterior alveolar area, but sufficient bone around the incisal foramen and adequate bone in the bicuspid area to accommodate three short and ultrashort implants.

Subsequently a 4.5 × 6.0 mm calcium phosphate-coated locking taper Integra CP implant (Bicon) was inserted into the area of the incisal foramen. In the premolar regions 4.0 × 5.0 mm calcium phosphate-coated locking taper Integra CP implants were inserted. The patient tolerated the procedure well and did not report any incisal nerve disturbance.

Approximately 6 months post-surgery a new CBCT showed good bone healing at all implant sites. The three implants were uncovered and full arch impressions were taken at the same time. Following a few days of healing, a bite registration was taken using the laboratory prepared wax-up. A week later a 12-unit metal-free fiber-glass-reinforced TRINIA bridge was inserted and fixed with screws [13] (Figs. 2.13, 2.14, 2.15, and 2.16).

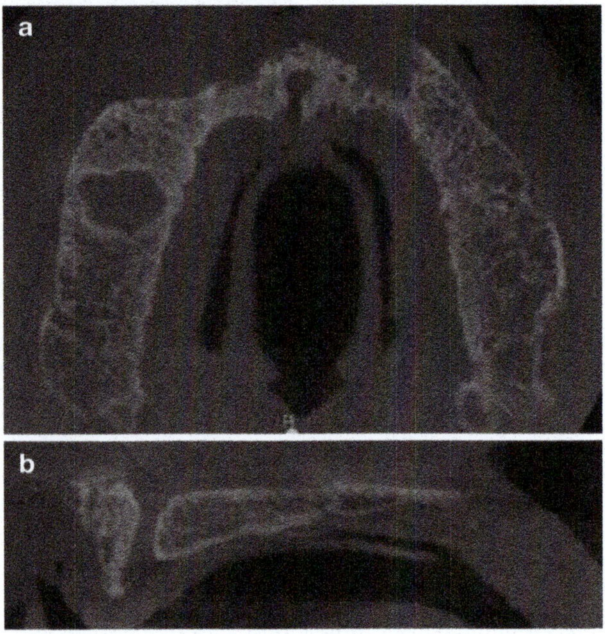

Fig. 2.13 (**a**, **b**) 65-year-old patient, 8 weeks following removal of the remaining maxillary teeth

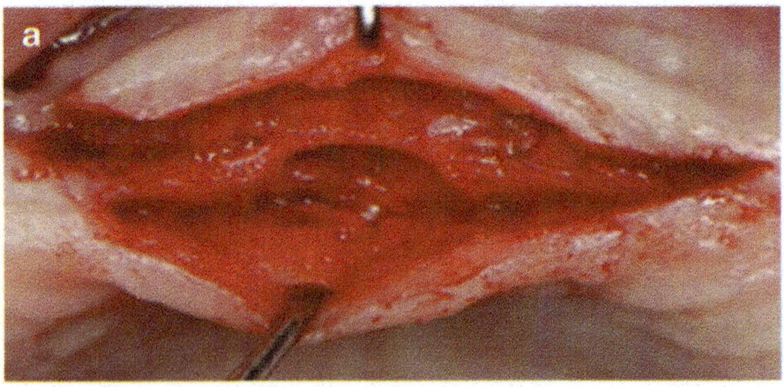

Fig. 2.14 (**a–c**) Placement of the 4.0 × 6 mm implant into the incisive foramen

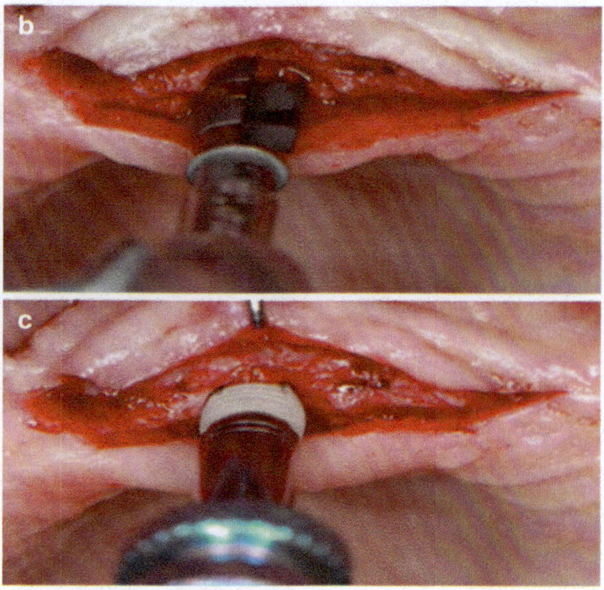

Fig. 2.14 (continued)

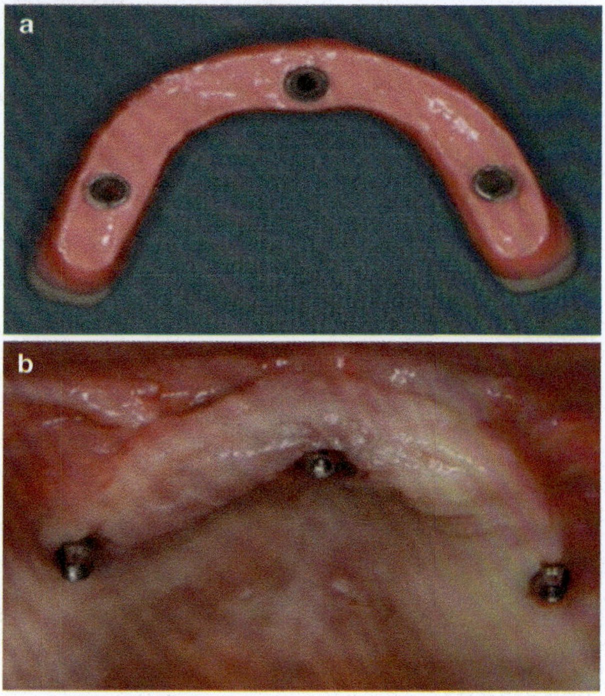

Fig. 2.15 (**a**–**c**) The uncovered implants with abutments in place and the final prosthesis

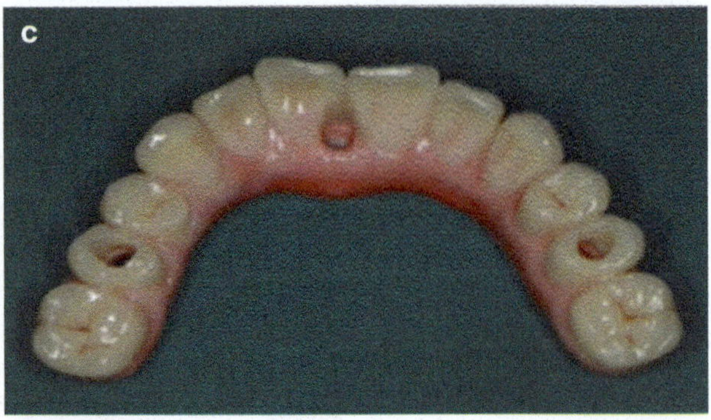

Fig. 2.15 (continued)

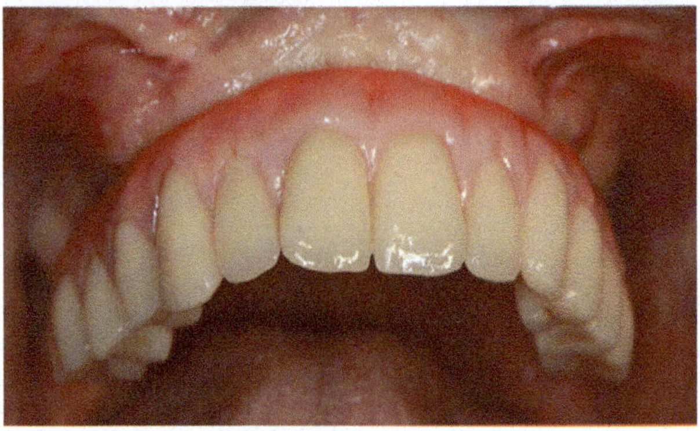

Fig. 2.16 The final prosthesis supported by three implants in place

The use of short and ultrashort implants in the highly atrophic maxilla in both the vertical and transversal dimensions allows the user to avoid extensive augmentations. The use of these implants shows good results comparable to those of standard implants with complex augmentations. The use of the incisal foramen has not led to any complications, and it seems to be an ideal implant site for short and ultrashort implants.

The indications and contraindications for short and ultrashort implants are similar to those of traditional length implants. The success rate of short and ultrashort implants is similar to traditional length implants [14]. However, specific instances such as described may make these implants preferable to those of traditional length. Short and ultrashort implants are indicated in some cases where implant placement is warranted in an adolescent. Using short and ultrashort implants when there is minimal residual bone height (RBH) and when the incisal foramen will be used as an implant site is another indication for usage.

References

1. Branemark PI, Hansson B, Adell R, et al. Osseointegrated implants in the treatment of the edentulous jaw. Experience from a 10 year period. Alqvist & Wiksell International: Stockholm; 1977.

2. Proceedings of the Toronto Conference on Osseointegration in Clinical Dentistry. J Prosthetic Dent, vol 49, 6 June 1983 and vol. 50, 1, 2 and 3 July, August and September 1983.
3. Ewers R. Maxilla sinus grafting with marine algae derived bone forming material: a clinical report of long term results. J Oral Maxillofac Surg. 2005;63(12):1712–23.
4. Friberg B, Jemt T, Lekholm U. Early failures in 4641 consecutively placed Branemark implants. Int J Oral Maxillofac Implants. 1991;6:142–6.
5. European consensus conference on short, angulated and diameter reduced implants. Cologne Germany 2017.
6. Marincola R, Ewers R, et al. Sinus elevations with short implants. Implants. 2017;2:20–4.
7. Makani N, et al. Osseointegrated implants in growing children: a literature review. J Oral Implantol. 2014;40(5):627–31.
8. Ewers R, Seeman R. Personal communication 2017.
9. Kendrick S, Wong D. Vertical and horizontal dimensions of implant dentistry: numbers every dentist should know inside dentistry 2009; July–August 2–5.
10. Friedrich R, Laumann F, Zrnc T, Assaf A. The nasopalatine canal in adults on cone beam computed tomograms—a clinical study and review of the literature. In Vivo. 2015;29(4):467–86.
11. Allard R, de Vries K, van der Kwast W. Persisting bilateral nasopalatine ducts: a developmental anomaly. Oral Surg Oral Med Oral Pathol. 1982;53:24–6.
12. De Mello JS, et al. Success rate and complications associated with dental implants in the incisive canal region: a systematic review. Int J Oral Maxillofac Surg. 2017;46(12):1584–91.
13. Ewers R, Seeman R. Trinia Trio—"all-on-three". Zahn Krone. 2017;3:11–7.
14. Lombardo G, et al. Cumulative success rate of short and ultrashort implants supporting single crowns in the posterior maxilla: a 3 year retrospective study. Int J Dent. 2017;2017:1–10. https://doi.org/10.1155/2017/8434281.

Short Implants and Early Brånemark Team Developments: Heritage Established at the Outset

3

Oded Bahat, Yvan Fortin, Martin L. Kolinski, Franck Renouard, and Richard M. Sullivan

Content

References.. 30

Per-Ingvar Brånemark's observation of bone fusing to a titanium surface in 1959 led to early evaluation as potential anchorage within bone for both loadbearing and passive prosthetic applications. Simultaneous research investigations within orthopedic, hand, ENT, and plastic surgery were all parallel to applications within dentistry and specialties for intraoral and extraoral maxillofacial anchorage solution potential. For the patient with unsolvable denture problems due to a highly resorbed maxilla and/or mandible, rehabilitation with a fixed, fully implant supported restoration was established in the 1970s as a routine treatment [1] (Fig. 3.1).

The early treatment focus on the edentulous patient with advanced resorption called for a jawbone anchorage system allowing for precisely fitting non-resilient full

O. Bahat
Private Practice Periodontology, Beverly Hills, CA, USA

Y. Fortin
Private Practice, Levis, QC, Canada

M. L. Kolinski
Midwest Dental Implantology, St. Charles, IL, USA

F. Renouard
Private Practice Oral and Maxillofacial Surgery, Paris, France

R. M. Sullivan (✉)
Clinical Technologies, Nobel Biocare, Yorba Linda, CA, USA
e-mail: rsulldds@aol.com

B. J. Tomasetti, R. Ewers (eds.), *Short Implants*,
https://doi.org/10.1007/978-3-030-44199-9_3

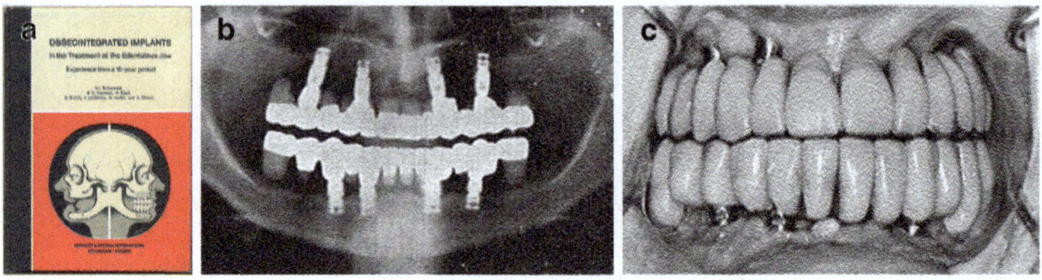

Fig. 3.1 (**a**) 1977 text on surgical and restorative experiences over a 10-year period. (**b**) Radiograph shows four implants 7 mm in length supporting fixed restorations with cantilevers. (**c**) Clinical photograph of denture teeth and screw-retained fixed restorations. Note similarity of treatment to logo on book cover

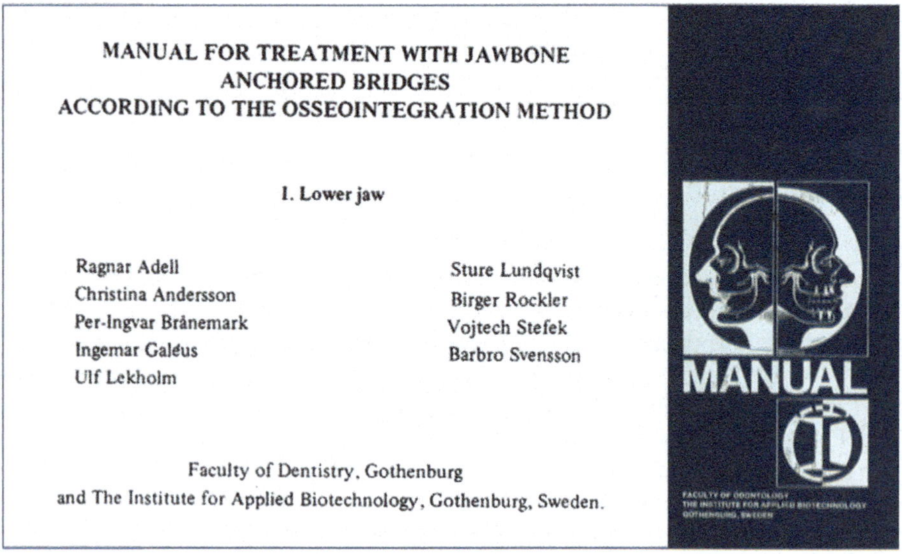

MANUAL FOR TREATMENT WITH JAWBONE ANCHORED BRIDGES ACCORDING TO THE OSSEOINTEGRATION METHOD

I. Lower jaw

Ragnar Adell
Christina Andersson
Per-Ingvar Brånemark
Ingemar Galéus
Ulf Lekholm
Sture Lundqvist
Birger Rockler
Vojtech Stefek
Barbro Svensson

Faculty of Dentistry, Gothenburg
and The Institute for Applied Biotechnology, Gothenburg, Sweden.

Fig. 3.2 Early surgical and restorative manual cover page listing faculty from Gothenburg, Sweden. Note again rehabilitative emphasis with logo, and "jawbone anchored bridges" terminology

arch prosthetic fixation (Fig. 3.2). The word "jawbone" with reference to implant anchorage is important to emphasize. Within the broad field of dental implants, the implant is often seen as a root replacement with a crown affixed on top. When treating individuals for "tooth loss" after decades of denture use and resorption, the patient typically presents with a composite defect, meaning that the patient is missing multiple tissues—clinical crowns and tooth roots; alveolar bone; soft tissue volume originally covering the bone. While the discussion with the patient may focus on replacing teeth, often significant volumes of bone and soft tissue deficiencies may also be present and require replacement [2]. What Brånemark and coworkers developed, among other things, was an implant system including short implant lengths developed around resorbed jaws. Time, possibly hastened by the introduction to the North American market, has led to the adaptation of this anchorage system for basal bone to dento-alveolar applications and replacement of also just one or a few teeth. This has led to other component designs on implant, abutment, biomaterial, and instrumentation fronts, with short implants always a consideration in the process.

In the situations with advanced resorption, the goal of the implant placement is to provide stable anchorage for a restoration that provides as ideal contours of prosthetic replacement as possible without oral hygiene compromises. The implants used at the time are only slightly varied between auricular, temporal, orbital, mid-face, finger joint, and maxillofacial designs. The 2 mm diameter for an abutment screw contained within an external hexagon delivery system (Fig. 3.3) to drive the implant to place has continued to this day and is fully compatible with current day prosthetics.

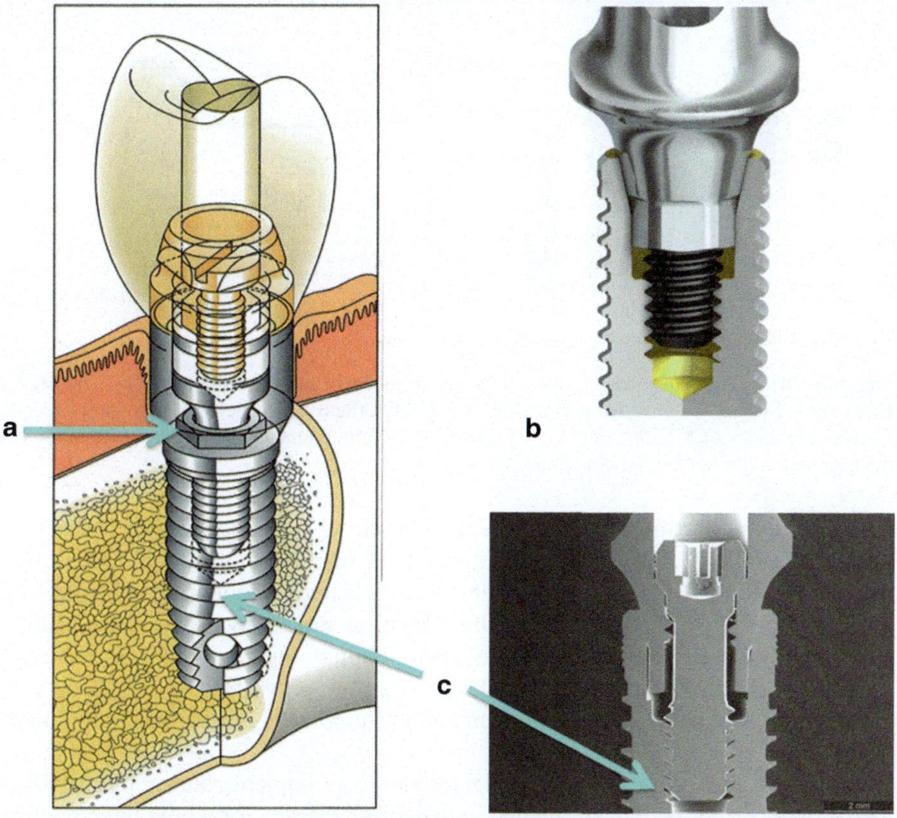

Fig. 3.3 The initial implant designs included an internal threaded aspect that was used to fixate an abutment cylinder dependent on soft tissue thickness. (**a**) The hexagon feature was present as a purchase point for the early implant drivers referred to as fixture mounts. Use of the hexagon feature for indexing purposes and anti-rotational capabilities came at a later time. (**b**) Clinical preference for conical connections is expanding, and there are many benefits for screw joint integrity. (**c**) As a practical matter, implant length is generally limited to the length of a compatible abutment screw that can be accommodated. A change in abutment screw length would introduce inventory incompatibilities and also require clinical validations

a

Fixture installation

Box 33053, S-40033 Gothenburg, Sweden.
Tel. 031-414560

B-01 = 10 mm × 3.75 mm (standard)
B-02 = 7 mm × 3.75 mm (short)
B-03 = 10 mm × 4.00 mm (extra large)
B-04 = 13 mm × 3.75 mm (extra long)

b

Components for Fixture Installation

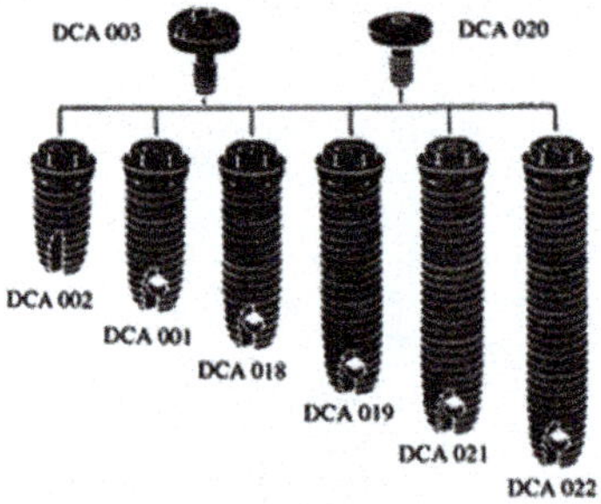

Art. No	Article	Pcs/pack
DCA 003	Titanium cover screw	20
DCA 020	Titanium cover screw, internal hexagon	20
DCA 002	Titanium fixture 3.75x 7 mm	11
DCA 001	Titanium fixture 3.75x10 mm	8
DCA 018	Titanium fixture 3.75x13 mm	6
DCA 019	Titanium fixture 3.75x15 mm	5
DCA 021	Titanium fixture 3.75x18 mm	4
DCA 022	Titanium fixture 3.75x20 mm	4
DCA 035	Titanium fixture 4.00x 7 mm (not shown)	1
DCA 023	Titanium fixture 4.00x10 mm (not shown)	1
DCA 036	Titanium fixture 4.00x13 mm (not shown)	1
DCA 037	Titanium fixture 4.00x15 mm (not shown)	1
DCA 038	Titanium fixture 4.00x18 mm (not shown)	1

Fig. 3.4 (**a**) Fixture installation form excerpt from early surgical manual. (**b**) The Biotes Brånemark System Catalog from Nobelpharma USA, effective January 1, 1986 shows recommended inventory of 3.75 diameter by 7 mm long and 4 mm diameter × 7 mm long implants. The 8.5 mm length did not begin being phased in until 1993

Throughout this time, external hexagon implants 7 mm in length (6.5 mm actual) have been available for management of advanced maxillary and mandibular resorption (Fig. 3.4a, b). Rather than functioning as replacement tooth roots, the implants were more often placed in residual host bone or grafted bone sites in positions where tooth roots were never located. The individual implant alignment needed to be viewed as part of an overall anchorage assembly providing the prosthetic platform for the missing tissue replacement and to support long-term physiologic function [3].

With consideration of the experimental nature of implants during this 1960s to 1980s time period, people unsatisfied with denture therapy for whom there were no other dental treatment alternatives were the first group of subjects reported on with 10-year results for both jaws published in 1977 [1]. The 15-year results of this group were presented in Toronto in 1982 [4] with the treatment results further explained and expanded upon with basic science, metallurgy, diagnosis, radiology, procedures, and complications in the textbook Tissue-Integrated Prostheses edited by Branemark, Albrektsson and Zarb in 1985 (Quintessence) (Fig. 3.5a, b).

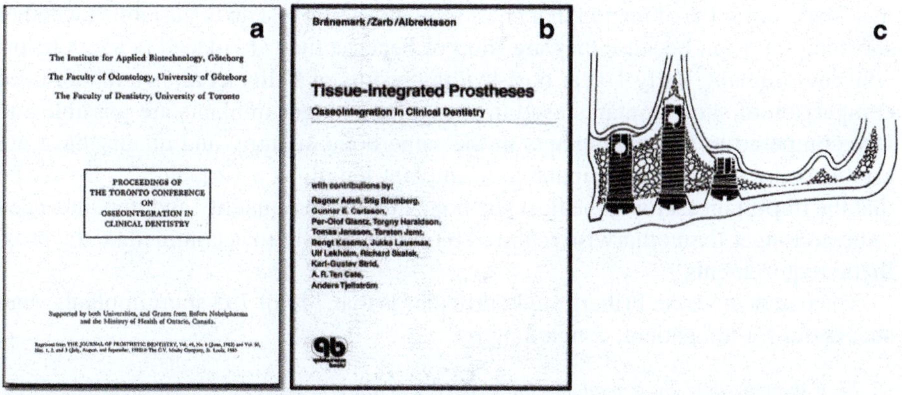

Fig. 3.5 (**a**) Treatment for the edentulous arch including work based on short implants was introduced to the North America academic community in Toronto, Canada 1982. (**b**) The findings of 15 years of human studies plus expanded basic science, diagnostic, radiographic, metallurgy, biomechanics, clinical procedural and complications' applications are published by Quintessence in 1985. (**c**) Short implants are shown, but are in no way singled out as a variable of clinical significance

Short implants of 7 mm length have passed 40 years of function as an edentulous arch anchorage unit for fixed full arch restorations in both jaws. While this group of patients has been followed and reported on in several publications, no attribution of implant loss or other complication was ever attributed to the 7 mm length itself. In 1991, Friberg et al. reported on 793 7 mm implants out of 4641 consecutively placed Brånemark System implants during a 3-year period [5]. The 44 short implants lost represented the highest percentage by length of all lost implants. There are several relevant observations that may be taken from the study that are applicable to clinical decisions today.

With 793 implants of 7 mm length reported out of 4641 implants placed over a 3-year period, this is not "occasional use" but represents a solid 17% of all implants placed. These were turned surface implants during 1985–1987. For the edentulous maxilla 7.1% (37/520) were lost and 3.1% (6/196) in the mandible. For a smaller number of partially edentulous applications, no implants were lost in the maxilla (0/11) and 1.5% (1/66) for the lower arch.

Measuring early results from implant placement through connection of the definitive restoration is an observation of whether a biologic process has occurred and survived with early stability. In 1981, Albrektsson et al. identified six factors contributing to lifelong osseointegration [6]. "Status of the implant bed" is a factor representing the local historical and current dynamic site conditions including blood supply, overall health and systemic effects of medication, blood sugar levels, and nicotine.

As the Friberg et al. study shows, minimal bone volume leads to short implants use and were indicated in 17% (793/4641) sites encountered. Within these sites often including soft bone quality as a compounding factor the distribution of 7.1%

maxillary and 3.1% of mandibular short implants being lost do not establish whether short implants fail because they are short or because they are placed in a less favorable environment. Early 1-year post-loading results of **Felice et al.** in a randomized comparison of short implants used in sites where longer implants are possible and also compared to longer implants in the same bone quantity and quality have not established a difference attributable to implant length as a variable [7]. It may be that the important factor is the host site bone quality and quantity and implants need to be no longer than otherwise required biomechanically to accommodate the prosthetic requirements.

The perspective the Friberg study provides is that 749 of 793 short implants were successful for the patient, concluding by

> *Even though some short implants failed during healing, it must be remembered that the majority of the 7 mm fixtures still became integrated and subsequently were used to support prosthetic restorations.*

Two recent studies by different Swedish investigators looked at different patient populations that included more partially edentulous patients and also now only implants with an oxidized surface [8, 9]. Combining the numbers from both studies, 54 of 511 implants would be classified as short, or over 10%. This shows that with long-term experience, the utilization of short implants by surgeons continues at a rate of 10% of all implants placed.

References

1. Brånemark P-I, Hansson B, Adell R, et al. Osseointegrated implants in the treatment of the edentulous jaw. Experience from a 10-year period. Alqvist & Wiksell International: Stockholm; 1977.
2. Bedrossian E, Sullivan R, Fortin Y, Malo P, Rangert B, Indersano T. Fixed-prosthetic restoration of the edentulous maxilla: a systematic pre-treatment evaluation method. J Oral Maxillofac Surg. 2008;66:112–22.
3. Brånemark P-I, Zarb G, Albrektsson T, editors. Tissue-integrated prostheses. Chicago: Quintessence; 1985. p. 60–8.
4. Proceedings of the Toronto Conference on Osseointegration in Clinical Dentistry. Reprinted from J Prosthetic Dent, vol. 49(6) (June 1983) and vol. 50(1, 2) and 3 (July, August, and September, 1983). St. Louis: The C.V. Mosby Company; 1983.
5. Friberg B, Jemt T, Lekholm U. Early failures in 4,641 consecutively placed Brånemark dental implants: a study from stage 1 surgery to the connection of completed prostheses. Int J Oral Maxillofac Implants. 1991;6:142–6.
6. Albrektsson T, Brånemark P-I, Hansson H-A, Lindström J. Osseointegrated titanium implants: requirements for ensuring a long-lasting direct bone-to-implant anchorage in man. Acta Orthop Scand. 1981;52:155–70.
7. Felice P, Cannizzaro G, Barausse C, Pistilli R, Esposito M. Short implants versus longer implants in vertically augmented posterior mandibles: a randomized controlled trial with 5-year after loading follow-up. Eur J Oral Implantol. 2014;7:359–69.

8. Östman P-O, Hellman M, Sennerby L. Ten years later. Results from a prospective single-centre clinical study on 121 oxidized (TiUnite™) Brånemark implants in 46 patients. Clin Implant Dent Relat Res. 2012;14:852–60.
9. Friberg B, Jemt T. Clinical experience of TiUnite™ implants: a 5-year cross-sectional, retrospective follow-up study. Clin Implant Dent Relat Res. 2010;12(Suppl 1):e95–e103.

The Short Implant Heritage Continues: The Possibility of Reduced Grafting Without Restorative Compromise

4

Oded Bahat, Yvan Fortin, Martin L. Kolinski, Franck Renouard, and Richard M. Sullivan

Contents

4.1 Approaching the Site with Minimal Bone Volume 34
4.2 The Most Important Part of the Implant 42
References 44

The expansion of implant support for partially edentulous and single tooth indications over the past 30 years has been remarkable, and usage of implants has changed to include more intact sites, placement at time of tooth extraction, and single tooth restoration. The use of short implants is evolving with these treatment applications (Fig. 4.1).

The clinical demands on a 4 × 7 mm implant coaxed within 5 mm height of posterior maxillary alveolar bone while supporting a 15 mm cantilever are far different than for an 11.5 mm implant in a maxillary lateral incisor site with minimal functional demands. Selection of implants by length appropriate for each patient needs to be evaluated for the most ideal structural support possible with the least

O. Bahat
Private Practice Periodontology, Beverly Hills, CA, USA

Y. Fortin
Private Practice, Levis, QC, Canada

M. L. Kolinski
Midwest Dental Implantology, St. Charles, IL, USA

F. Renouard
Private Practice Oral and Maxillofacial Surgery, Paris, France

R. M. Sullivan (✉)
Clinical Technologies, Nobel Biocare, Yorba Linda, CA, USA
e-mail: rsullddds@aol.com

B. J. Tomasetti, R. Ewers (eds.), *Short Implants*,
https://doi.org/10.1007/978-3-030-44199-9_4

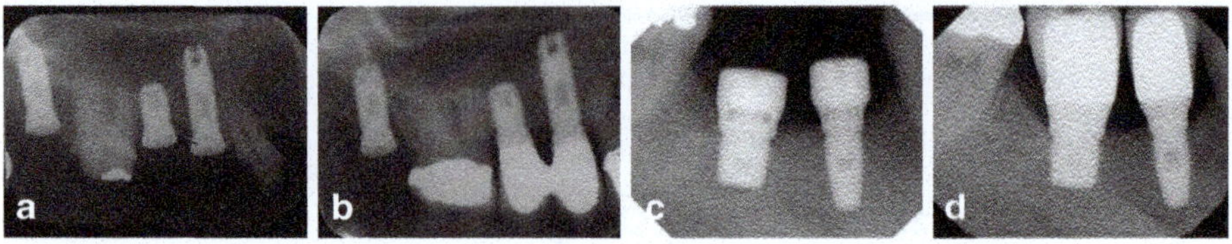

Fig. 4.1 (**a, b**) Twenty-three year follow-up of short implant used as splinted support for two unit screw-retained maxillary restoration. (**c, d**) Seventeen year follow-up of freestanding short posterior implant

compromise and potential risk. Each implant in each potential site is based on the assessment of benefits and risks as it contributes to achievement of overall treatment objectives. If an additional implant in a pontic site could be a potential benefit over a projected 30 years and present minimal additional risk to the patient, this is a consideration for which a definitive answer cannot be known.

For an individual patient choosing between a long implant and bone graft versus a short implant the consideration goes beyond the success rates of the different options to include also associated morbidity, cost, treatment time, and the individual realistic feasibility of outcome.

To assist the clinician with the research foundation supporting decisions about how short implants can fit into today's practice, the editors of the International Journal of Oral & Maxillofacial Implants have provided two topical reviews on this subject [1, 2]. Numerous Journal articles discuss the biomechanical aspects, including the crown/implant ratio of short implants [3–10]. There are several recent relevant publications on short implants [3–13]. The decision of either the recommendation or inadvisability of short implants on the patient's behalf will largely be based on the perception of compromise in results. This decision will likely occur as the patient is deciding on perceived invasiveness, prognosis, and time required during planning of bone grafting approaches to treatment results achieved using other methods. This subject has been researched and published with an attempt to provide an objective assessment of support there is for clinical decisions today [14]. As a brief but highly worthwhile departure from the traditional textbook format you are able to take advantage of this QR Code to bring you a presentation by one of the authors, Dr. Franck Renouard on the "Risks and Rewards of Not Grafting" presented at the Academy of Osseointegration Meeting in February 2016 (Fig. 4.2).

4.1 Approaching the Site with Minimal Bone Volume

The functional interface of the implant of importance for the patient is:

- the horizontal plane of the implant platform,
- the perpendicular axial plane extending through the implant center and extending through the occlusal or incisal interface,

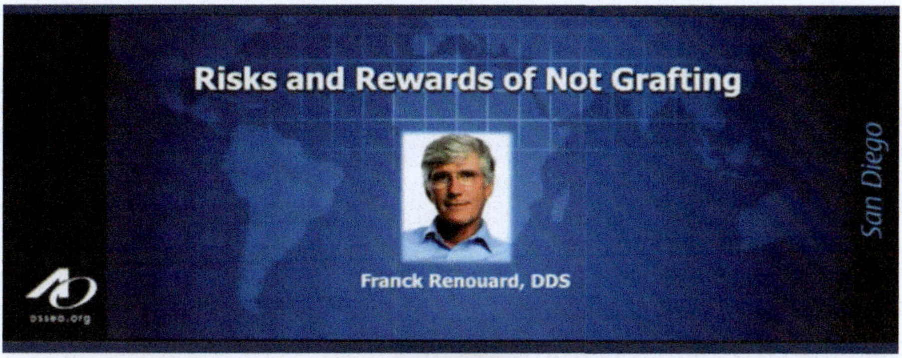

Fig. 4.2 Please use the QR code to access a video discussing short implants as a bone grafting alternative

- the 3D positioning of the platform to receive long-term functional loads within stable soft tissue utilizing optimal restorative emergence profile established in planning stages.

This means that positioning of the implant interface is ideally based on having already established a restorative plan that is able to be integrated into the patient's scan of bone and capture of soft tissue information (Fig. 4.3).

Details that are important for all implants may have potential for even greater cumulative benefit or compromise when short implants are used. For patient safety reasons, limited available bone indicating the use of short implants means that the surgeon needs accurate information to allow maximum short-term and long-term utilization of available bone (Figs. 4.4, 4.5 and 4.6).

Within Nobel Biocare, the shortest implants have always been listed as 7 mm in the external hexagon Brånemark System and NobelSpeedy compatible systems. The length of the implant itself however is 6.5 from the base to the top of the platform; going to the top of the hexagon exceeds 7 mm. The Mk III design also has a 0.8-mm machined collar (Figs. 4.4 and 4.7) This means that with 6 mm of available bone, the threaded oxidized surface is able to be fully submerged and have available an almost 1 mm supra-osseous connection that can accept titanium or zirconia directly for either screw-retained or cemented restorations (Fig. 4.8). It is possible to view the 7 mm/6.5 mm actual length Brånemark System or NobelSpeedy implants as 5.5 mm threaded implants with a built-in almost 1 mm abutment. This Regular Platform external hexagon implant interface allows attachment of both single and multiple unit zirconia restorations as well as all titanium abutments and splinting frameworks or bars.

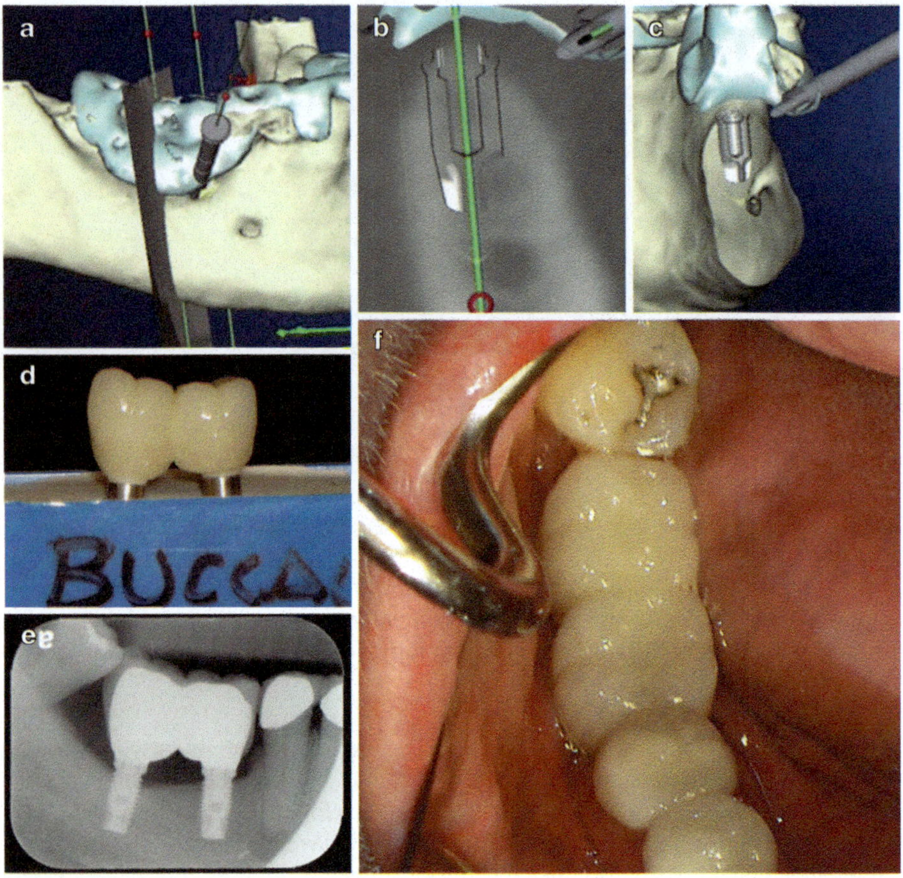

Fig. 4.3 (**a–c**) Advances in digital diagnosis allow us to add tooth position and soft tissue thickness to the patient's pre-operative scan for optimal placement planning; producing a surgical template from this planning helps deliver a straightforward restoration. (**d–f**) NobelProcera porcelain-to-zirconica screw-retained restoration on Brånemark System 8.5 mm Mk III implants with collar left deliberately supraosseous to function as an abutment. There is a 30° draw for path of insertion at the implant interface level for restoration of Nobel Biocare implants with non-engaging components such as this restoration

The turned-surface finish of the Brånemark System implant existed in the 6.5 mm ("7 mm") height and 9.5 mm ("10 mm") since the 1960s. In 1993, an 8.5 mm (*8.0 actual)* length was added to the 3.75 and 4 mm Brånemark System and both 7 and 8.5 mm lengths continued with wide diameter and NobelSpeedy implants (Fig. 4.7). The design properties of the self-tapping Mk III implant, the tapered designs of the Mk IV and NobelSpeedy implant, and the conical connection abutment interface have all been combined in the development of the NobelParallel CC implant [15] (Fig. 4.8).

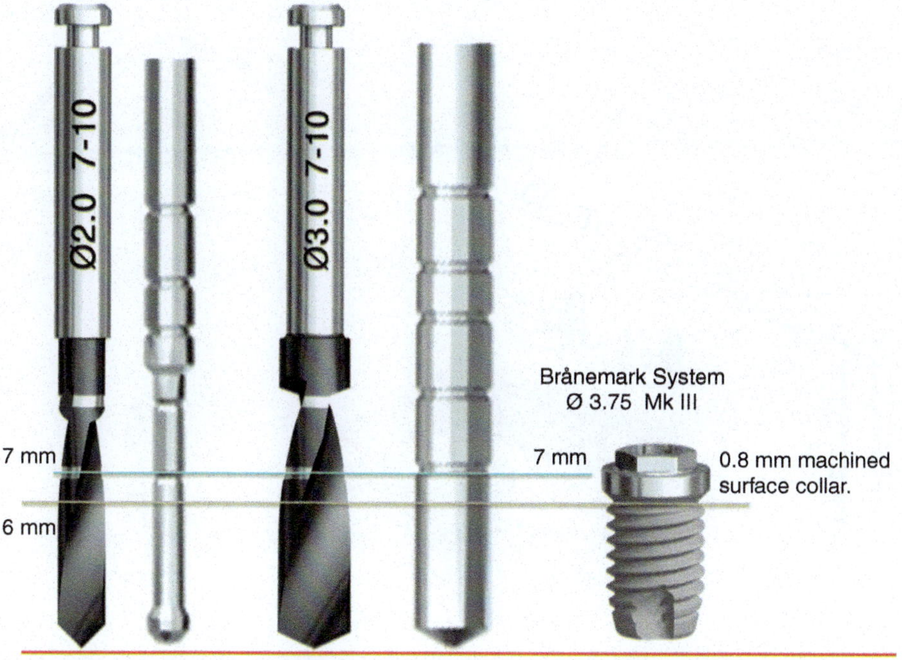

Fig. 4.4 Six millimeter of available osseous site depth (+ appropriate safety margin) is sufficient to place a 7 mm implant with the collar supraosseous. There are single and splinted multiple unit screw-retained zirconia restorations emerging directly from the implant platform to accommodate a wide range of restorative needs or preferences

Steri-Oss implants had always been available in both 8 and 10 mm lengths and share abutment compatibilities. This trend has continued with the Replace Select and NobelReplace Tapered System using the tri-channel connection (Figs. 4.9 and 4.10).

With both the external hexagon and tri-channel connections esthetic emergence profile is able to begin atop the implant with shaded zirconia. The starting point of esthetic emergence profile is an additional consideration with conical connection implants. With the conical connection interface, the implant platform needs to be placed 1.5 mm deeper to achieve the same soft tissue starting point with restorative shade material (Fig. 4.11). This means 3 mm submersion of the implant interface below the anticipated stable soft tissue crest will provide a zirconia restorative starting point 1.5 mm subgingival from this crest.

If there has been an application where short implants have been improved upon it is as terminal support in the posterior maxilla with full maxillary restoration. It has been the combination of limited bone volume and softer bone qualities that have presented a challenge for anchorage and unfavorable cantilever function. The introduction of zygomatic implants, trans-sinus and tilted implants as alternatives for both short implants and sinus grafts have become predictable foundations for full

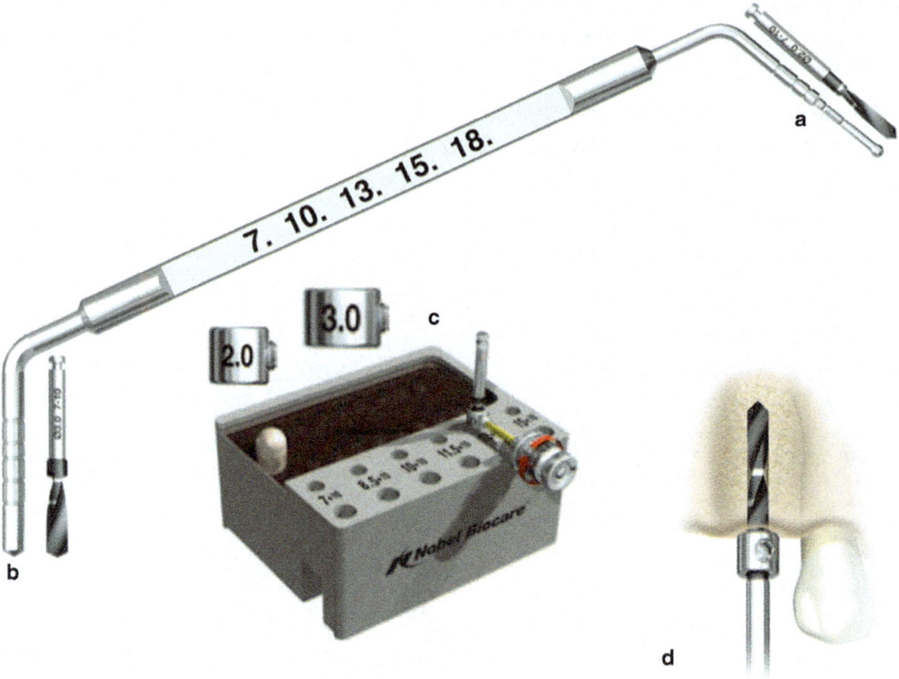

Fig. 4.5 Patient safety first. Patient injury is a risk with implant site preparation above, below or alongside structures susceptible to injury. More important than implant length is exact knowledge of drilling depths and safety margins, with the appropriate size implant to follow. Use of a depth gauge to verify intended site preparation helps assure intraoperative drilled depth required for full implant seating is achieved. (**a**) 2 mm end of Depth Gauge has round ball at end to minimize trauma elevating mucous membrane. Shown with a 7–10 mm length / 2 mm diameter twist drill as often used with short implants, it is useful from 7 to 18 mm lengths. (**b**) 3 mm end of depth gauge 7–10 mm diameter 3 mm twist drill. The Depth Gauge (32948) is included with all non-guided surgical kits except Replace Tapered Systems. (**c**) Drill Stops are available for varied twist drill diameters. (**d**) Whether used with surgical templates or freehand, use of drill stops can be valuable working with short preparation depths and difficult access.

arch maxillary restorations [16–20]. These examples reposition the originally recommended parallel implant alignment to instead take advantage of available bone to decrease cantilever function with the ability to position the implants more posteriorly and in to more dense bone despite resorption or anterior maxillary sinus pneumatization (Figs. 4.12 and 4.13).

From the patient, dental technician and restorative dentist perspective, the important part of an implant is how the platform is best positioned to withstand or even thrive in an environment of challenge. The optimal positioning of this interface is foremost be the implant 7 mm or 45 mm in length, with soft tissue health and volume, ideal restorative contours and optimal three-dimensional positioning all taken in to account.

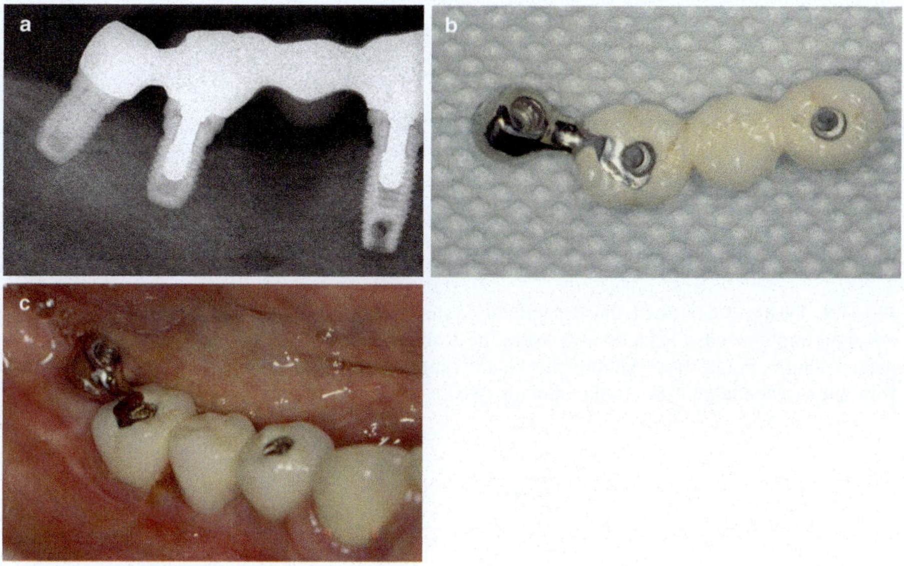

Fig. 4.6 (**a–c**) Two 7 mm implants combined with a 10 mm implant. By extending the framework and thereby distributing load to a third implant there is an additional possibility for improved biomechanical function

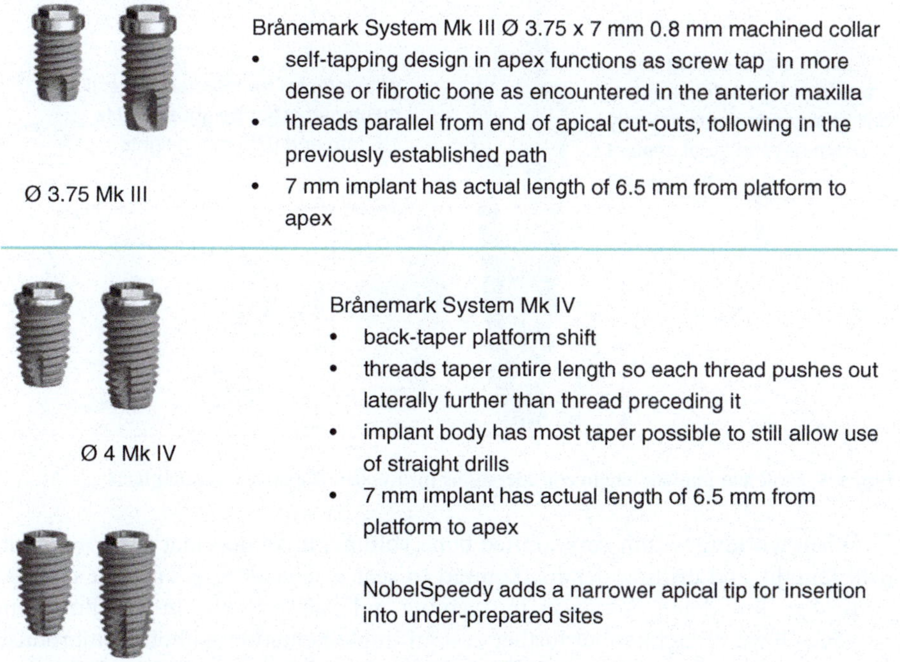

Fig. 4.7 Summary of Brånemark System and NobelSpeedy short 7 and 8.5 mm implants

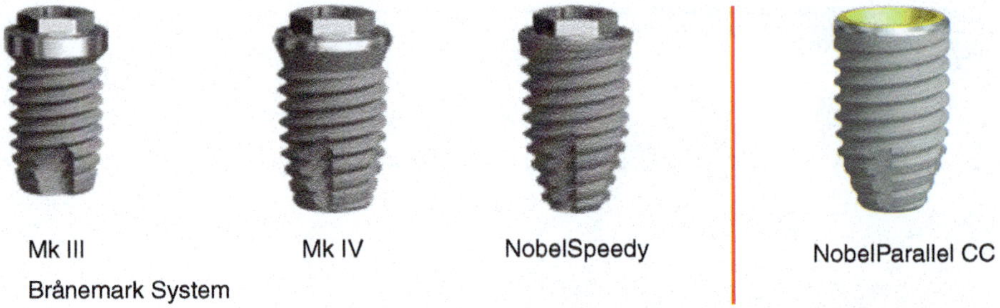

Fig. 4.8 Design features of the Brånemark System Mk III, MK IV and NobelSpeedy external hexagon implants have been considered in the NobelParallel CC that incorporates a conical connection abutment interface. All implants have a 7 mm stated length with an actual length of 6.5 mm from the prosthetic platform to the implant apex

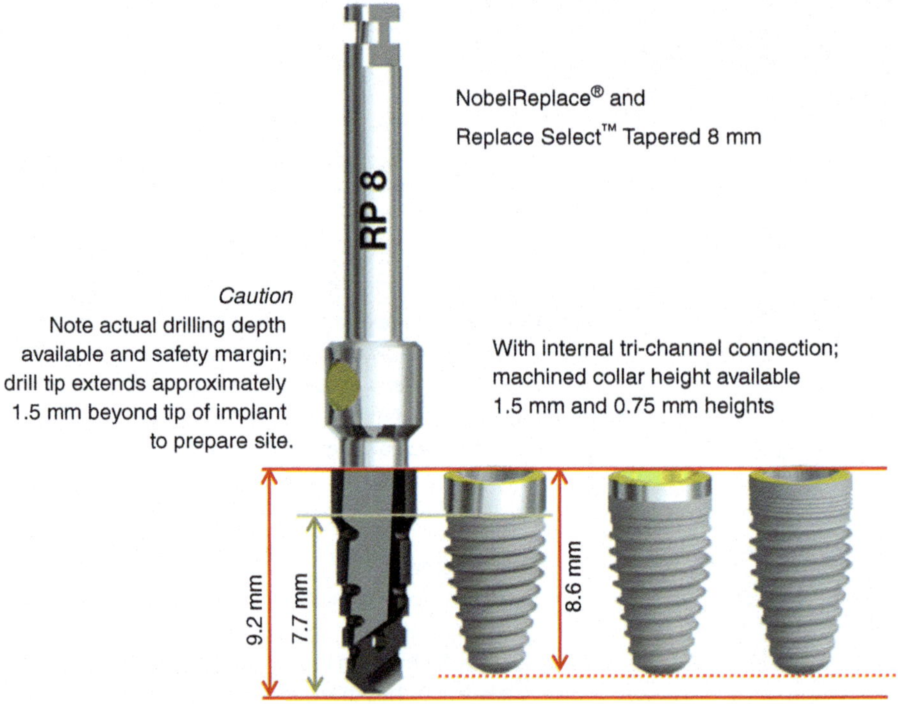

Fig. 4.9 Drill and implant length considerations for Replace Tapered 8 mm implants

When working within very limited bone volume, it is important to know actual drill lengths and drilling depths required to seat a selected implant to a selected vertical seating depth. Advances in scanning and true synergies in workflow convergence have brought about further ease of implementation without compromise in patient safety. NobelProcera, DTX Implant planning software, NobelGuide surgical templates and dynamic navigation all help the patient receive the most value

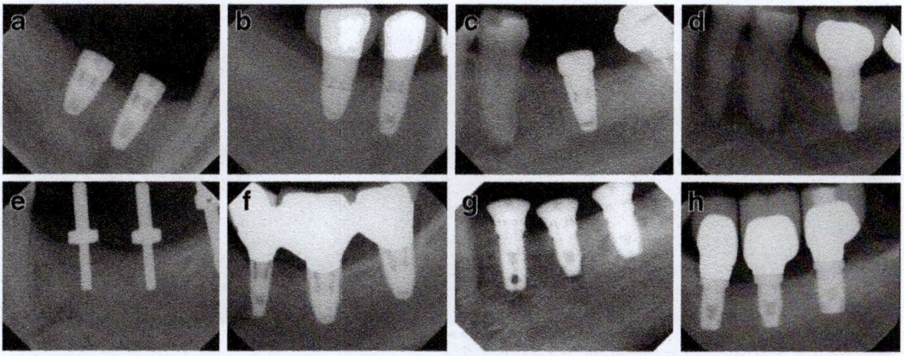

Fig. 4.10 Eight millimeter length Replace Tapered Implants are routinely used with limited space over the inferior alveolar canal. This is a routine treatment indication, and here patient expectations are high. Use of short implants in more minimal bone volumes can be technically challenging, and is considered by many to be an advanced procedure. (**a, b**) 8 mm posterior and 10 mm anterior Replace Tapered Implants at placement and 5 year follow-up. (**c, d**) 8 mm Replace Tapered Implant in site 20 at placement and 6 year follow-up. Splinting or not-splinting posterior implants for biomechanical loading considerations is largely a matter of preference for a given patient. (**e, f**) Site preparation and 5 year follow-up of a splinted restoration (**g, h**) placement and 16 year follow-up of freestanding 8 mm implants

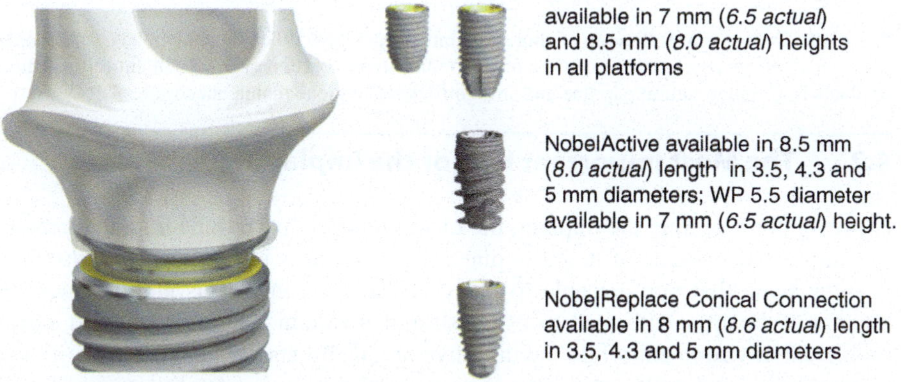

Fig. 4.11 All conical connection implants carry an additional seating consideration of depth of placement. The conical connection back taper and platform shift area require 1.5 mm vertical space from the implant platform to begin to develop any restorative emergence profile. For the external hexagon and tri-channel connections, this esthetic development is able to be controlled directly from the top of the implant. The conical connection implants require 1.5–2 mm further seating depth to equal the same restorative starting point as the external hexagon and tri-channel connection implants

from their scan through providing more planning information that can be used to plan and achieve treatment results. While surgical and restorative hardware are important, optimal results of their use are achieved when appropriate advantage is taken of data pre-operatively.

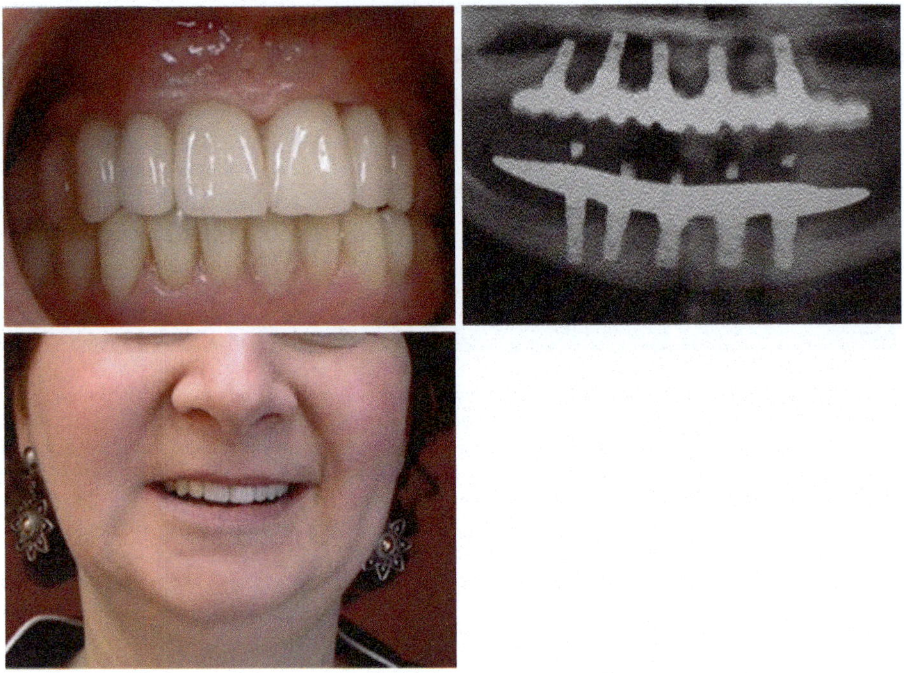

Fig. 4.12 Twelve year follow-up of short implants in each jaw. When the patient has a tooth-only deficiency, the appropriate treatment plan is a tooth-only restoration even if built entirely on short implants to give her natural papillae and straightforward hygiene maintenance

4.2 The Most Important Part of the Implant

However short or long the implant, the most important part of the implant is really the empty space inside of it. An implant in this sense is just a receptacle installed into the bone that you are able to fixate restorations into. This empty space for restorative fixation will need to establish and maintain a harmonious and stable biological environment while having physiologically stable and functioning "life requirements" in an also easy to maintain prosthetic design facilitating and minimizing required dental hygiene interventions.

The short implants utilizing limited amounts of residual host bone or grafted bone can be viewed as instruments to minimize compromise. It may be that a treatment could proceed without an additional short implant; however, it is clear in a well-fitting restoration the implant will lessen the load and could just make the difference in the long-term function of the overall restoration. Implants are prescribed for structural support. Short implants as supplemental support in pontic areas are a valid consideration.

Short implant can be considered in instances of

1. supplemental biomechanical support with and without splinting to other implants,
2. when medical conditions indicate a grafting alternative,

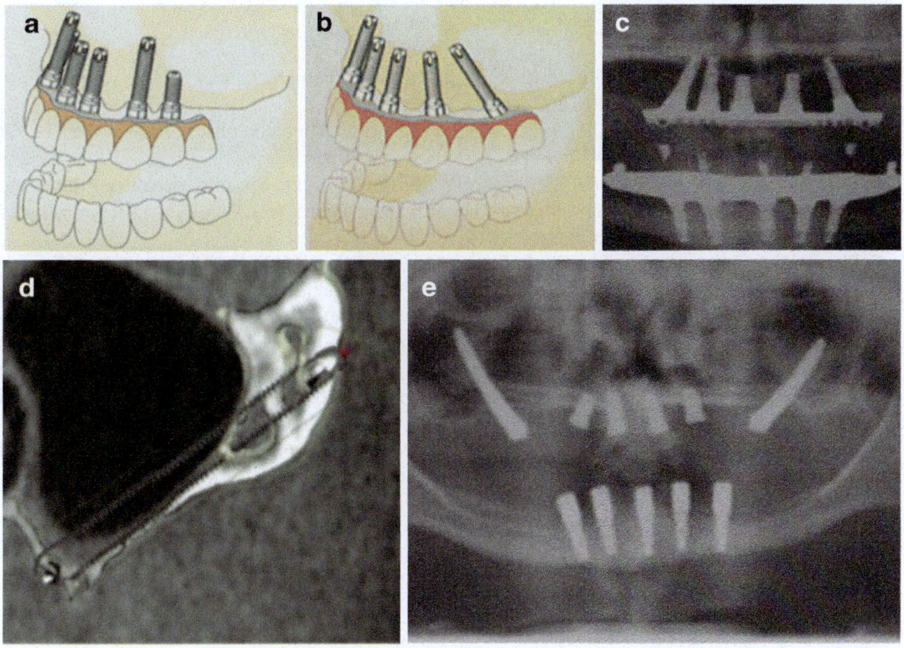

Fig. 4.13 Management of implant anchorage with limited bone in the posterior maxilla for the edentulous patient is a situation commonly encountered after many years of denture wear. The form of the maxillary sinus made the treatment approach shown in (**a**) understandable as a consideration. However the combination of poor bone quality in limited volume with necessity for cantilever support has been a strong motivation for avoiding short implants in this particular application. This is where the sinus graft for the edentulous maxilla became so popular, as an alternative for a short terminal implant supporting a maxillary fixed restoration. Today we consider it a successful development that there are now two very predictable alternatives to either a short implant in the posterior maxilla or the sinus graft alternative. When bone is present in the maxillary premolar area an implant tilted along the anterior wall of the maxillary sinus (**b**, **c**) allows use of a longer implant in better quality of bone with a reduction of cantilever length. For situations when there is no bone present in either the molar or premolar area, a zygomatic implant may be used for posterior support (**d**, **e**) combined with short implants in the anterior maxilla

3. decreased arch length is an acceptable alternative to minimize loads without the introduction of cantilevers,
4. extreme mandibular atrophy,
5. extreme anterior maxilla atrophy; for posterior maxillary advanced resorption the alternatives of tilted, trans-sinus [18], and zygomatic implants can all be considered,
6. to engage available bone anchorage independent of prosthetic design,

Recognize your immediate ability to take further advantage of 5, 6, 7, and 8 mm available site opportunities for osseous anchorage to benefit so many more patients without bone grafts but also without restorative compromise by taking full advantage of the diagnostic and planning software available and their utilization through delivery of the provisional and definitive restoration.

References

1. Estafanous E. Short implants: more long term data. Thematic abstract review. Int J Oral Maxillofac Implants. 2015;30:1237–40.
2. Huynh-Ba G. Crown-to-implant ratio: what is the latest? Thematic abstract review. Int J Oral Maxillofac Implants. 2015;30:259–61.
3. Romeo E, Storelli S, Casano G, Scanferla M, Botticelli D. Six-mm versus 10-mm long implants in the rehabilitation of posterior edentulous jaws: a 5-year follow-up of a randomized controlled trial. Eur J Oral Implantol. 2014;7:371–81.
4. Bulaqi HA, Mousavi Mashhadi M, Safari H, Samandari MM, Geramipanah F. Effect of increased crown height on stress distribution in short dental implant components and their surrounding bone: a finite element analysis. J Prosthet Dent. 2015;113:548–57.
5. Sanz M, Donos N, Alcoforado G, Balmer M, Gurzawska K, Mardas N, Milinkovic I, Nisand D, Rocchietta I, Stavropoulos A, Thoma DS, Torsello F. Therapeutic concepts and methods for improving dental implant outcomes. Summary and consensus statements. The 4th EAO consensus conference 2015. Clin Oral Implants Res. 2015;26(Suppl 11):202–6.
6. Esposito M, Pistilli R, Barausse C, Felice P. Three-year results from a randomized controlled trial comparing prostheses supported by 5-mm long implants or by longer implants in augmented bone in posterior atrophic edentulous jaws. Eur J Oral Implantol. 2014;7:383–95.
7. Torsiglieri T, Raith S, Rau A, Deppe H, Hölzle F, Steiner T. Stability of edentulous, atrophic mandibles after insertion of different dental implants. A biomechanical study. J Craniomaxillofac Surg. 2015;43:616–23.
8. Pommer B, Hingsammer L, Haas R, Mailath-Pokorny G, Busenlechner D, Watzek G, Fürhauser R. Denture-related biomechanical factors for fixed partial dentures retained on short dental implants. Int J Prosthodont. 2015;28:412–4.
9. Quaranta A, Piemontese M, Rappelli G, Sammartino G, Procaccini M. Technical and biological complications related to crown to implant ratio: a systematic review. Implant Dent. 2014;23:180–7.
10. Garaicoa-Pazmiño C, Suárez-López del Amo F, Monje A, Catena A, Ortega-Oller I, Galindo-Moreno P, Wang H. Influence of crown/implant ratio on marginal bone loss: a systematic review. J Periodontol. 2014;85:1214–21.
11. Mezzomo L, Miller R, Triches D, Alonso F, Shinkai R. Meta-analysis of single crowns supported by short (<10 mm) implants in the posterior region. J Clin Periodontol. 2014;41:191–213.
12. Anitua E, Piñas L, Begoña L, Orive G. Long-term retrospective evaluation of short implants in the posterior areas: clinical results after 10–12 years. J Clin Periodontol. 2014;41:404–11.
13. Malchiodi L, Cucchi A, Ghensi P, Consonni D, Nocini P. Influence of crown-implant ratio on implant success rates and crestal bone levels: a 36-month follow-up prospective study. Clin Oral Implants Res. 2014;25:240–51.
14. Nisand D, Renouard F. Short implant in limited bone volume. Periodontology 2000. 2014;66:72–96.
15. Villa G, Stavola L, Fincato A, Guida A, Magliano A, Merli M, Polizzi G, Karl M. Short, parallel-walled, conical-connection implants for a broad range of indications in the maxilla and mandible: retrospective multicenter study with up to 33 months of follow-up. Qunitessence Int. 2018;49(8):645–51.
16. Fortin Y, Sullivan R, Rangert B. The Marius implant bridge: surgical and prosthetic rehabilitation for the completely edentulous upper jaw with moderate to severe resorption: a 5-year retrospective clinical study. Clin Implant Dent Relat Res. 2002;4:69.
17. Fortin Y, Sullivan R. Terminal posterior tilted implants planned as a sinus graft alternative for fixed full-arch implant-supported maxillary restoration: a case series with 10- to 19-year results on 44 consecutive patients presenting for routine maintenance. Clin Implant Dent Relat Res. 2017;19(1):56–68.

18. Brånemark P-I, Gröndahl K, Ohrnell L-O, Nilsson P, Petruson B, Svensson B. Zygoma fixture in the management of advanced atrophy of the maxilla: technique and long-term results. Scand J Plast Reconstr Surg Hand Surg. 2004;38:70–85.
19. Maló P, Nobre M, Lopes A. Immediate loading of 'All-on-4' maxillary prostheses using trans-sinus tilted implants without sinus bone grafting: a retrospective study reporting the 3-year outcome. Eur J Oral Implantol. 2013;6(3):273–83.
20. Fortin Y. Placement of zygomatic implants into the malar prominence of the maxillary bone for apical fixation: A Clinaical Report of 5 to 13 Years. Int J Oral Maxillofac Implants. 2017;32(3):633–41.

The Straumann Short Implants

5

Waldemar D. Polido and Dean Morton

Contents

5.1 Introduction 47
5.2 The Straumann 6 mm Implant 48
5.3 The Straumann 4 mm Implant 50
5.4 Conclusions 56
References 56

5.1 Introduction

Prosthetic rehabilitation using dental implants in edentulous and partially edentulous patients with adequate bone condition is usually a safe treatment with predictable results, showing long term survival rates around 98% [1]. Anatomical limitations, such as reduced bone width and height, generate significant surgical difficulties in the installation of dental implants. In situations involving limited remaining bone, advanced surgical techniques were developed to make possible the installation of the implant, in a simultaneous or staged fashion. [2].

With the development of bone augmentation techniques, it became possible to rehabilitate many of these cases with implant supported prosthesis. However, clinical results show that vertical bone augmentation techniques, such as guided bone regeneration, distraction osteogenesis, interpositional bone grafts, onlay bone grafts, and the use of growth factors, are technique-sensitive, requiring significant

W. D. Polido (✉) · D. Morton
Indiana University School of Dentistry, Indianapolis, IN, USA
e-mail: wdpolido@iu.edu; deamorto@iu.edu

B. J. Tomasetti, R. Ewers (eds.), *Short Implants*,
https://doi.org/10.1007/978-3-030-44199-9_5

surgical experience, and producing unpredictable results. Moreover, they also increase treatment time, morbidity, complications, and cost [3, 4]. For the posterior maxilla, the sinus floor elevation is a predictable and well-documented technique, but also requires more time and a staged approach in severe atrophies [5]. The vertically deficient posterior mandible remains a challenging anatomic area to restore with implant-supported fixed prosthesis [6].

In the last decade, the use of short implants (<8 mm) became of great interest among professionals [7]. Rehabilitation using short implants in areas with limited bone height offers a less complex, less costly, and less traumatic treatment for patients. It has been demonstrated by several systematic reviews, RCTs, prospective, and retrospective clinical series publications that the use of short implants is a safer option for edentulous areas with limited bone height, when compared to the advanced and complex vertical augmentation techniques [8–13].

Some aspects should be considered of influence in the short- and long-term survival rates of short implants, such as achieving good primary stability, adequate bone to implant contact, potentially a high crown-to-implant ratio, and the effect on the marginal bone loss after loading. Those factors are directly influenced by the implant design, surface, and implant/abutment connection [14].

The Straumann Dental Implant System (Straumann Group, Basel, Switzerland) has a 6 mm and a 4 mm length implant available, both in the classic Soft-Tissue Level (STL) level design. The combination of a well-documented surface with a body design aimed at obtaining good primary stability, and a polished collar neck with an internal conical connection, allow this short implant designs to obtain predictable results when addressing the factors described above.

Our chapter will discuss characteristics and indications for these two short implants.

5.2 The Straumann 6 mm Implant

The utilization of short (6 mm) Straumann implants with the TPS surface goes back to the late-1980s, and favorable clinical results were first reported in the late 1990s [15, 16]. By the end of 1998, the "SLA—Sandblasted Large-Grit, Acid-etched" surface was launched on the 6 mm length and the "SLActive" surface was made available for the same length by the year 2005. Since then, the Straumann 6 mm implants are available in both "SLA" and "SLActive" surfaces. The SLActive surface brought the possibility of reducing osseointegration time and improving bone-to-implant contact. The SLA surface is considered one of the best documented implant surfaces in the market [1].

Recently, the Roxolid alloy (TiZi) was introduced with improved results not only in the strength of the alloy (it was initially launched with emphasis on reduced diameter implants), but also on the faster and improved osseointegration. It was then expanded to the whole line of the Straumann implants, with both the SLA and SLActive surface treatments [17].

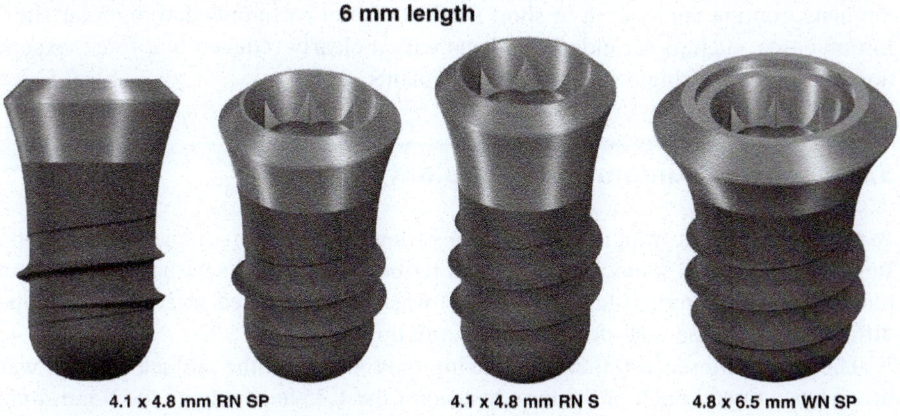

Fig. 5.1 The 6 mm implants

The 6-mm implants are available in Standard (2.8 height of polished collar) and Standard Plus (1.8 mm height of polished collar) designs, with 4.1 and 4.8 mm body diameters, in both regular (4.8) and wide (6.5 mm) neck configurations. The implant body itself has a solid screw parallel-wall configuration, with the thread pitch of the 6 mm implant having a distance of 1.25 mm between them, and a rounded apex. Once the body has 4.1 mm, and the neck has 4.8 (for the RN design), the "tulip-shaped" design helps to improve the primary stability at the neck of the implant, especially in the posterior maxilla sites (Fig. 5.1).

The polished collar neck provides a crown-to-implant connection at a supragingival (Soft Tissue) level, allowing for less crestal bone loss and an excellent peri-implant tissue stability. Since these short implants are usually positioned in the posterior region, esthetics are a minor concern, and the benefits of the polished tissue level collar surpass the possible show of a small portion of its grayish appearance. It is important to emphasize that the surgical length considered is the rough surface covered area, and the polished collar adds another 1.8 or 2.8 mm to the whole implant length.

The Tissue Level design also has an internal morse-taper conical connection (synOcta), providing a biological seal and excellent mechanical stability [18]. This characteristic may also be beneficial when dealing with short implants, giving more stability and helping to decrease the crown-to-implant ratio.

The use of short implants has been regarded as an effective alternative to approach the posterior atrophic maxilla with minimal invasiveness [19–21]. A recent prospective 1-year study on patient-reported outcomes has highlighted the high satisfaction obtained with the use of short implants compared to SFE, as it decreases morbidity, treatment time, and cost [11].

It is noteworthy, however, that one must differentiate between single standing implants and multiple adjacent implants, which can be splinted. In the case of multiple implants, short (6 mm) implants have been utilized in the posterior maxilla with good clinical outcomes, but they should be splinted. For single standing implants, routine application of short implants is not recommended in molar sites. In rare cases, such as for elderly patients with a clearly reduced bite force, exceptions are made for single standing short implants [22].

5.3 The Straumann 4 mm Implant

A novel Straumann implant with 4 mm of length (4.1 mm–diameter Straumann Regular Neck, solid screw, SLActive soft tissue level implants with 0.8-mm thread pitch and 4-mm length, titanium grade-4) was first introduced in 2009, with some differences from the well-documented 6 mm implant.

The main difference (other than having only 4 mm on the surface length), was that it has a thread pitch of 0.8 mm, instead of the 1.25 available on the 6-mm-long implant. It was launched commercially only in the Roxolid (Titanium-Zirconium alloy), and in an SLActive surface, with the SP (Standard Plus) 1.8 polished collar neck, in three different configurations: 4.1 (diameter) with 4.8 Neck (Regular Neck); 4.8 diameter with 4.8 neck (Wide-body), and 4.8 diameter with a 6.5 neck (Wide Neck) (Fig. 5.2).

The same surgical steps are utilized, with a 4 mm mark present on all the drills and depth gauges (Fig. 5.3). Extreme care should be taken to not overdrill the site in both vertical and horizontal directions, since it can lead to nerve damage and/or loss of primary stability. In the atrophic posterior mandible, usually all the alveolar bone is resorbed, and the implant has to be placed in a more cortical bone. Due to the reduced thread pitch, the primary stability obtained is very high. Hence, the use of tapping is highly recommended in order to avoid excessive insertion torque, which can potentially lead to lack of osseointegration.

A publication of Slotte et al. [23], reported on 24 patients (87 implants) examined for 2 years post-loading. All implants were found to be stable [survival rate

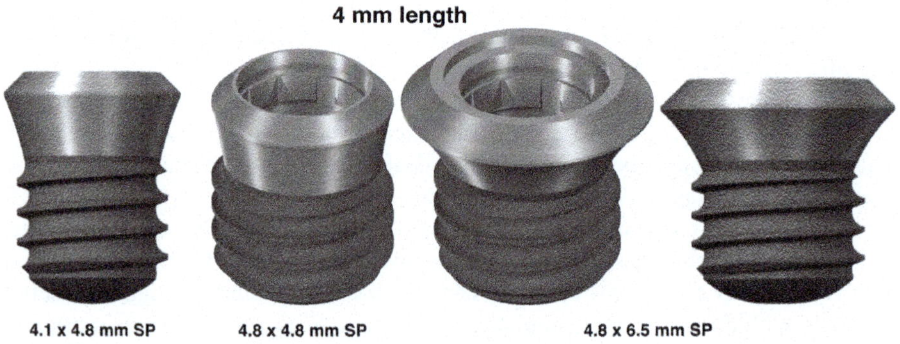

Fig. 5.2 The 4 mm implants

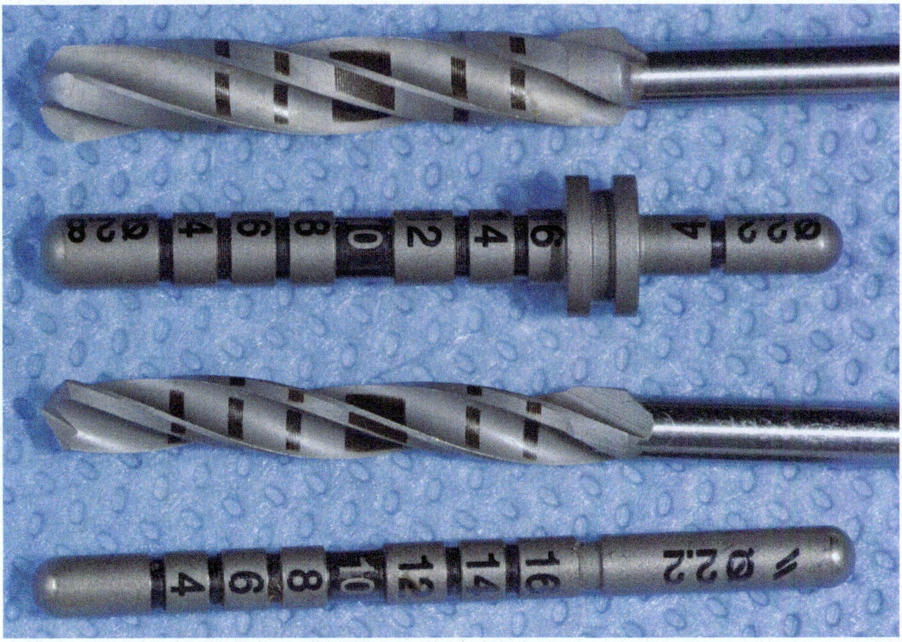

Fig. 5.3 Drills and direction indicators for the 4 mm implant

95.7% (confidence interval, CI 88.8–98.3) after 1 year and 92.3% (CI 84.5–96.2) after 2 years. The mean change from BL to 12 months was—0.43 mm (CI 0.31–0.59; $p < 0.001$) and from 12 to 24 months—0.11 mm (CI –0.01–0.23; $p = 0.056$).

The same group was followed for 5 years, and reported on a second publication [24], with 24 subjects and 71 implants still active at the 5-year follow-up (92.2% survival).

Calvo-Guirado et al. [25] reported on the use of forty 4 mm implants (4.1 × 4.8 RN, Roxolid, TiZi SLActive), placed in the posterior mandible of fully edentulous patients and splinted with longer (4.1 × 10 mm RN TiZi SLActive) implants to support a fixed prosthesis. After 1-year follow-up, the survival rate was 97.5%.

Polido and Nunes [26] present the outcomes after 2 years of follow-up of 50 implants with 4 mm of length placed in the posterior mandible of 25 patients. Implants were all titanium-zirconium SLActive surface, with 4 mm of length and 4.1 mm of diameter. Results showed that 5 out of the 50 implants failed in 4 patients, all before obtaining osseointegration (early failures). After an average follow-up period of 27 months (12–42 months), the implant survival rate was 90%. After restoration, no implants were lost, leading to a restoration survival rate of 100% of the restored implants. No patients reported neurosensory deficits.

The implants should be always splinted with another implant (of 4 mm or more in length), with flat occlusal surfaces, reduced occlusal area (premolarization), good occlusal contacts and adjustment, and without cantilevers, in order to obtain predictable results (Fig. 5.4).

Slotte et al. [24] conclude that with careful selection, treatment, and follow-up are carried out, 4-mm-long titanium implants, with the SLActive surface, can be safely and successfully used to support an FDP in severely resorbed posterior mandibles for at least 5 years, with healthy peri-implant conditions. Limited evidence is available for the use of this 4 mm implants for the posterior maxilla. However, short implants may be considered a reasonable alternative for rehabilitation of severely resorbed maxillae with reduced height to avoid a more invasive and less predictable bone reconstruction before implant placement. Papaspyridakos and cols. [27] performed a sistematic review and meta-analysis on the use of short implants (≤ 6 mm). Their clinical implications suggest the use of short implants as a valid alternative in selected cases where bone quantity precludes the use of longer implants, which would potentially require extensive bone grafting that can increase morbidity and risks. They also point that short implants may be a viable alternative for the posterior mandible, where vertical augmentation tends to be a more challenging procedure.

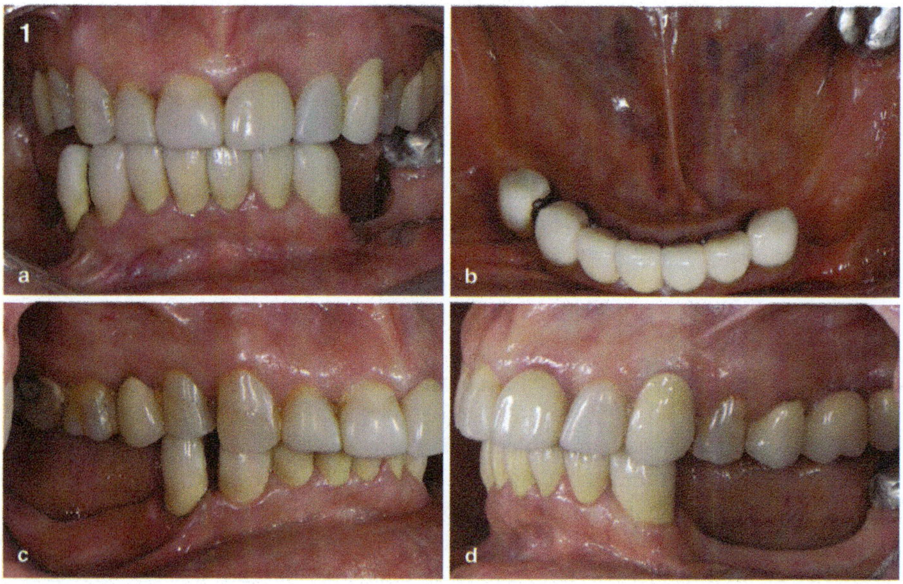

Fig. 5.4 Clinical case. (4.1) Initial clinical images: (**a**) Frontal. (**b**) Occlusal. (**c**) Right and (**d**) Left. (4.2) Preop CBCT images. (**a**) Right side, with cross cuts (**b**). (**c**) Left side, with (**d**) cross cuts. (4.3) (**a**) Transoperatory—notice tap and (**b**) 4 mm implant. (4.4) (**a**) Immediate post-op CBCT. (**b**) Right. (**c**) Left. (4.5) (**a**) Final right and (**b**) left. (4.6) Final occlusal. (**a**) Right and (**b**) left. (4.7) Final panoramic—1-year follow-up. Surgery: Dr. Waldemar D. Polido; Restorative work: Dr. Paulo Eduardo Pittas do Canto

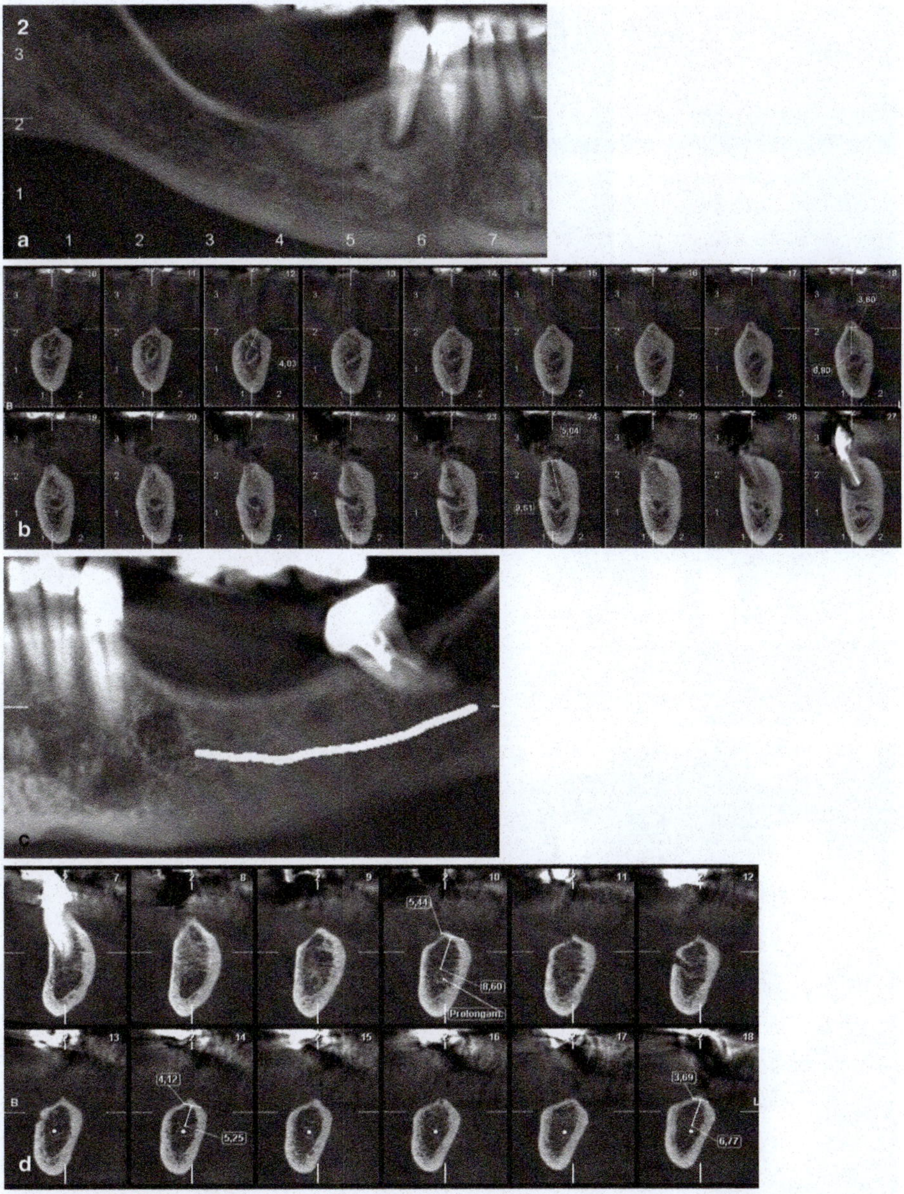

Fig. 5.4 (continued)

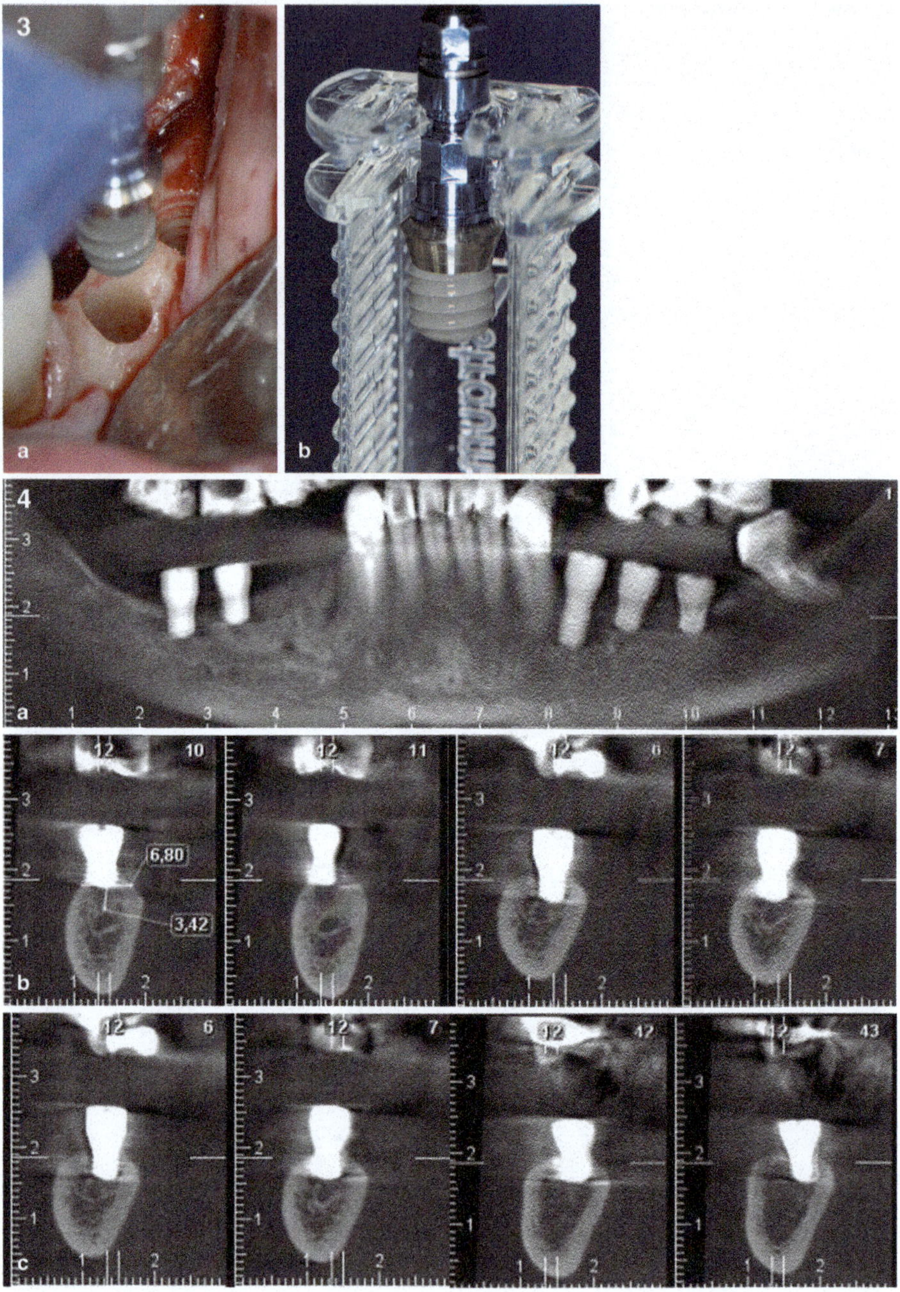

Fig. 5.4 (continued)

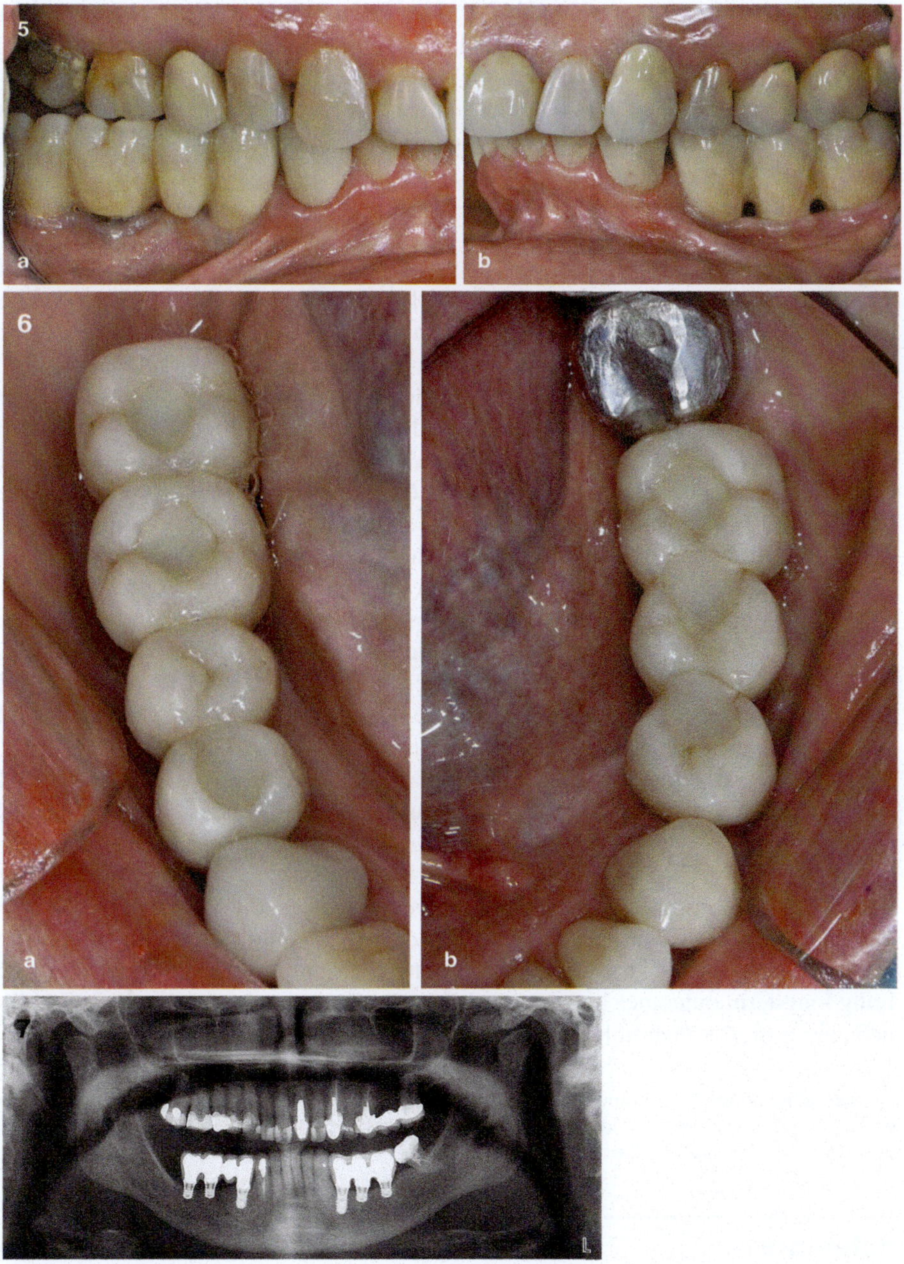

Fig. 5.4 (continued)

The 4 mm implant is available on the European, South American, and Oceania markets since 2010, and although it has limited evidence published in the literature, it is considered a less invasive and more predictable alternative to restore the posterior region with better patient outcomes when compared to more invasive and less predictable vertical augmentation techniques, especially for the mandible.

5.4 Conclusions

The surgical steps to place an ultrashort implant are similar to those used to place a regular implant, and although they require a good level of surgical expertise to be placed, it is technically less demanding than any vertical augmentation technique.

The reported survival rate of 90–95% is lower than the average survival rate for regular length implants (>8 mm). However, this procedure should be compared with the more invasive surgical procedures routinely utilized for vertical augmentation of the posterior mandible that show a failure rate ranging from 20 to 70%. When native bone is available, the use of longer implants should be the first choice of treatment.

The use of the Straumann short (6 mm) has been extensively documented, with good long-term survival rates. Recently the ultrashort (4 mm) has also been the object of attention, and many clinical studies are currently underway, to assess the use of this interesting tool. The characteristics that contribute to the success of this implant are the excellent surface treatment (SLActive), applied at the novel Titanium-Zirconium alloy (Roxolid), and the well-documented tissue level polished collar neck design, that carries a strong and stable internal conical connection. Detailed restorative care and recommendations (should be used splinted, reduced occlusal surface-premolarization, and low cusp occlusal tables) should be followed to optimize long-term results.

With the increasing trend to a minimally invasive surgical treatment with dental implants, especially with the elderly patients' population, the Straumann short and ultrashort implants should be considered when treating posterior vertically atrophic areas of the maxilla and the mandible. Current undergoing and future studies should bring long-term outcomes and stronger evidence for its use, specially for vertically deficient posterior mandibles.

Acknowledgements The authors would like to acknowledge and thank Dr. Paulo Eduardo Pittas do Canto, DDS, at Contento Odontologia, Porto Alegre, Brazil, for his contribution on the restorative work for the case that illustrates this chapter.

References

1. Buser D, Janner SFM, Wittneben J-G, Brägger U, Ramseier CA, Salvi GE. 10-Year survival and success rates of 511 titanium implants with a sandblasted and acid-etched surface: a retrospective study in 303 partially edentulous patients. Clin Implant Dent Relat Res. 2012;14(6):839–51.
2. Aghaloo TL, Moy PK. Which hard tissue augmentation techniques are the most successful in furnishing bony support for implant placement? Int J Oral Maxillofac Implants. 2007;22(Suppl):49–70.

3. Chiapasco M, Casentini P, Zaniboni M. Bone augmentation procedures in implant dentistry. Int J Oral Maxillofac Implants. 2009;24(Suppl):237–59. https://doi.org/10.1097/ID.0b013e3181ad8c6c.
4. Esposito M, Grusovin MG, Felice P, Karatzopoulos G, Worthington HV, Coulthard P. The efficacy of horizontal and vertical bone augmentation procedures for dental implants: a Cochrane systematic review. In: Evidence-based practice: toward optimizing clinical outcomes. Berlin: Springer; 2010. p. 195–218. https://doi.org/10.1007/978-3-642-05025-1_13.
5. Buser D, Monje A, Polido W. Treatment options for the posterior edentulous jaw: surgical options for implant therapy in the posterior maxilla of partially edentulous patients. ITI Forum Implantologicum. 2017;13(1):4–17.
6. Plonka AB, Urban IA, Wang H-L. Decision tree for vertical ridge augmentation. Int J Periodontics Restorative Dent. 2018;38(2):269–75. https://doi.org/10.11607/prd.3280.
7. Srinivasan M, Vazquez L, Rieder P, Moraguez O, Bernard J-P, Belser UC. Survival rates of short (6 mm) micro-rough surface implants: a review of literature and meta-analysis. Clin Oral Implants Res. 2014;25(5):539–45. https://doi.org/10.1111/clr.12125.
8. Camps-Font O, Burgueño-Barris G, Figueiredo R, Jung RE, Gay-Escoda C, Valmaseda-Castellón E. Interventions for dental implant placement in atrophic edentulous mandibles: vertical bone augmentation and alternative treatments. A meta-analysis of randomized clinical trials. J Periodontol. 2016;87(12):1444–57. https://doi.org/10.1902/jop.2016.160226.
9. Nisand D, Picard N, Rocchietta I. Short implants compared to implants in vertically augmented bone: a systematic review. Clin Oral Implants Res. 2015;26:170–9. https://doi.org/10.1111/clr.12632.
10. Thoma DS, Cha J-K, Jung U-W. Treatment concepts for the posterior maxilla and mandible: short implants versus long implants in augmented bone. J Periodontal Implant Sci. 2017;47(1):2–11. https://doi.org/10.5051/jpis.2017.47.1.2.
11. Thoma DS, Zeltner M, Hüsler J, Hämmerle CHF, Jung RE. EAO Supplement Working Group 4—EAO CC 2015 short implants versus sinus lifting with longer implants to restore the posterior maxilla: a systematic review. Clin Oral Implants Res. 2015;26:154–69. https://doi.org/10.1111/clr.12615.
12. Tong Q, Zhang X, Yu L. Meta-analysis of randomized controlled trials comparing clinical outcomes between short implants and long implants with bone augmentation procedure. Int J Oral Maxillofac Implants. 2017;32(1):e25–34. https://doi.org/10.11607/jomi.4793.
13. Uehara PN, Matsubara VH, Igai F, Sesma N, Mukai MK, Araújo MG. Short dental implants (≤7 mm) versus longer implants in augmented bone area: a meta-analysis of randomized controlled trials. Open Dent J. 2018;12(1):354–65. https://doi.org/10.2174/1874210601812010354.
14. Gonçalves TMSV, Bortolini S, Martinolli M, Alfenas BFM, Peruzzo DC, Natali A, et al. Long-term short implants performance: systematic review and meta-analysis of the essential assessment parameters. Braz Dent J. 2015;26(4):325–36. https://doi.org/10.1590/0103-6440201300265.
15. Atieh MA, Zadeh H, Stanford CM, Cooper LF. Survival of short dental implants for treatment of posterior partial edentulism: a systematic review. Int J Oral Maxillofac Implants. 2012;27(6):1323–31.
16. Ten Bruggenkate CM, Asikainen P, Foitzik C, Krekeler G, Sutter F. Short (6-mm) non-submerged dental implants: results of a multicenter clinical trial of 1 to 7 years. Int J Oral Maxillofac Implants. 1998;13(6):791–8.
17. Gottlow J, Dard M, Kjellson F, Obrecht M, Sennerby L. Evaluation of a new titanium-zirconium dental implant: a biomechanical and histological comparative study in the mini pig. Clin Implant Dent Relat Res. 2012;14(4):538–45. https://doi.org/10.1111/j.1708-8208.2010.00289.x.
18. Scacchi M. The development of the ITI DENTAL IMPLANT SYSTEM. Part 1: a review of the literature. Clin Oral Implants Res. 2000;11(Suppl 1):8–21. https://doi.org/10.1034/j.1600-0501.2000.011S1008.x.
19. Fugazzotto PA. Shorter implants in clinical practice: rationale and treatment results. Int J Oral Maxillofac Implants. 2008;23(3):487–96.

20. Nedir R, Nurdin N, Abi Najm S, El Hage M, Bischof M. Short implants placed with or without grafting into atrophic sinuses: the 5-year results of a prospective randomized controlled study. Clin Oral Implants Res. 2017;28(7):877–86. https://doi.org/10.1111/clr.12893.
21. Rodrigo D, Cabello G, Herrero M, Gonzalez D, Herrero F, Aracil L, et al. Retrospective multicenter study of 230 6-mm SLA-surfaced implants with 1- to 6-year follow-up. Int J Oral Maxillofac Implants. 2013;28(5):1331–7.
22. Rossi F, Botticelli D, Cesaretti G, De Santis E, Storelli S, Lang NP. Use of short implants (6 mm) in a single-tooth replacement: a 5-year follow-up prospective randomized controlled multicenter clinical study. Clin Oral Implants Res. 2015;27(4):458–64. https://doi.org/10.1111/clr.12564.
23. Slotte C, Grønningsaeter A, Halmøy A-M, Öhrnell LO, Stroh G, Isaksson S, et al. Four-millimeter implants supporting fixed partial dental prostheses in the severely resorbed posterior mandible: two-year results. Clin Implant Dent Relat Res. 2011;14:e46–58. https://doi.org/10.1111/j.1708-8208.2011.00346.x.
24. Slotte C, Grønningsaeter A, Halmøy A-M, Öhrnell LO, Mordenfeld A, Isaksson S, Johansson L-Å. Four-millimeter-long posterior-mandible implants: 5-year outcomes of a prospective multicenter study. Clin Implant Dent Relat Res. 2015;17:e385–95. https://doi.org/10.1111/cid.12252.
25. Calvo-Guirado JL, López Torres JA, Dard M, Javed F, Pérez-Albacete Martínez C, Maté Sánchez de Val JE. Evaluation of extrashort 4-mm implants in mandibular edentulous patients with reduced bone height in comparison with standard implants: a 12-month results. Clin Oral Implants Res. 2016;27(7):867–74. https://doi.org/10.1111/clr.12704.
26. Polido WD, Nunes LSS. Ultra-short implants for rehabilitation of the edentulous posterior mandible: outcomes after 1-3 years. Accepted for presentation, AAOMS Annual Meeting 2018, October 2018, Chicago; 2018.
27. Papaspyridakos P, Souza A, Vazouras K, Gholami H, Pagni S, Weber HP. Survival rates of short dental implants (≤6 mm) compared with implants longer than 6 mm in posterior jaw areas: A meta-analysis. Clin Oral Implants Res. 2018;29(S16):8–20. https://doi.org/10.1111/clr.13289.

Short Implants: Historical Perspectives

6

Clarence Lindquist

Contents

6.1 What Is a Short Implant? ... 74
6.2 Implant Design ... 77
6.3 Rational for Short Implants, Why Do They Work? ... 77
6.4 Summary and Conclusion ... 78
References ... 78

My experience with implant dentistry started in September of 1982. At that time, Dr. P. I. Branemark came to my office to treat five cases. Dr. Paul Krogh, Dr. Daniel Sullivan, and Dr. Lloyd Vakay also participated in this event. In October of 1983 I went to the "The Institute for Applied Biotechnology" in Gothenburg, Sweden to study their method of implant technology. At that time, the Nobelpharma implants that they used, ranged in length from 7.0 to 20.0 mm. The only width available at that time was 3.75 mm in the implant body with a 4.1-mm-diameter platform [1, 2]. I never had any experience with the 20.0 mm length at any time in my practice and used the 18.0 mm length in a few cases in the maxillary tuberosity and pterygoid plate. I used a number of 7.0 mm implants to avoid injury to the inferior alveolar neurovascular bundle or to avoid penetrating the maxillary sinus. We were advised at the Institute not to use the 7.0 mm implants unless it was necessary. My own personal experience with the 7.0 mm implants was favorable and several are in function after more than 30 years (Cases #1 and #2).

C. Lindquist (✉)
Chevy Chase Oral and Implant Surgery, Chevy Chase, MD, USA
e-mail: drl@omsusa.com

B. J. Tomasetti, R. Ewers (eds.), *Short Implants*,
https://doi.org/10.1007/978-3-030-44199-9_6

Case #1

Failed vestibuloplasty with skin graft done in 1970s. Retreated with visor osteotomy in 1983 that was unsuccessful. Retreated again with 6, 3.75 × 7.0 mm implants in 1989. Ten millimeter long abutments (3.0 mm longer than the implants) were used due to tissue thickness. Implants are in place and functioning well with no identifiable bone loss 30 years later (Figs. 6.1, 6.2, 6.3, 6.4, 6.5, and 6.6).

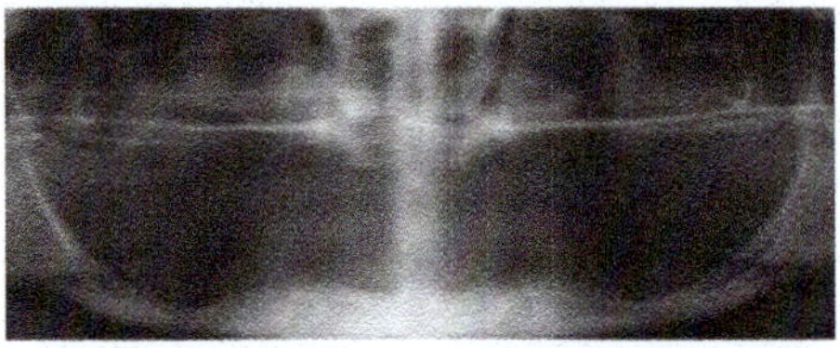

Fig. 6.1 Pre-op 12–13–83

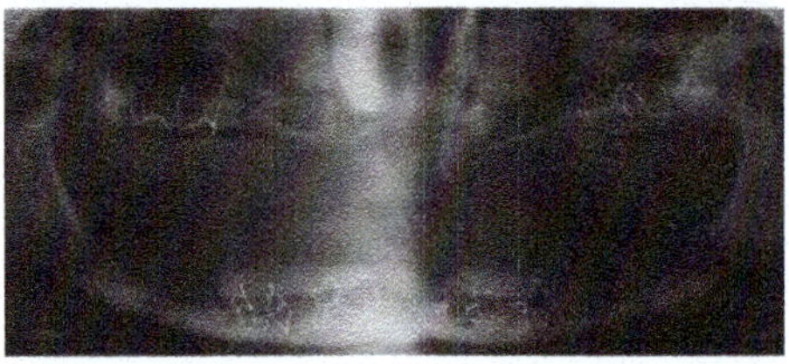

Fig. 6.2 Post-op iliac crest grafts 2–24–84

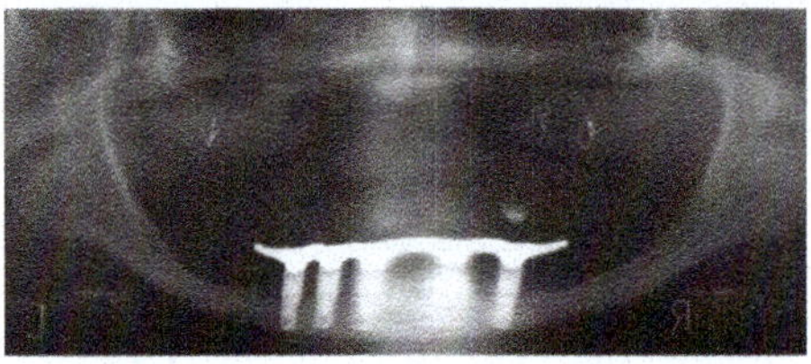

Fig. 6.3 Hybrid bridge in place 1–30–90

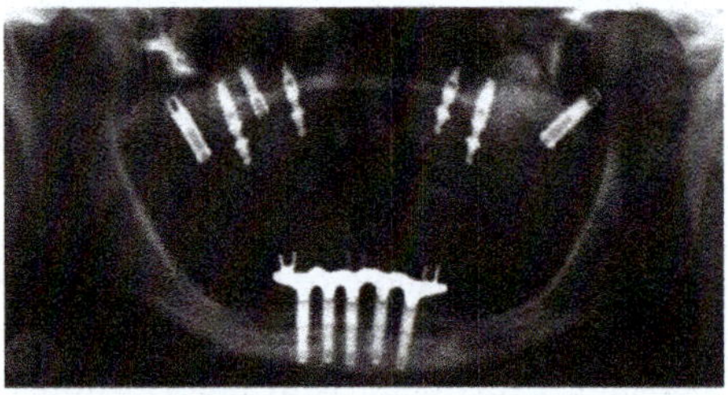

Fig. 6.4 Original mandibular hybrid bridge, 2–15–02

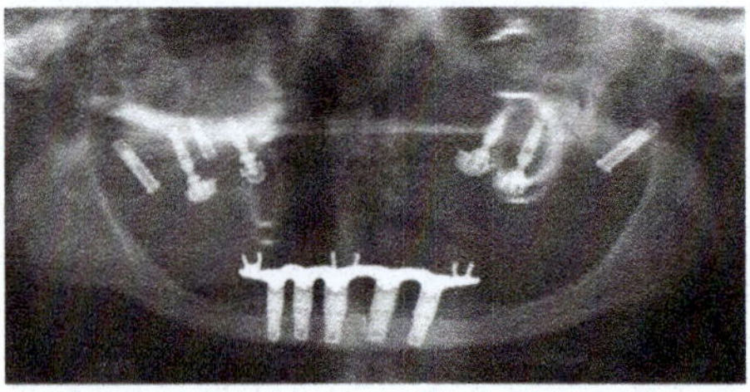

Fig. 6.5 Thirty-year post-op hybrid bridge

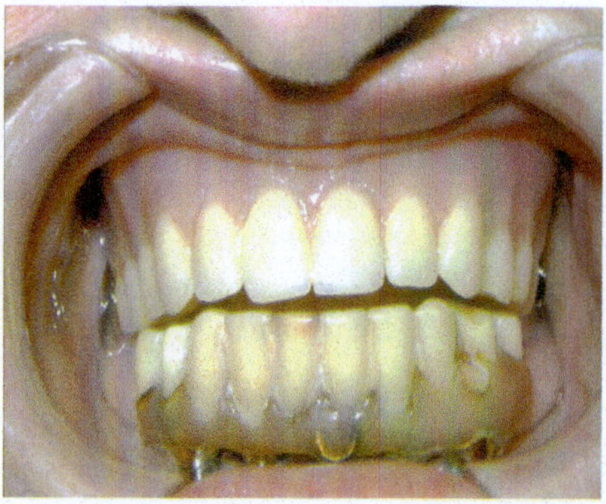

Fig. 6.6 Twenty-five-year post-op clinical photo

Case #2

2, 5.0 × 6.0 mm implants placed in missing #19 and #20 sites in 2009, 10-year post-op. (Courtesy Bicon Corporation) (Figs. 6.7, 6.8, and 6.9)

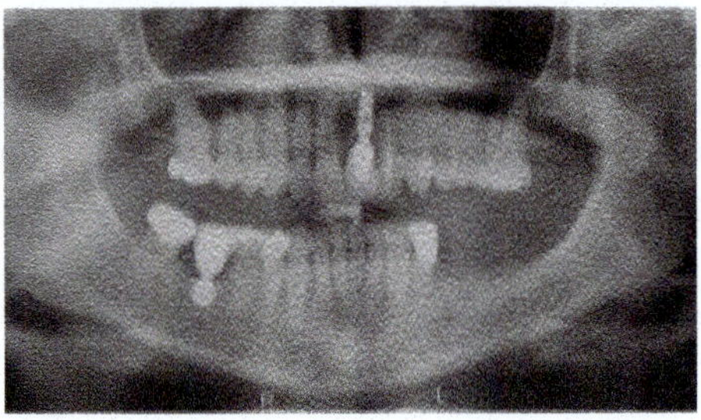

Fig. 6.7 Pre-op, 2009

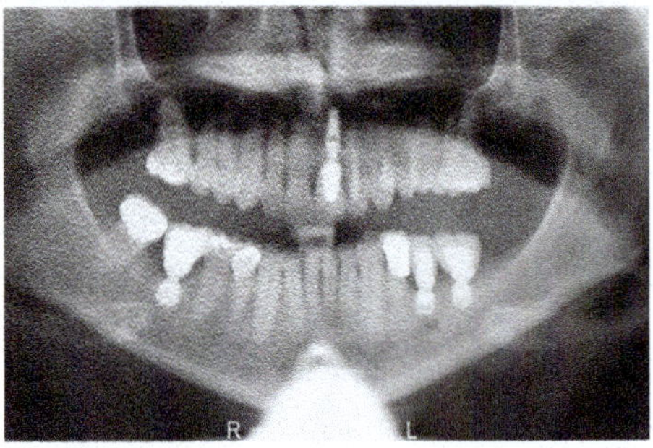

Fig. 6.8 Post-op 2011

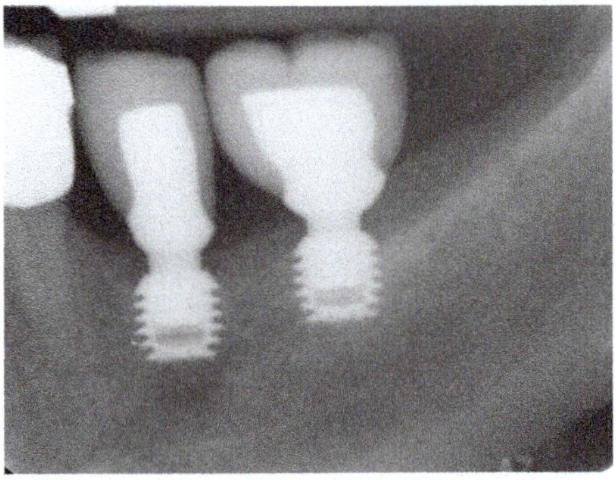

Fig. 6.9 Post-op

Dental implants represent a significant segment of the treatment modalities for the replacement of missing teeth. Barriers to successful implant placement are anatomic and physiologic. Physiologic barriers include medical problems such as bisphosphonate therapy (either previously or at the time of placement), radiation therapy, infection, bone diseases such as malignancies, congenital bone deficiencies, metabolic disease such as hyperparathyroidism, osteoporosis, and idiopathic reasons [3, 4].

Anatomic barriers exist in both the maxilla and the mandible. Mandibular barriers may be transverse deficiencies, (narrow, knife-edged ridges), deficient vertical height, deep lingual undercuts, and superior mandibular nerve position (caused by bone resorption or anatomically high nerve placement). Maxillary barriers consist of transverse deficiencies (knife-edged, narrow ridges), deficient vertical height, and encroachment of the maxillary sinus into the alveolar ridge for anatomic reasons or bone resorption [5] (Cases #3 to #5).

Case #3

Failed bridge, lower left quadrant, 2009. #19 replaced with a 4.5 × 6.0 mm and #20 with a 4.5 × 8.0 mm implant above neurovascular bundle, 10-year follow-up (Figs. 6.10, 6.11, 6.12, 6.13, 6.14, and 6.15).

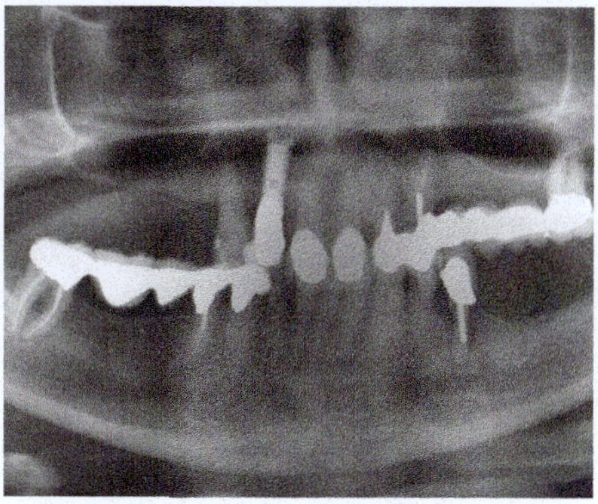

Fig. 6.10 Pre-op high nerve

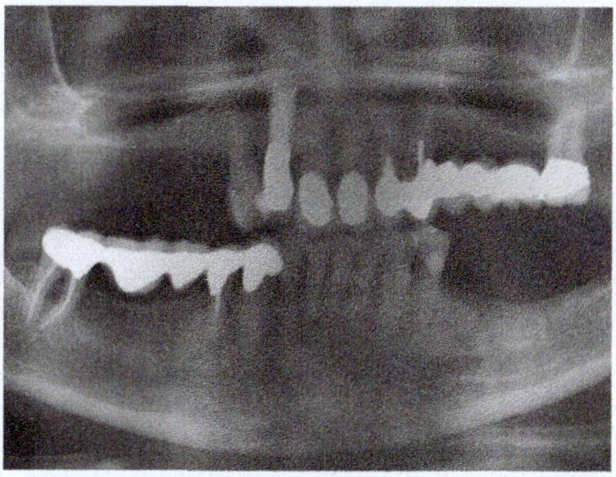

Fig. 6.11 Pre-op implant placements #19, #20

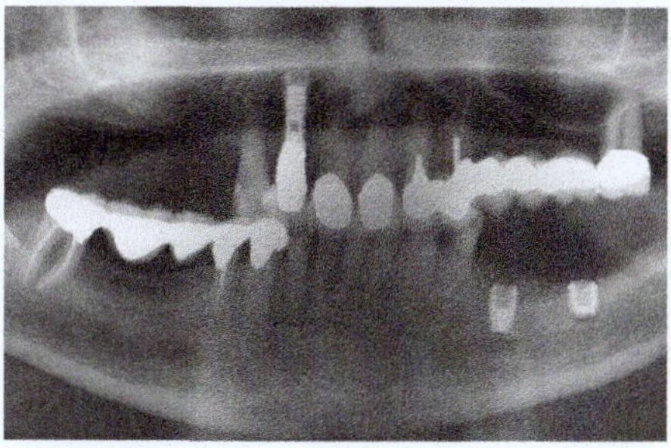

Fig. 6.12 Stage 1, 6.0 mm #19, 8.0 mm #20

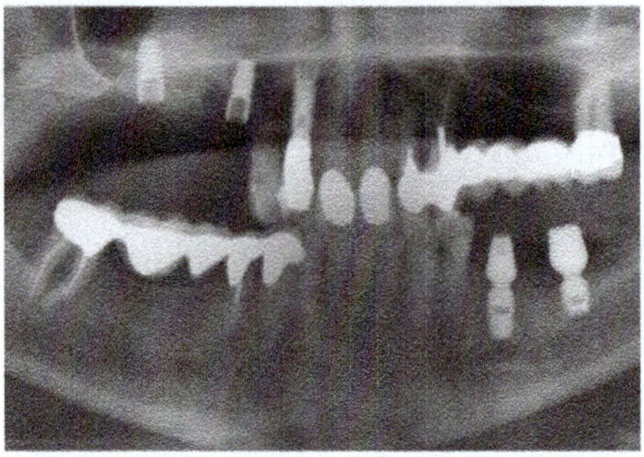

Fig. 6.13 Stage 2

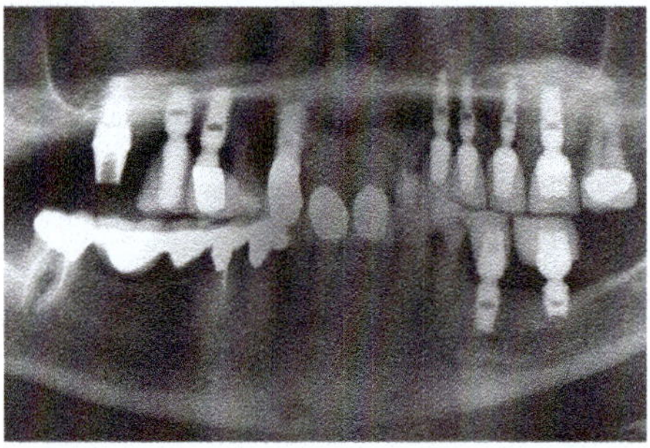

Fig. 6.14 Restorations

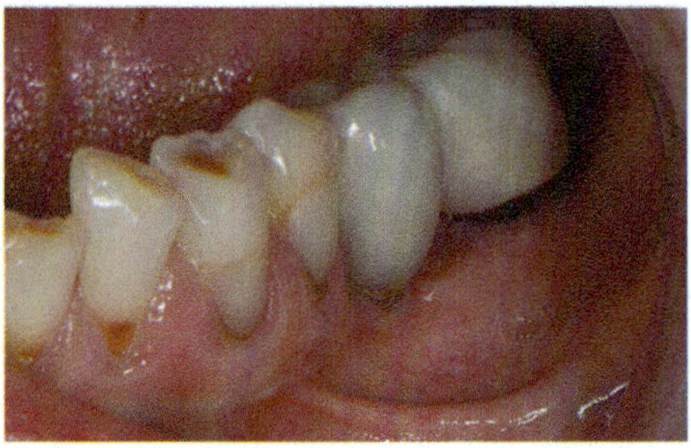

Fig. 6.15 Restoration

Case #4

Compromised alveolar ridges with high inferior neurovascular bundle position on right side. 2, 4.5 × 6.0 mm implants inserted above neurovascular bundle in #30 and #31 sites on 6–7–2011 (Figs. 6.16, 6.17, and 6.18).

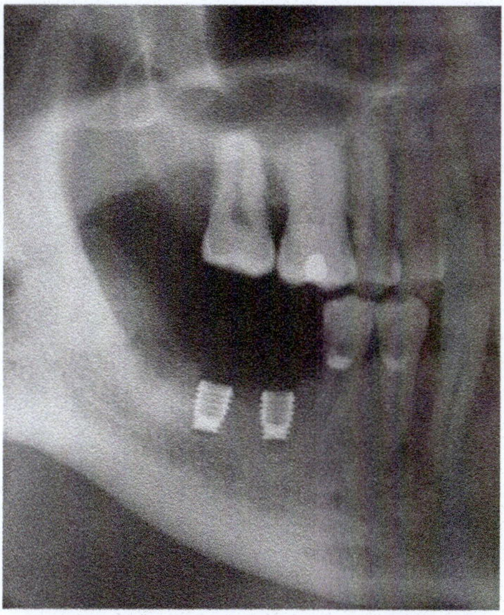

Fig. 6.16 Stage 1 implants, high nerve position

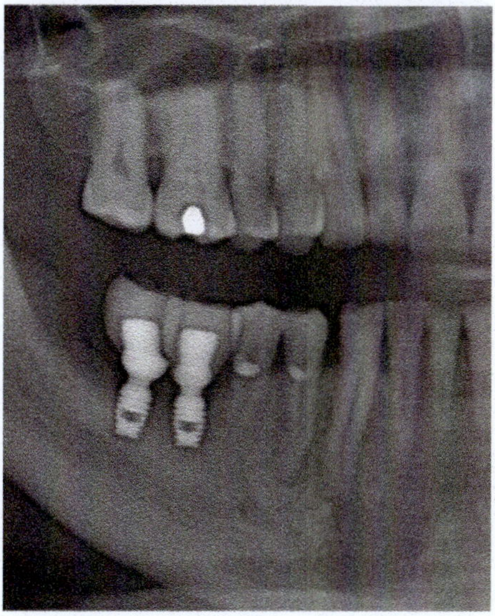

Fig. 6.17 Restored

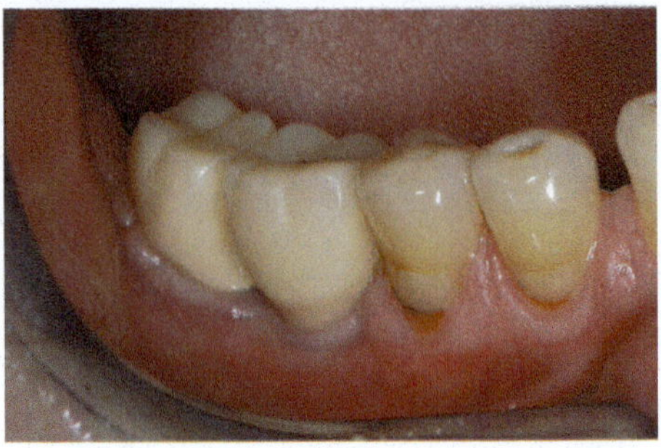

Fig. 6.18 Restored clinical

Case #5

Failed implant #3 site due to fracture-removed. Vertical ridge deficiency below maxillary sinus, tooth #3 site. 5.0 × 6.0 mm implant inserted in 2008, 11-year follow-up. No bone loss (Figs. 6.19, 6.20, 6.21, 6.22, and 6.23).

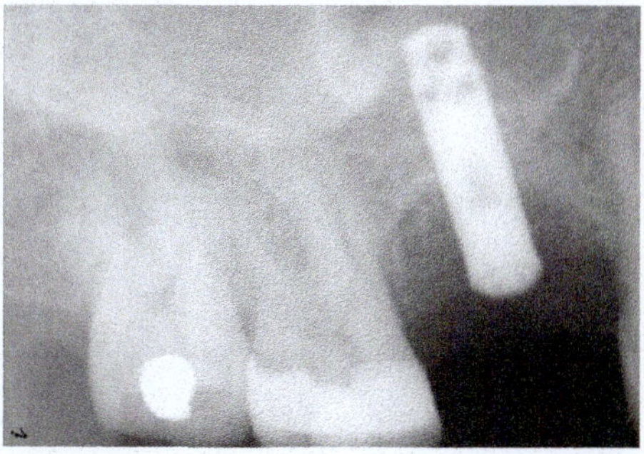

Fig. 6.19 Pre-op, removal fractured implant

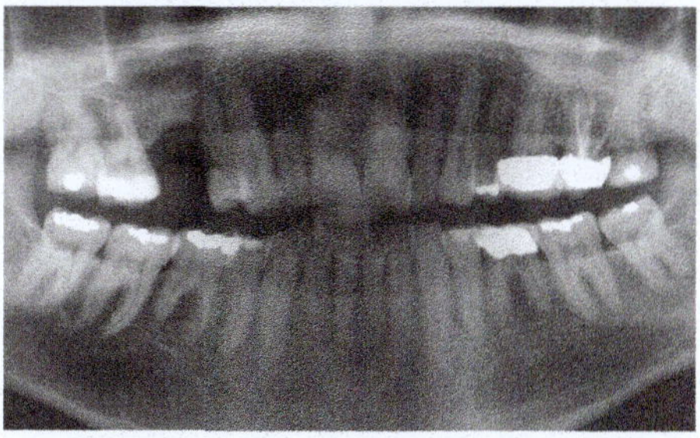

Fig. 6.20 Pre-op stage 1 implant

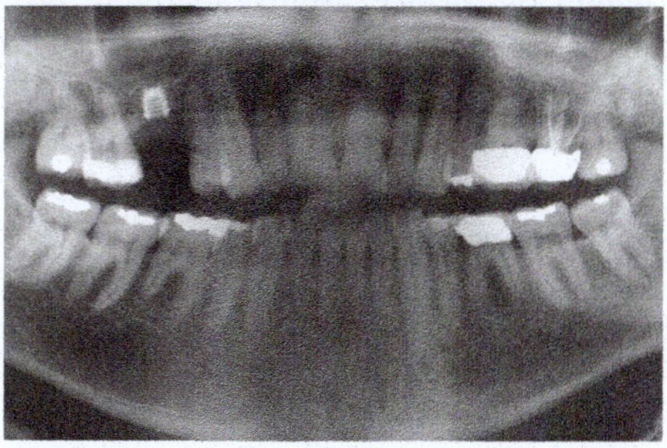

Fig. 6.21 Stage 1 6.0 mm length implant, 2008

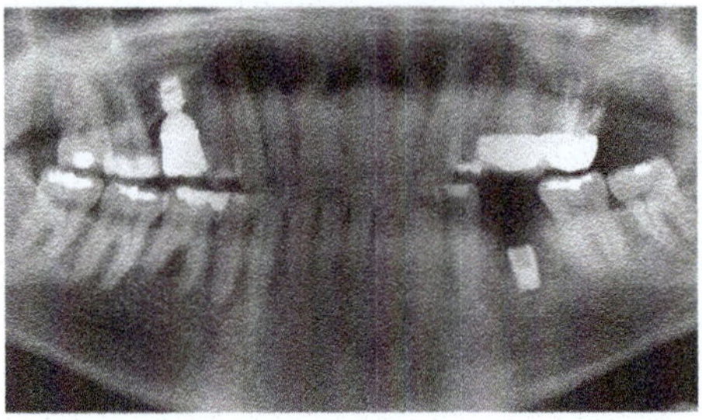

Fig. 6.22 Four-year post-op, restored

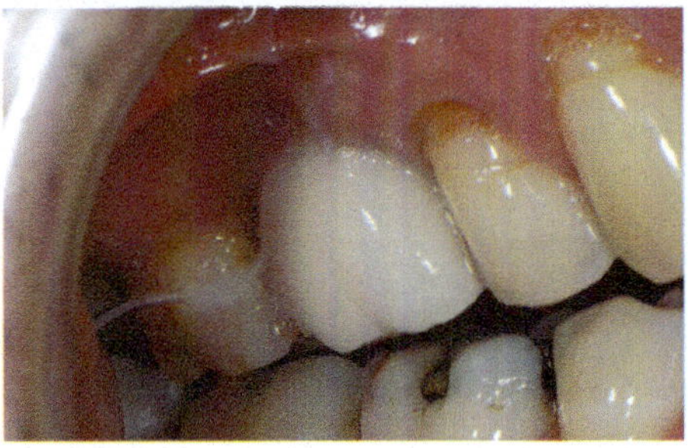

Fig. 6.23 Post-op restoration

Problems caused by bone physiology cannot be addressed by changing implant length or surface. Many anatomic problems can be overcome by using shorter implants, bone grafting, or ridge expansion techniques. Vertical deficiencies have been treated by augmentation grafting using autogenous bone grafts, either particulate or cortical blocks. They have also been treated with allografts and xenografts in particulate or block form. BMP (bone morphogenic protein) has been used alone or in combination with the other methods. All of these approaches are invasive and/or expensive. Current literature shows that treatment outcomes are good but are not better than traditional implant placement techniques in native bone [6, 7] (Case #6).

Case #6

Original implants placed in Europe 2009. Implants placed into maxillary sinus. They failed and were removed by the surgeon. CBCT scan showed extensive vertical and horizontal deficiencies. Treated with bilateral iliac crest and bilateral open sinus grafts. Restored with eight implants including, 3, 3.5 × 8.0 mm implants and 1, 4.5 × 8.0 mm implant on 4–26–2010 (Figs. 6.24, 6.25, 6.26, 6.27, 6.28, 6.29, 6.30, 6.31, and 6.32).

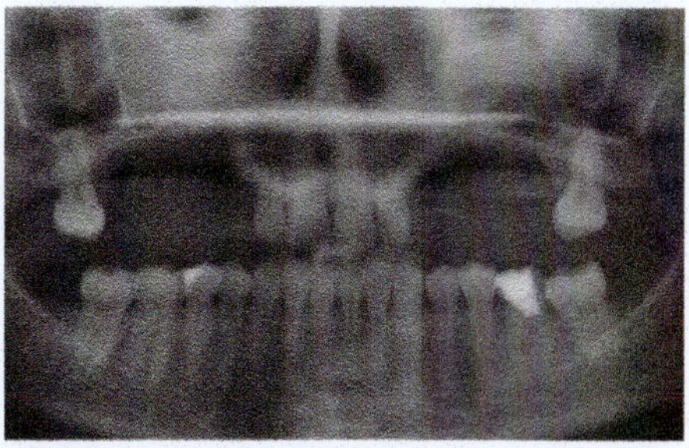

Fig. 6.24 Pre-op iliac crest and sinus grafts

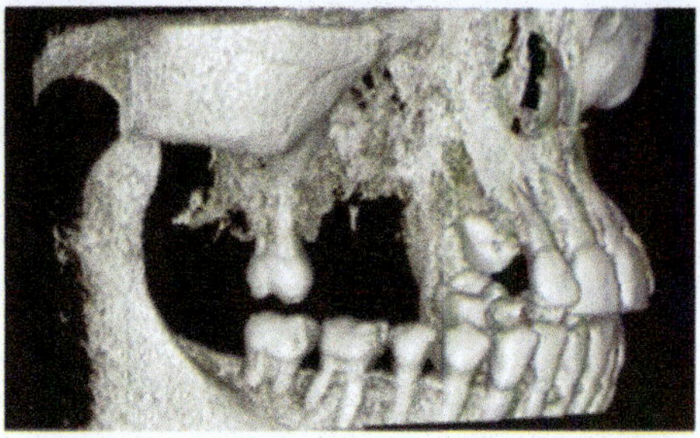

Fig. 6.25 Pre-op CT

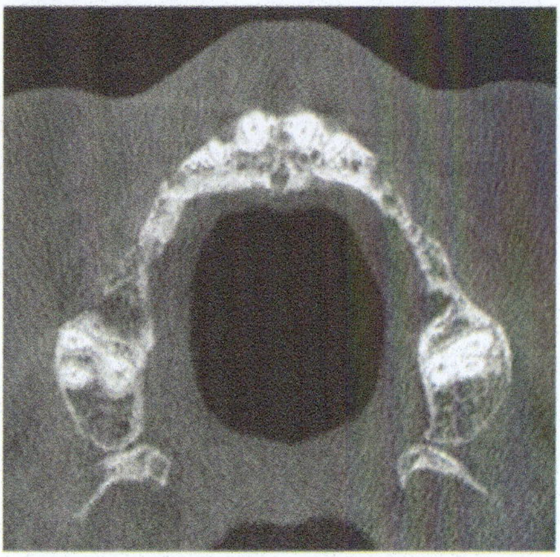

Fig. 6.26 Pre-op CT

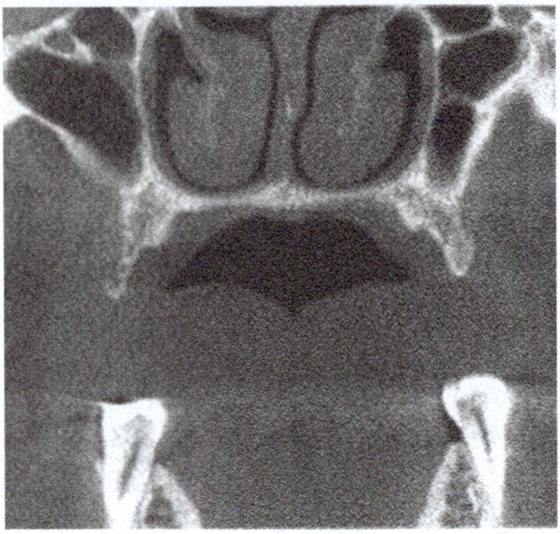

Fig. 6.27 Pre-op CT

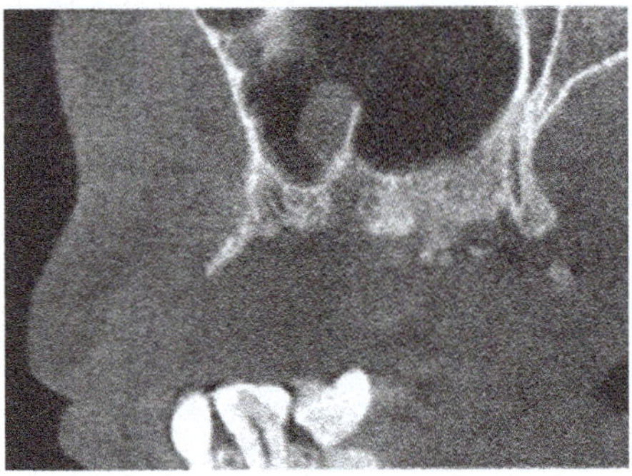

Fig. 6.28 Pre-op CT

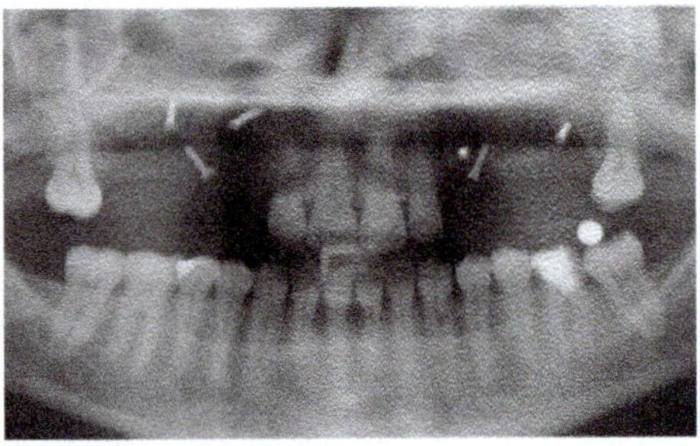

Fig. 6.29 Post-op iliac and sinus grafts

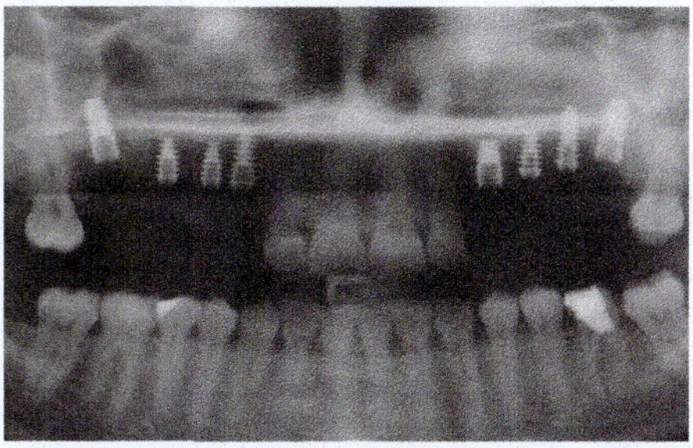

Fig. 6.30 Stage 1 implants, 4 8.0 mm length implants placed

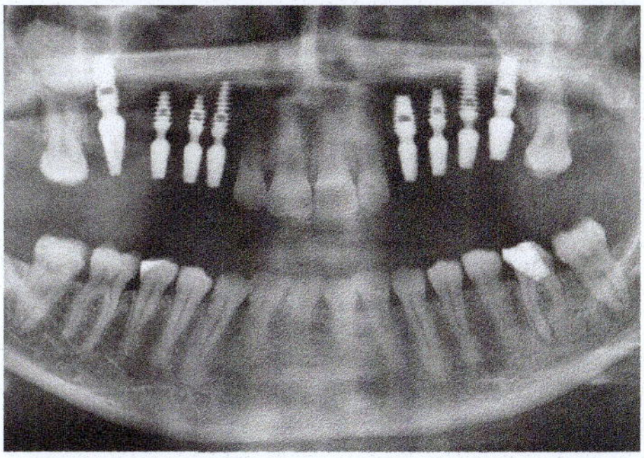

Fig. 6.31 Post-op stage 2

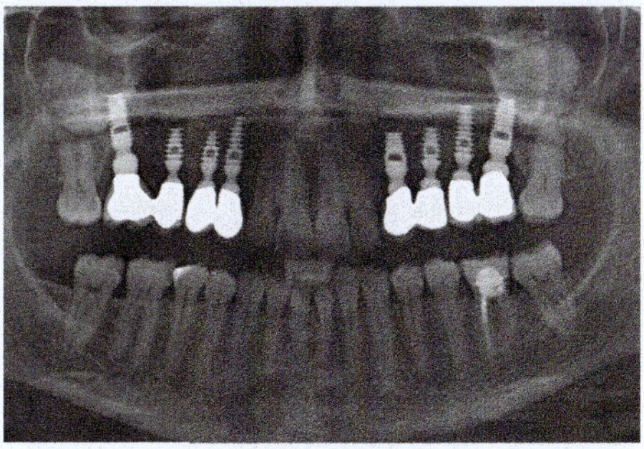

Fig. 6.32 Six-year post-op

The advantage of short implants is obvious. They are minimally invasive and they are flexible. They can be used in all areas of the jaws. For the patient, it means shorter treatment time and less pain and morbidity [8]. From an economic standpoint, the advantages are significant. By eliminating expensive complex bone grafting and minimizing risks of nerve injury or sinus penetration, patient acceptance is increased. If you can place an implant that has as good, if not better, prognosis than the longer implant why use a longer implant? (Cases #7 and #8).

Case #7

Vertical bone deficiency under maxillary sinus, tooth #14 site. 5.0 × 5.0 mm implant inserted on 2010, 9-year follow-up after stage 2 (Figs. 6.33, 6.34, 6.35, and 6.36).

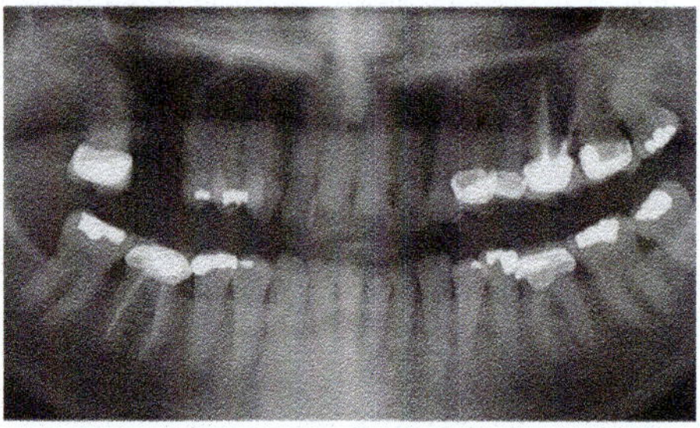

Fig. 6.33 Short vertical height, tooth #3 pre-op

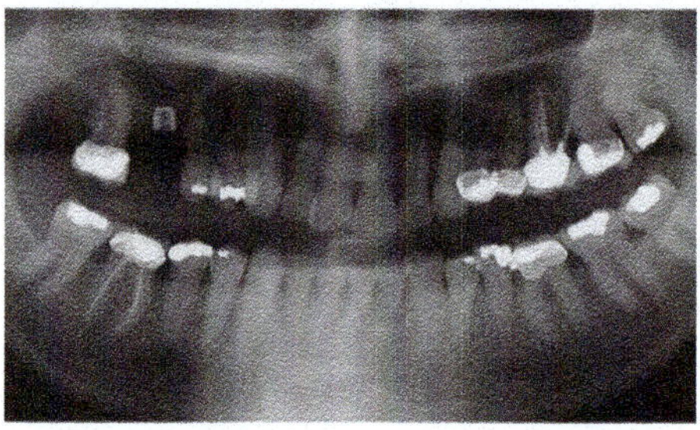

Fig. 6.34 Stage 1, 5 × 5.0 mm

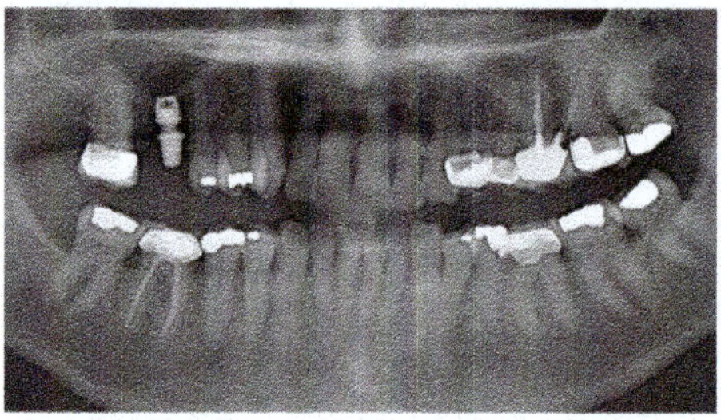

Fig. 6.35 Eleven months stage 2

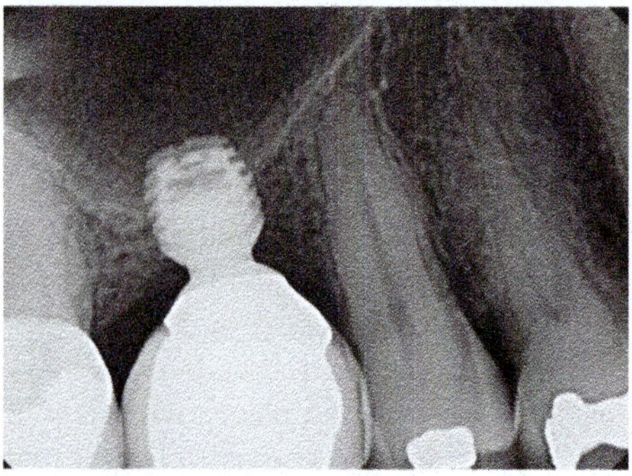

Fig. 6.36 Tooth #3 restored

Case #8

Vertical bone deficiency under maxillary sinus, tooth #14. 5.0 × 5.0 mm inserted successfully in 2011, 8-year follow-up (Figs. 6.37, 6.38, 6.39, and 6.40).

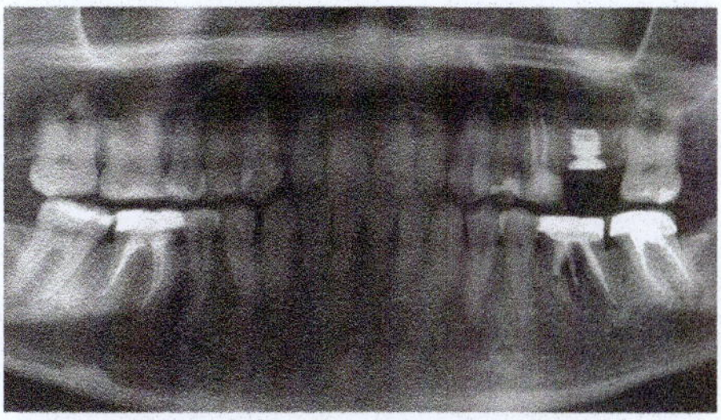

Fig. 6.37 Stage 1, short vertical bone height, #14, 5x5 mm

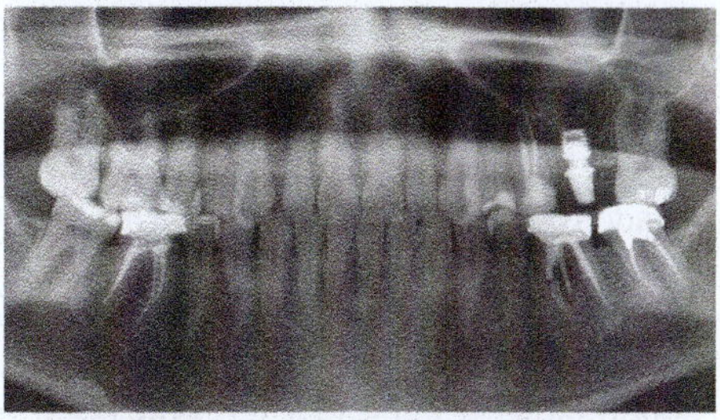

Fig. 6.38 Stage 2

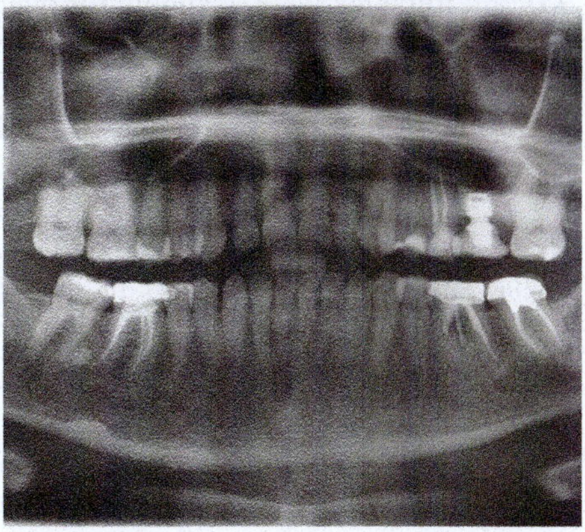

Fig. 6.39 Post-op, restored

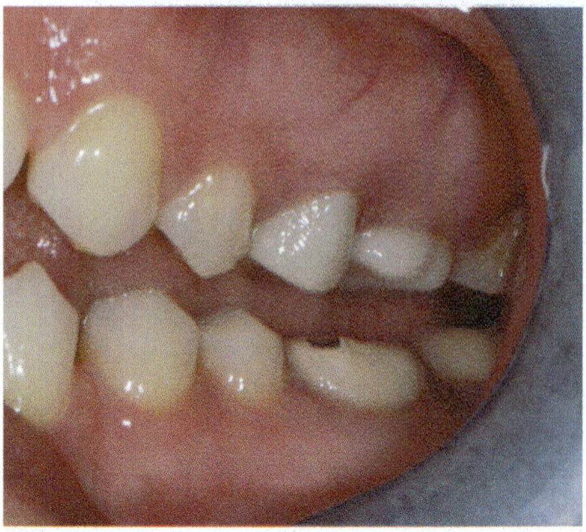

Fig. 6.40 Post-op #14 restored 2

6.1 What Is a Short Implant?

The SSID (State of the Science in Implant Dentistry) Conference sponsored by the Academy of Osseointegration, in Chicago, Illinois in August of 2006 defined a "short" implant as one 8.0 mm or less in Designed Intrabony Length (DIL) [9]. The length of the implant body in the bone is what defines a "short implant." This definition was arrived at after evaluating previous articles. Most contemporary implant manufacturers have had 8.0-mm-long implants in their inventory for many years. 7.0 mm implants were available for over 30 years, from at least one manufacturer. 6.0 mm length implants have been available since 1997 and 5.0 mm lengths since 2008.

Although root form implants fitting this definition may have been available for some time, the scientific history begins with the original Nobelpharma implant, designed by Dr. Branemark and his team in the 1960s and 1970s. This implant worked well in mandibles and maxillae with D-1 or D-2 bone but not as well in the posterior maxilla in D-3 and D-4 bone [10]. This study showed overall that the mandibular implants had a prognosis of 93.7% and the maxillary implants had a prognosis of 90.2%. The 7.0-mm-long implants had the lowest success rates, especially in the posterior maxilla.

At the 2009 Annual Meeting of the Academy of Osseointegration Dr. Tomas Albrektsson commented that the 7.0 mm Nobelpharma implants had a poor prognosis in the posterior maxilla. He was surprised to see that an article by Arun Garg showed consistent success rates in the 90% range. When he read the article, the Garg team had made just one variation in the protocol. The countersinking was eliminated which improved the initial stability and the outcomes (The author attended this lecture). These comments showed that survival rates of implants can be technique sensitive. The 7.0 mm implants could survive in an area in which the previous success rates were poor. This implant is no longer available from the manufacturer. Sometimes, implants need a full redesign to improve survival (Case #9).

Case #9

3.5 × 7.0 mm length implants placed in #3 and #14 sites on 6–22–1989. 30-year follow-up with no visible bone loss (Fig. 6.41).

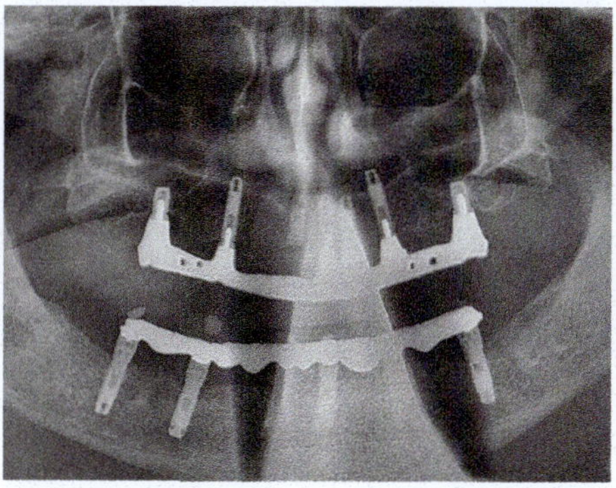

Fig. 6.41 7.0 mm implants in #3 and #14, 30-year follow-up

Short implants do not have greater failure rates as a result of the reversal of traditional crown-to-root ratios [11, 12]. Bicon corporation introduced a 6.0 mm wide by 5.7 mm long implant in 1997. This implant has had a success rate of 92.2% [3]. Currently, implants of 6.0 mm length, 5.0 mm length, and 4.0 mm length are marketed [8]. In response to the documented success of the short implants, several manufacturers are now marketing 6.0 mm and shorter length implants (Case #10).

Case #10

6.0 × 5.7 mm implant placed into #3 site in 1997, 13-year follow-up, X-ray taken in 2010. (Courtesy Bicon Corporation) (Figs. 6.42 and 6.43)

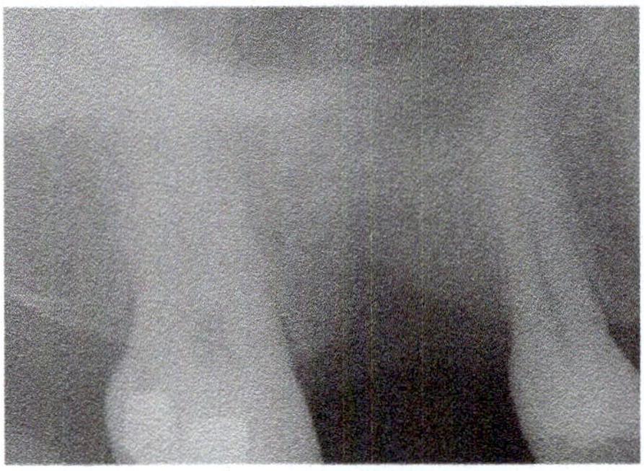

Fig. 6.42 Pre-op 1997, short vertical bone height

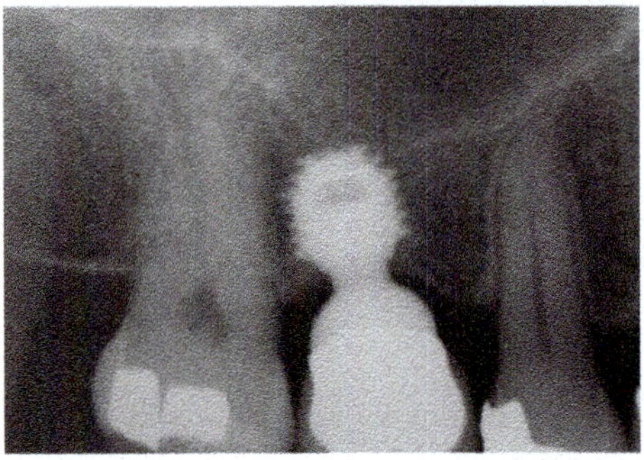

Fig. 6.43 Post-op restored, 13-year follow-up, 6.0 × 5.7 mm implant

6.2 Implant Design

Not all existing implants can be successfully shortened to 6.0 mm or less. An implant consists of a macro design, which is the easily visible geometry of the implant, and a surface treatment or coating which needs magnification to be evaluated. The most important factor seems to be the macro design of the implant. The original osseointegrated implants had smooth surfaces. Roughened surface treatments in many forms have evolved. Contemporary implants mostly have roughened surfaces of various types [13–15].

6.3 Rational for Short Implants, Why Do They Work?

The effect of the forces on an integrated implant has been well understood for many years. Analyses of these forces reveal that the greatest lateral forces occur within the coronal 3.0 mm of the implant body [16] (Fig. 6.44) [17]. This is where the axis of rotation of an integrated implant occurs. This differs from a natural tooth where the axis of rotation is at the junction of the apical one-third and the coronal two-thirds. The difference is caused by the space created by the periodontal ligament [16]. Consequently, the greatest lateral forces on an implant are in the crestal bone in the coronal area of the implant. The coronal

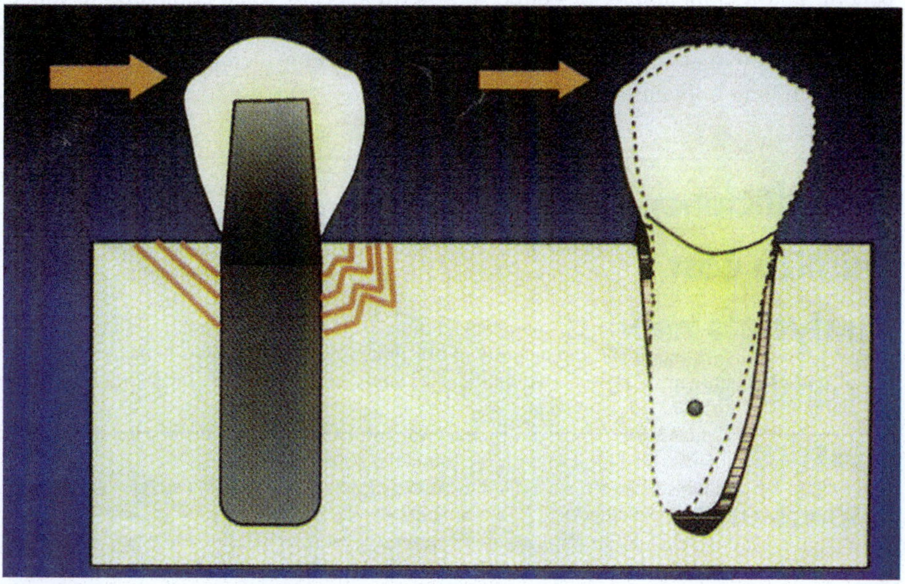

Fig. 6.44 An implant captures the stresses at the crest of the bone. A tooth rotates away from the load and distributes the stresses to the root, periodontal membrane, and cribiform plate. (Dentistry Today, 1999: courtesy of Misch Implant Institute)

area was the site of many early implant fractures, particularly with older design implants of 4.0 mm diameter or less which did not have enough strength to resist these forces.

If the greatest need of an implant is to be strong enough to resist lateral forces in the coronal 3.0 mm, why did most implants, longer than 8.0 mm, in older studies show better success rates? The answer is unclear, and the rational for using longer implants is not evidence based.

The final question is how short can an implant be manufactured and still work? Less 4 mm in DIL will encroach upon the internal implant length that will support the detachable, restorative components. An implant shorter than 4.0 mm could be a one-piece implant-abutment unit but that could affect restorative flexibility.

6.4 Summary and Conclusion

Short implants as defined by the SSID and documented by the literature have been an effective and reliable adjunct to treatment with dental implants. Reports in the 1980s and earlier in the Branemark literature started the evolutionary process. The first short implants were 7.0 mm and 8.0 mm in length and were used infrequently. As of this writing, 6.0 mm length implants are in common use. Literature has shown that the 6.0-mm-long implants have a better success rate than the longer implants [18]. I have used 5.0-mm-long implants since 2007 with no difference in outcomes. Short implants benefit dental patients by minimizing morbidity, greater economic benefit, and a comparable, or better, long-term success when compared to longer implants. Given the fact that "short implants" have a comparable success rate when compared to longer implants, should they really be considered as a separate category from long implants?

References

1. Albrektsson T, Zarb G, Worthington P, Eriksson A. The long-term efficiency of currently used dental implants. A review and proposed criteria of success. Int J Periodontics Restorative Dent. 1986;1:11–25.
2. van Steenberghe D, Lekholm U, Bolender C, Folmer T, Henry P, Hermann I, Higuchi K, Laney W, Linden U, Astrand P. The applicability of osseointegrated oral implants in the rehabilitation of partial edentulism: a prospective multicenter study of 558 fixtures. Int J Oral Maxillofac Implants. 1990;5:272–81.
3. Gentile MA, Chuang SK, Dodson TB. Survival estimates and risk factors for failure with 6X5.7-mm implants. Int J Oral Maxillofac Implants. 2005;20(6):930–7.
4. Tsolaki IN, Madainos PN, Vrostsos JA. Outcomes of dental implants in osteoporotic patients. A literature review. J Prosthodont. 2009;18(4):D309–23.
5. Renouard F, Nisand D. Short implants in the severely resorbed maxilla: a 2-year retrospective clinical study. Clin Implant Dent Relat Res. 2005;7:104–10.
6. Anitua E, Orive G. Short implants in maxillae and mandibles: a retrospective study with 1 to 8 years of follow-up. J Periodontol. 2010;81(6):819–26.

7. Felice P, Checci V, Pistilli R, Scarano J, Pellegrino G, Esposito M. Bone augmentation versus 5-mm dental implants in posterior atrophic jaws, four-month post loading results from a randomized controlled clinical trial. Eur J Oral Implantol. 2009;2(4):267–28.
8. Deporter D, Ogiso B, Sohn D-S, Ruljancich K, Pharoah M. 'Ultrashort' sintered porous-surfaced dental implants used to replace posterior teeth: a case series report. J Periodontol. 2008;79:1280–6.
9. Renouard R, Nisand D. Impact of implant length and diameter on survival rates. Clin Oral Implants Res. 2006;17(Suppl 2):35–51.
10. Lekholm U, Gunne J, Henry P, Higuchi K, Linden U, Bergstrom C, van Steenberghe D. Survival of the Branemark implant in partially edentulous jaws: a 10 year prospective study. J Oral Maxillofac Implants. 1999;14(5):639–45.
11. Birdi H, Schulte J, Kovacs A, Weed M, Chuang SK. Crown to-root ratios of short length implants. J Oral Implantol. 2010;36(6):425–33.
12. Urdaneta RA, Rodriguez S, McNeil DC, Weed M, Chuang SK. The effect of increased crown-to-root ratio on single tooth locking-taper implants. Int J Oral Maxillofac Implants. 2010;25(4):729–43.
13. Coelho PG, Granjeiro JM, Romanos GE, Suzuki M, Silva NRF, Cardaropoli G, Thompson VP, Lemons JE. Basic research methods and current trends of dental implant surfaces. J Biomed Mater Res. 2009;888:579–96.
14. Gotfredsen K, Nimb L, Hjorting-Hansen E, Jensen JS, Holmen A. Histomorphometric and removal torque analysis for TiO_2 blasted titanium implants. An experimental study on dogs. Clin Oral Implants Res. 1992;3:77–84.
15. Kotosovillas S, Fourmousis I, Karoussis IK, Bamia C. A systematic review and meta-analysis on the effect of implant length on the survival of rough surface dental implants. J Periodontol. 2009;80(11):1700–18.
16. Misch C. Functional surface area: short vs long implant. Dent Today. 1999;18:60–5.
17. Rangert B, Jemt T, Jornas L. Forces and moments on Branemark implants. Int J Oral Maxillofac Implants. 1989;4(3):241–7.
18. Urdaneta RA, Daher S, Leary J, Emanuel K, Chuang SK. The survival of ultrashort locking taper implants. Int J Oral Maxillofac Implants. 2012;27:644–54.

Significance of Bone–Implant Contact in Short Implants and Clinical Impact

7

Reha S. Kisnisci and Ismail Doruk Kocyigit

Contents

7.1 Bone Biology, Osseointegration, Bone–Implant Contact, and Physics.................... 82
7.2 Assessment of Osseointegration.. 84
7.3 Clinical Osseointegration and Short Implants.. 86
7.4 Conclusion Statements.. 90
References.. 90

The introduction of dental implants has resulted in many new developments in modern dentistry. The long-term clinical success of dental implants among other factors depends on understanding the interaction between bones and implants under various conditions and locations [1–3].

In cases of vertical bone height deficiencies various simultaneous or staged surgical procedures may be needed for implant placements. Despite favorable outcomes of such oral reconstructive surgical procedures, increased costs and associated morbidities may be unavoidable. For this reason the use of short implants are evidently emerged as another option in resorbed or atrophied bones for oral rehabilitation. Once there was a publicized opinion among clinicians that short implants considered to have lower success rates. However evidence has shown that success rates are similar with those of standard implants. In fact short (≤8–10 mm) and standard (>10 mm) implants statistically show the same success rate [4, 5]. This

R. S. Kisnisci (✉)
Department of Oral and Maxillofacial Surgery, School of Dentistry, Ankara University, Ankara, Turkey

I. D. Kocyigit
Department of Oral and Maxillofacial Surgery, Former Resident in Ankara University, School of Dentistry, Kirikkale University, Kirikkale, Turkey

B. J. Tomasetti, R. Ewers (eds.), *Short Implants*,
https://doi.org/10.1007/978-3-030-44199-9_7

section discusses osseointegration, osseointegration of short implants, the bone–implant contact, and its clinical impact on long-term success.

7.1 Bone Biology, Osseointegration, Bone–Implant Contact, and Physics

According to "disuse physiological phenomena" lacking functional loads or under exceeding pressures bone undergo resorptive patterns. This may be reversed biomechanically and physiologically if functional forces are restored thus transmitted mechanically to the bone to disrupt resorption. This may even result in bone deposition whereby this phenomenon is called bone remodeling. In general, the bone density changes are affected and vary due to the bone site, age, gender, and associated systemic health problems. It was shown that the bone density estimate varies between 1.7–2.0 g/cm^3 for cortical bone and 0.2–1.0 g/cm^3 for cancellous bone [6, 7]. Once an implant or implants are inserted into the bone, the mechanical properties of the bone undergo changes and according to Wolff's law, the internal structure of the bone is remodeled to adapt not only for the implant but for the loads applied upon the implant.

The type of force when applied to the tissue activates the mechanism that induces control at cellular levels remains unclear. Whether implant success is affected by loading or not loading still remains unclear or at least a controversial topic. Genetically, bone is coded to bear only a portion of the load and in theory, 100% bone–implant contact can be achieved through such remodeling [8, 9]. However, it manifests itself as resorption when the bone encounters deviations in stress generated by exceeding loads [10].

Irrespective of length all dental implants expected to reveal osseointegration, which by definition bone growth occurs toward the entire implant surface. Osseointegration is defined as a clinically asymptomatic and stable bone–implant contact in which force is directly transmitted to the bone without the presence of a histological soft tissue interface. This structural connection facilitates enhanced formation of bone–implant contact [4, 5, 11, 12].

Bones healing in terms of osseointegration of dental implants occur in three phases: primary stability, secondary stability, and tertiary stability. Primary stability is the mechanical hold of dental implant following insertion, depending multitude of factors including the macro/micro design of the implant, bone density, and the type of osteotomy. Secondary stability takes place by a complete and direct connection between the implant surface and bone. There is a latency period during the healing process to take place between primary and secondary stability phases in order that bone–implant union would be maximized for a favorable secondary healing [8, 9, 11]. It is due to this reason that therefore, ongoing researches focus on implant designs and surface features to further enhance the strength of this unification. Tertiary stability is essentially the functional adaptation created by assumed loads to the dental implant which then transmits to the surrounding bone. The quality of tertiary stability largely depends on the primary but mostly secondary stability, and the sustainability of tertiary stability facilitates long-term success [13–15].

Primary stability is the fundamental step for a successful osseointegration. This is facilitated by a minimum torque of 30 Nm that is the value of dental implant placement torque. It is reported that up to 32% of all implant failures, are caused by inadequate primary stability [16]. Factors ensuring attainment of primary stability are multivariate including most notably the bone density and quantity as the local determinant factors. Implant design and surgical technique do attribute to the initial stability but available options enable adaptability to overcome complicating bony conditions [17]. The dental implant related identifiable and distinguishable characteristics including length, diameter, surface structure, and groove configuration are other major factors that affect the primary stability. Many studies have shown that enhanced surface topography by increasing the surface area facilitate the bone–implant contact relationship at the time of insertion. As the implant size decreases in length and diminishes in diameter, this issue becomes even much more crucial [18, 19]. It can readily be explained by the higher success rates of rough surfaces as opposed to machined surfaces in terms of bone–implant interface by the fact that the wettability of rough surfaces is proved to be much higher resulting in spontaneous recognition of protein deposits such as fibronectin by osteoblasts. Moreover, rough surfaces enhance osteogenic cell line proliferation and differentiation [20, 21]. It has been identified that implants with circular shapes and designs with smooth grooves yield more favorable results in terms of bone–implant contact (Fig. 7.1) [22, 23]. However, the biomechanical contact between bone and implant contact does not always get increased through surface roughness as dental implant with machined surfaces may tolerate micro movements up to 100 nm whereas dental implants with roughened surfaces such movements range in between 50–150 nm [24, 25]. Current knowledge emphasis more on the importance of the properties and control of occlusal surfaces and well achieved primary stability of dental implants with respect to a successful osseointegration.

Tertiary stability and long-term success is the preservation of bone–implant functional stability under bite forces certainly within functional limits. Many clinical studies have shown that the forces implant-supported prostheses are subjected to

Fig. 7.1 Machined and rough surfaces of an implant

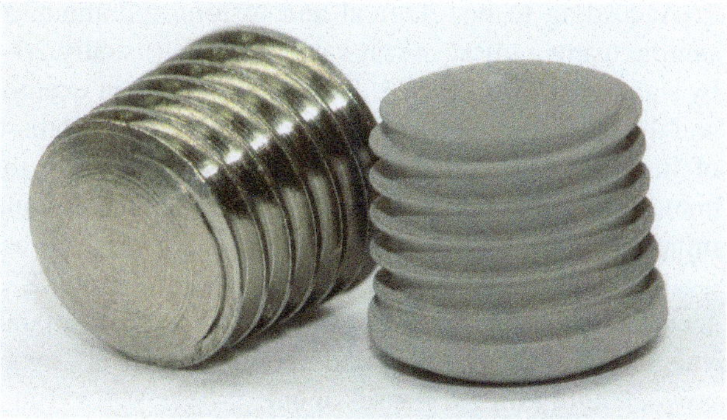

are within the range of 15–50 N which is equivalent to or slightly lower than the forces in dentate cases [26, 27]. The transmitted energy generated by bite forces to the bone via dental implant should be at such a level that bone remodeling and reorganization can take place in a permanent fashion to ensure long-term dental implant stability. As can be expected the bite forces may be multidirectional in nature including mainly axial or oblique directions and both the magnitude and the generation of repetitive excessive loads resulting from these forces may lead to microfractures in surrounding bone. Such continuing forces if are higher than normal levels, or if not timely unloaded than the bone induces osteoclastic activity [28].

Conclusively implant stability is more dependent on osseointegration hence the effect of implant length has not been clearly identified. Moreover 100% osseointegration will never be possible following dental implant placements and at subsequent stages. Currently therefore implants in which more than 50% clinical osseointegration has occurred in other words by the presence of bone–implant contact it is considered as a successful outcome. Despite the osseointegration rate was found to be fewer than 50% in early studies in terms of bone–implant contact, more recent studies have reported rates of 80%. It is still debated which percentage should be considered as a criterion for success [29–31] is yet to be conclusive.

7.2 Assessment of Osseointegration

Several methods can be used to assess to quantify osseointegration and may fall into invasive and noninvasive categories as well as in-vivo and ex-vivo methods. In vivo methods include various radiographic examinations and resonance frequency (ISQ) measurements that are performed without removing the implant out from the bone. Resonance frequency analysis provides information about the implant stability rather than the degree of osseointegration; however, it is not possible at all to obtain any unbiased data when using such measurements.

In ex-vivo methods, the implant is explanted un-bloc with the surrounding bone tissue and mechanical assessments such as push and pull tests, reverse torque tests, in addition to radiological and histological analysis such as confocal laser scanning electron microscopy (CLSM) and scanning electron microscopy (SEM) can be performed for further assessments.

According to histological and histomorphometrical analysis, 3–4 slices of the sample using a microsaw at various levels (usually 20–30 μm) is obtained followed by staining (Fig. 7.2) [32]. These slices are then examined under a light microscope and the bone–implant contact is calculated and expressed as percentile. The amount of fibrous tissue contact surface is discarded from the calculation and hence the contact of dental implant along its entire length with encasing bone would be determined (Fig. 7.3). However, currently this particular assessment technique is being gradually replaced by other means such as SEM, CLSM, and backscattered electron scanning electron microscopy (BS-SEM) due to mainly resultant lower resolution images. The technique is also cannot completely avoid bias and require considerably a lengthy time for assessment.

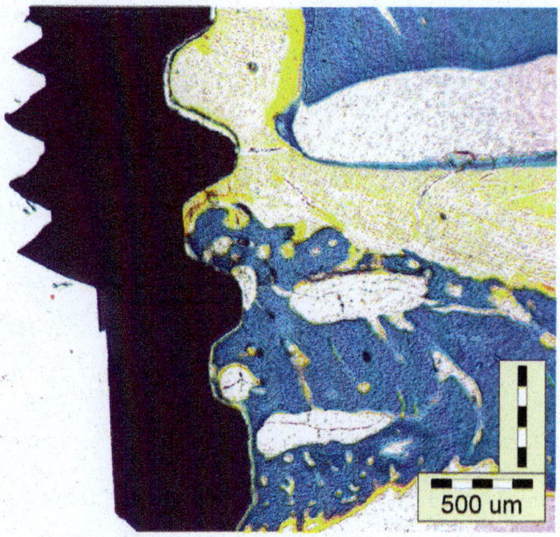

Fig. 7.2 Masson Goldner's Trichrome staining to provide superior identification between osteoid and mature bone matrix

$$\mathrm{BIC\%} = \frac{\text{implant surface length in contact with osseous tissue}}{\text{total length of implant}} \times 100$$

Fig. 7.3 Calculation of bone–implant contact (BIC) percentage based on histological data

The CLSM method is used to perform evaluations through high-contrast visual data without applying any additional procedures for the assessment of bone tissue and the implant [33–35]. Bone–implant contact evaluations are performed using SEM with secondary and backscattering electrons and particularly useful for the evaluation of implant surfaces [36–41].

In the BS-SEM method the sample is covered with evaporated carbon and fixated with colloidal silver and the obtained image is evaluated by means of using software. As the entire analysis of the image is standardized thereby rule out bias renders it one of the most reliable methods for the assessment of bone–dental implant contact. As the contrast difference between the implant and the bone can be achieved quite sharply owing to the high image resolution it enables to examine the implant in its entirety rather than only a portion of it.

Currently another major concept for assessment in terms of long-term success is the evaluation of the bone–implant volume (Fig. 7.4). This evaluation is basically based on the quantification of the contact bone volume that is formed between the implant grooves using synchrotron radiation microcomputed tomography (SCμCT) method [42]. This notable aspect of assessment of bone–implant volume also enables calculation of thickness of the new bone formed between the implant and the bone cavity. Although various studies to elaborate correlation between histomorphometrical and biomechanical data are performed, reliable results are yet to be obtained [43, 44]. Because SCμCT is a nondestructive method it can be used to simulate the implant–bone volume in three dimensions and to embody histomorphometrical and biomechanical aspects. In addition, finite element analyses can also be included to allow elaborations to be made related to bone–implant contact and implant stability.

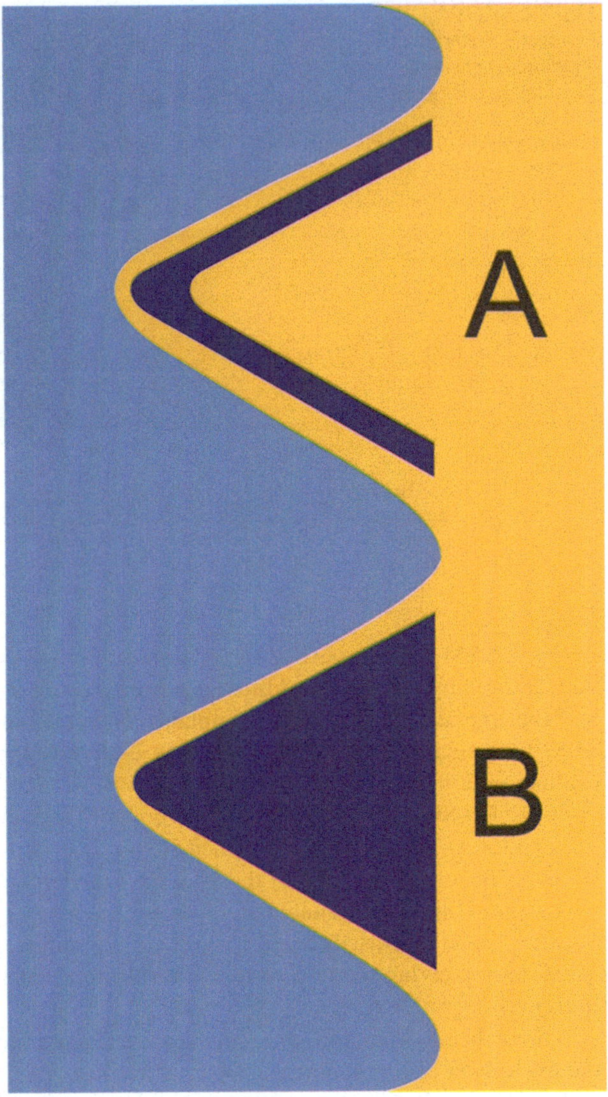

Fig. 7.4 (**a**) Bone–implant contact. (**b**) Bone–implant volume

7.3 Clinical Osseointegration and Short Implants

The forces generated in the crestal region of an implant are always stronger as compared to apically transmitted forces. Therefore preservation of the bone–implant contact in the crestal region against axial forces is of paramount importance for long-term success. Furthermore, oblique forces accentuate the generated stress within the bone–implant surface interface by 5–20 folds, and these loads also require intense consideration during the planning stage [45].

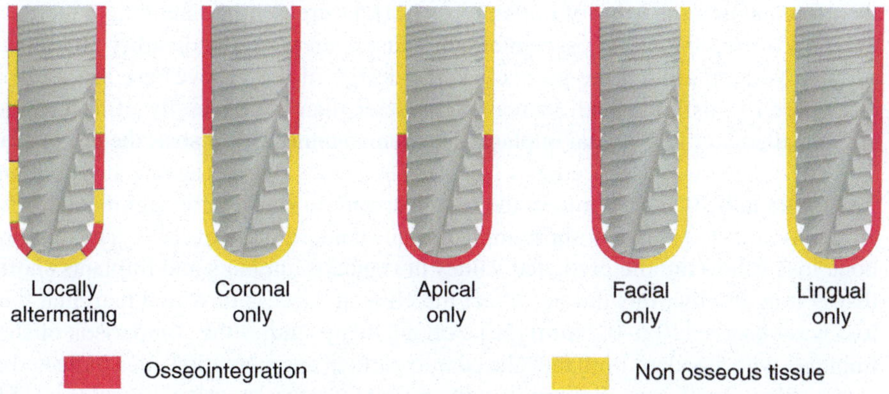

Fig. 7.5 Different patterns of bone–implant contact

Fig. 7.6 Immediate short implant placement into a poor bone quality following fresh extraction socket and curettage

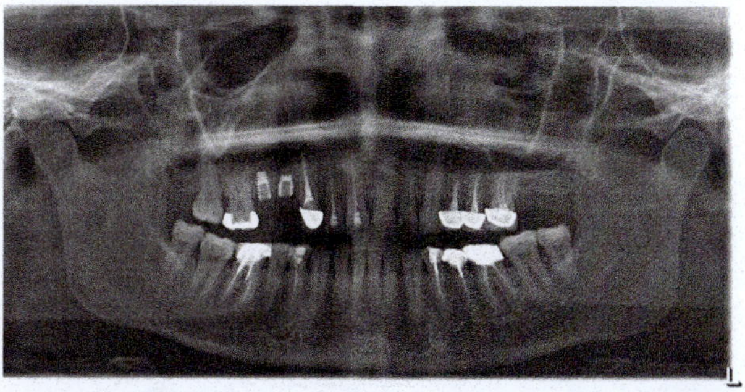

In case of short implants, the bone implant formation pattern is more evident and remarkable than the bone–implant contact percentile (Fig. 7.5). This new bone pattern can present along the entire and all around crestal, apical, lingual, and palatal regions of the implants. The response of the bone is more intense to impaction loads around the crestal region being generally of compact bone type as compared to apical region although there are exceptions of bone type at the crestal region [10]. Bone–implant contact forms at higher rates in compact bone than does in cancellous type bone hence success is much lower in implants placed in type-4 cancellous bone particularly if regular groove-typed short and smaller diameter implants are preferred. Otherwise the success of standard and short implants is nearly equivalent in all other bone types (Fig. 7.6).

The transmission of forces applied in apical direction from above to the implant and generated stress at the surrounding bone occurs at most in the first 3 mm at the superior region and gradually tapers off toward apical direction. In other words stress accumulation is concentrated in the crestal bone where it leads to gradual bone resorption at this region accordingly [46, 47]. Short implants with grooves alike a normal length dental implant (>8 mm) with added inevitable increase of crown/root ratio in most cases potentially leads to increased marginal bone loss and therefore an increased risk of implant loss [48]. Decreased implant length increases the clinical importance of osseointegration and even more the quantity and quality of bone volume around the grooves. If the design of the grooves are as described elsewhere in this book with increased diameter than the necessity of accustomed size and diameter type dental implants are deemed unnecessary so as the pre-implant surgical reconstructive procedures. Marginal bone loss even in regular short implants was found to be 0.5–1.37 mm in the first year and no statistically significant difference was detected between short implants and standard implants [49]. The marginal bone loss values are the predicted values in standard implants and implants shorter than 9 mm and that this did not affect the clinical success in which marginal bone loss was observed (0.6–0.7 mm) [50]. Among many studies the comparison of short implants with standard implants placed into vertical augmentation sites indicated no statistically significant difference with respect to the marginal bone loss [51]. However those with specific plateau type grooves and treads of short and wide implants can be used obviating the preparatory reconstructive surgical phase for secondary implant placements (Fig. 7.7).

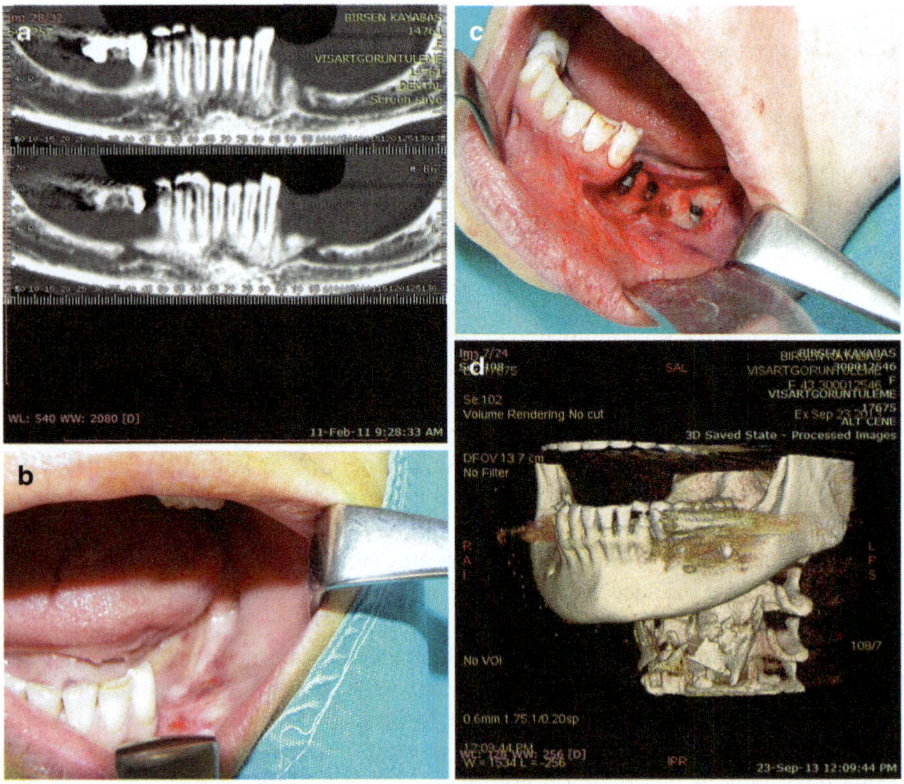

Fig. 7.7 (**a**) Pre-op CT. (**b**) Clinical pre-op. (**c**) Intra-op placement of short implants. (**d**) Six-year post-op CT

It is reported that long-term (5–10 years) success is remarkable in short implants on supporting single crowns. However, it should be noted that several factors that may be detrimental upon standard implants do also apply on short implants such as including bone type-4 and load characteristics [52, 53]. Based on current implant-supported prosthetics principles, the ideal crown-root ratio should be 1:2 and the minimum crown-implant ratio should be 1:1 although the crown-implant ratio is updated as 2:1 in the EAO consensus report [54]. In certain cases, especially with short implants, this ratio cannot be achieved. But the importance of crown-implant ratio is discredited where the crown height distance is proposed to be more determinant and that each 1-mm increase in the crown height length increases the magnitude of load in the cervical area by 20% [55, 56]. The cut-off crown height is found to be 15 mm and the maximum ideal crown height distance is also suggested to be around 15 mm (Fig. 7.8). Bone–implant contact may also adversely affected in terms of marginal bone loss caused by the opposing implant-supported occlusion against short implants that leads to more marginal bone loss than tooth-supported or other types of occlusions (Fig. 7.9) [57].

Immediate loading is not advised for implants shorter than 10 mm however when placed with additional standard implants the success rate increases with immediate or early loading so as low quality bone as a confounding factor [58]. Overall it is recommended that in order to achieve a long-term success, the bone–implant contact should not be under 50% in short implants. Similar outcome is reported

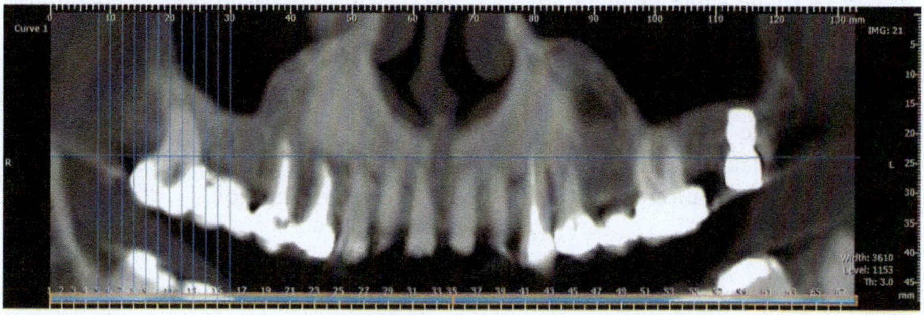

Fig. 7.8 Maximum ideal crown height distance must be taken into consideration

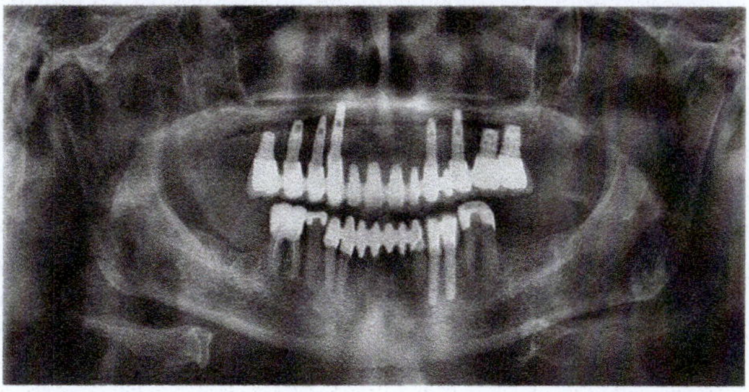

Fig. 7.9 Proper planning must be instituted to minimize marginal bone loss caused by the opposing or implant-supported occlusion

following immediate loading on the degree of osseointegration and clinical success between short implants connected with standard implants when compared to standard implants only.

7.4 Conclusion Statements

1. The bone–implant contact with a crestal bone increases the success rate.
2. The implant volume and its pattern on the implant surface are found as important as the bone–implant contact ratio.
3. Short implants with rough surfaces are more successful with respect to bone–implant contact than those with machined surfaces.
4. In short implants, primary stability must be provided with a torque of at least 25 Nm.
5. The success of short implants in type-4 bone is low and such conditions should be well considered ahead of time at planning.
6. Short implants with appropriate grooves increase the primary stability in soft bones and will therefore facilitate the desirable formation of bone–implant contact.
7. Histological-histomorphometrical methods are still the golden standard as invasive methods in bone–implant contact research. BS-SEM also provides extremely detailed and standardized results. Moreover the utilization of SCμCT method can facilitate finite element analysis and provide improved bone–implant contact data.
8. Crown height distances of 15 mm or shorter are safe for prosthetic rehabilitations for short implants to avoid marginal bone loss also by ensuring perseverance of bone–implant contact percentile.
9. Although data on early loading in short implants is rather limited, there is no untoward correlation between splinting and osseointegration.

References

1. Balshi TJ, Wolfinger GJ, Slauch RW, Balshi SF. A retrospective analysis of 800 Branemark system implants following the all-on-four protocol. J Prosthodont. 2014;23(2):83–8.
2. Buser D, Schenk RK, Steinemann S, Fiorellini JP, Fox CH, Stich H. Influence of surface characteristics on bone integration of titanium implants. A histomorphometric study in miniature pigs. J Biomed Mater Res. 1991;25:889–902.
3. Den Hartog L, Slatter JJ, Vissink A, Meijer HJ, Raghoebar GM. Treatment outcome of immediate early and conventional single-tooth implants in the aesthetic zone : a systematic review to survival, bone level, soft tissue, aesthetics and patient satisfaction. J Clin Periondontol. 2008;35:1073–86.
4. Piatelli A, Pontes AE, Degidi M, Iezzi G. Histologic studies on osseointegration soft tissues response to implant surfaces and components. A review. Dent Mater. 2011;27:53–60.
5. Branemark PI. Osseointegration and its experimental background. J Prosthet Dent. 1983;50:399–410.

6. Doblare M, Garcia JM. Anisotropic bone remodelling model based on a continuum damage-repair theory. J Biotech. 2002;35:1–17.
7. O'Mahony AM, Williams JL, Katz JO, Spencer P. Anisotropic elastic properties of cancellous bone from human edentulous mandible. Clin Oral Implants Res. 2000;11:415–21.
8. Chou HY, Jagodnik JJ, Müftü S. Prediction of bone remodelling around dental implant systems. J Biotech. 2008;41:1365–73.
9. Dominiak M, Lysiak-Drwal K, Solski L, Zywicka B, Rybak Z, Gedrange T. Evaluation of healing processes of intraosseous defects with and without guided bone regeneration and platelet rich plasma. An animal study. Ann Anat. 2012;194:549–55.
10. Rubin CT, Lanyon LE. Regulation of bone mass by mechanical strain magnitude. Calcif Tissue Int. 1985;37:411–7.
11. Sagırkaya E, Kucukkekenci AS, Karasoy D, Akca K, Eckert SE, Cehreli MC. Comparative assessments, meta-analysis and recommended guidelines for reporting studies on histomorphometric bone-implant-contact in humans. Int J Oral Maxillofac Implants. 2013;28:1243–53.
12. Javed F, Ahmed HB, Crespi R, Romanos GE. Role of primary stability for successful osseointegration of dental implants: factors influence and evaluation. Invert Med Appl Sci. 2013;5:162–7.
13. Esposito M, Grusovin MG, Chew YS, Coulthard P, Worthington HV. One-stage versus two-stage implant placement. A cochrane systematic review of randomized controlled trials. Euro J Oral Implantol. 2009;2:91–9.
14. Hasan I, Dominiak M, Blaszczyszyn A, Bourauel C, Gedrange T, Heinemann F. Radiographic evaluation of bone density around immediately loaded implants. Ann Anat. 2015;199:52–7.
15. Botzenhart U, Kunert-Keil C, Heinemann F, Gredes T, Seiler J, Berniczei-Royko A, Gedrange T. Osseointegration of short titan implants: a pilot study in pigs. Ann Anat. 2015;199:16–22.
16. Friberg B, Jemt T, Lekholm U. Early failures in 4641 consecutively placed Branemark dental implants: a study from stage 1 surgery to the connection of completed prostheses. Int J Oral Maxillofac Implants. 1991;6:142–6.
17. Friberg B, Ekestubbe A, Sennerby L. Clinical outcome of Brenamark system implants of various diameters: a retrospective study. Int J Oral Maxillofac Implants. 2002;17:671–7.
18. Heinemann F, Bourauel C, Hasan I, Gedrange T. Influence of the implant cervical topography on the crystal bone resorption and immediate implant survival. J Physiol Pharmacol. 2009;60(Suppl. 8):99–105.
19. Heinemann F, Mundt T, Biffar R, Gedrange T, Götz W. A 3 year clinical and radiographic study of implants placed simultaneously with maxillary sinus floor augmentation using a new nano crystalline hydroxyapatite. J. Physiol. Pharmacol. 2009b;60(Suppl. 8):91–7.
20. Kieswetter K, Schwartz Z, Dean DD, Boyan BD. The role of implant surface characteristics in the healing of bone. Crit Rev Oral Bill Med. 1987;7:329–45.
21. Degasne B, Basle MF, Demais V, Hure G, Lesourd M, Grolleau B, Mercier L, Chappard D. Effects of roughness, fibronectin and vitronectinon attachment, spreading, and proliferation of human osteoblast like cells (Saos-2) on titanium surfaces. Calico Tissue Int. 1999;64:499–507.
22. Hansson S, Norton M. The relation between surface roughness and interfacial shear strength for bone-anchored implants. A mechanical model. J Biotech. 1999;32:829–36.
23. Vaillancourt H, Piliar RM, McCammond D. Finite element analysis of crestal bone loss around porous coated dental implants. J Appl Biomater. 1995;6:267–82.
24. Thakur AJ. The elements of fracture fixation. New York: Churchill Livingstone; 1997. p. 27–56.
25. Esposito M, Grusovin MG, Coulthard P, Worthington HV. Different loading strategies for dental implants. A cochrane systematic review of randomized controlled trials. Eur J Oral Implantol. 2008;1:259–76.
26. Lundgren CG. In vivo fracture of a basket-type osseointegration dental implant: a case report. Int J Oral Maxillofac Implants. 1989;4:255–6.

27. Falk H, Laurell L, Lundgren D. Occlusal force pattern in dentitions with mandibular implant-supported fixed cantilever prostheses occluded with completed dentures. Int J Oral Maxillofac Implants. 1989;4:55–62.
28. Smith E, Raab DM. Osteoporosis and physical activity. Acta Med Scand Suppl. 1987;5(Suppl):149–56.
29. Roberts WE. Bone tissue interface. J Dent Educ. 1988;52:804–9.
30. Block MS, Finger LM, Fontenot MG, Kent JN. Loaded hydroxylapatite-coated and grit-blasted titanium implants in dogs. Int J Oral Maxillofac Implants. 1989;4:219–25.
31. Bart E, Johansson C, Albrektsson T. Histologic comparison of ceramic and titanium implants in cats. Int J Oral Maxillofac Implants. 1990;5:227–331.
32. Donath K, Brauner G. A method for the study of undecalcified bones and teeth with attached soft tissues. The Säge-Schliff (sawing and grinding) technique. J Oral Path. 1982;11:318–26.
33. Grötz KA, Piepkorn B, Al-Nawas B, Duscher H, Bittinger F, Kann P, Beyer J, Wagner W. Confocal laser scanning microscopy: a non destructive subsurface histotomography of healthy human bone. Calcif Tissue Int. 1999;65:8–10.
34. Al-Nawas B, Götz H. Three dimensional topographic and metrologic evaluation of dental implants by confocal laser scanning microscopy. Clin Implant Dent Relat Res. 2003;5:176–83.
35. Orsini G, Piatelli M, Scarano A, Petrone G, Kenaly J, Piatelli A, Caputi S. Randomized, controlled histological and histomorphometric evaluation of implants with nanometer-scale calcium phosphate added to the dual acid-etched surface in the human posterior maxilla. J Periodontol. 2007;78:209–18.
36. Marin C, Granato R, Suzuki M, Gil JN, Piatelli A, Coelho PG. Removal torque and histomorphometric evaluation of bioceramic grit-blasted/acid etched and dual acid etched, implant surfaces: an experimental study in dogs. J Periodontol. 2008;78:209–18.
37. Fontana F, Rocchietta I, Addis A, Schupbach P, Zanotti G, Simion M. Effects of a calcium phosphate coating on the osseointegration of endosseous implants in a rabbit model. Clin Oral Implants Res. 2011;22:760–6.
38. Chang CS, Lee TM, Chang CH, Liu JK. The effect of microrough surface treatment on miniscrews used as orthodontic anchors. Clin Oral Implants Res. 2009;20:1178–84.
39. Lee J, Sieweke JH, Rodriguez NA, Schupbach P, Lindstrom H, Susin C, Wikesjo UM. Evaluation of nano-technology modified zirconia oral implants: a study in rabbits. J Clin Periodontol. 2009;36:610–7.
40. Vidigal GM, Groisman M, Gregorio LH, Soares GDA. Osseointegration of titanium alloy and HA coated implants in healthy and ovariectomized animals. A histomorphometric study. Clin Oral Implants Res. 2009;20:1272–7.
41. Manresa C, Bosch M, Manzanares MC, Carvalho P, Echeverria JJ. A new standardized-automatic method for bone-to-implant contact histomorphometric analysis based on backscattered scanning electron microscopy images. Clin Oral Implants Res. 2014;25:702–6.
42. Bernhardt R, Kuhlisch E, Schulz MC, Eckelt U, Stadlinger B. Comparison of bone-implant contact and bone-implant volume between 2D histological sections and 3D SRμCT slices. Eur Cells Mater. 2012;23:237–48.
43. Buser D, Broggini N, Wieland M, Schenk RK, Denzer AJ, Cochran DL, Hoffmann B, Lussi A, Steinemann SG. Enhanced bone apposition to a chemically modified SLA titanium surface. J Dent Res. 2004;83:529–33.
44. Ferguson SJ, Broggini N, Wieland M, deWild M, Rupp F, Geis-Gerstorfer J, Cochran DL, Buser D. Biomechanical evaluation of the strength of a chemically modified sandblasted and acid etched titanium surface. J Biomed Mater Res. 2006;78:291–7.
45. Papavasiliou G, Kamposiora P, Bayne SC, Felton DA. 3d-FEA of osseointegration in percentages and patterns on implant-bone interfacial stresses. J Dent. 1997;25:485–91.
46. Bouaruel C, Aitlahrach M, Heinemann F, Hasan I. Biomechanical finite element analysis of small diameter and short dental implants: extensive study of commercial implants. Biomed Tech. 2012;57:21–32.
47. Hassan I, Bourauel C, Mundt T, Heinemann F. Biomechanical finite element analysis of small diameter and short dental implant. Biomed Tech. 2013;55:341–55.

48. Morand M, Irinakis T. The challenge of implant therapy in the posterior maxilla: providing a rationale for the use of short implants. J Oral Implantol. 2007;33:257–66.
49. Sivolella S, Stellini E, Testori T, Di Fiore A, Berngo M, Lops D. Splinted and unsplinted short implants in mandibles: a retrospective evaluation with 5 to 16 years follow-up. J Periodontol. 2013;84:502–12.
50. Draenert FG, Sagheb K, Baumgardt K, Kammerer PW. Retrospective analysis of survival rates and marginal bone loss on short implants in the mandible. Colin Oral Implants Res. 2012;23:1063–9.
51. Esposito M, Pistilli R, Barausse C, Felice P. Three year results from a randomized controlled trial comparing prostheses supported by 5mm long implants or by longer implants in augmented bone in posterior edentulous jaws. Eur J Oral Implantol. 2014;7:383–95.
52. Lai H-C, Si M-S, Zhuang LF, Shen H, Liu YL, Wismeijer D. Longterm outcomes of short dental implants supporting single crowns in posterior region: Z clinical retrospective study of 5 to 10 years. Clin Oral Implants Res. 2013;24:230–7.
53. Bidez MW, Misch CE. Clinical biomechanics in implant dentistry. In: Misch CE, editor. Contemporary implant dentistry. St. Louis: Mosby; 2008. p. 543–55.
54. Sanz M, Naert I. Biomechanics/risk management (Working Group 2). Clin Oral Implants Res. 2009;4:107–11.
55. Nissan J, Ghelfan O, Gross O, Priel I, Gross M, Chaushu G. The effect of crown/implant ratio and crown height space on stress distribution in unsplinted implant supporting restorations. J Oral Maxillofac Surg. 2011;69:1934–9.
56. Nissan J, Gross O, Ghelfan O, Priel I, Gross M, Chaushu G. The effect of splinting implant-supported restorations on stress distribution of different crown-implant ratios and crown height spaces. J Oral Maxillofac Surg. 2011;69:2990–4.
57. Anitua E, Alkhraist MH, Pinas L, Begona L, Orive G. Implant survival and crestal bone loss around extra-short implants supporting a fixed denture: the effect of crown height space, crown to implant ratio, and offset placement of the prosthesis. Int J Oral Maxillofac Implants. 2014;29:682–9.
58. Anitua E, Flores J, Flores C, Alkhraisat MH. Longterm outcomes of immediate loading of short implants: a controlled retrospective cohort study. Int J Oral Maxillofac Implants. 2016;31:1360–6.

The Survival of Short and Ultrashort Plateau Root Form Implants

8

Rainier A. Urdaneta and Sung-Kiang Chuang

Contents

8.1 Introduction ... 95
8.2 Survival Studies on Plateau Root Form Implants ... 102
8.3 Statistical Models ... 103
8.4 Data Sample ... 103
8.5 Factors Associated with Failures of Osseointegration ... 104
8.6 Smoking Impairs Osseointegration in the Maxilla ... 105
8.7 One-Stage Surgical Protocol and Osseointegration ... 106
8.8 Immediate Implant Placement and Higher Failures in the Mandible ... 107
8.9 Implant Size and Osseointegration ... 108
8.10 Failure to Survive after Loading ... 109
8.11 Long-Term Performance of Ultrashort Implants in Posterior Maxilla ... 111
8.12 Long-Term Performance of Ultrashort Implants in Posterior Mandible ... 113
References ... 124

8.1 Introduction

This chapter will evaluate the scientific evidence supporting the survival rates of short and ultrashort implants as well as present the different risk factors that may affect the performance of plateau root form implants. For the purpose of this discussion, *Short* implants will be defined as those implants ≤8 mm in length, implants 5 and 6 mm long will be considered *Ultrashort* and implants longer than 8 mm will be considered of conventional length or *Long*.

R. A. Urdaneta (✉)
Private Practice, Shrewsbury, MA, USA

S.-K. Chuang
Department of Oral Health Policy and Epidemiology, Harvard School of Dental Medicine, Boston, MA, USA
e-mail: schuang@hsph.harvard.edu

B. J. Tomasetti, R. Ewers (eds.), *Short Implants*,
https://doi.org/10.1007/978-3-030-44199-9_8

Conventional restoring protocols recommend to splint implants in order to improve their long-term survival. This rationale assumes that bone loss surrounding dental implants is inevitable and thus a certain amount of bone loss should be considered acceptable. Accordingly, the longer the implant, the longer it will survive in bone. The current understanding also assumes that osseointegration may degenerate overtime and that masticatory forces will dislodge *Short* implants during function. Concluding, without scientific evidence to support it, that protecting bone from masticatory loads is conducive to better survival rates. The case presented in Fig. 8.1 illustrates the conventional approach.

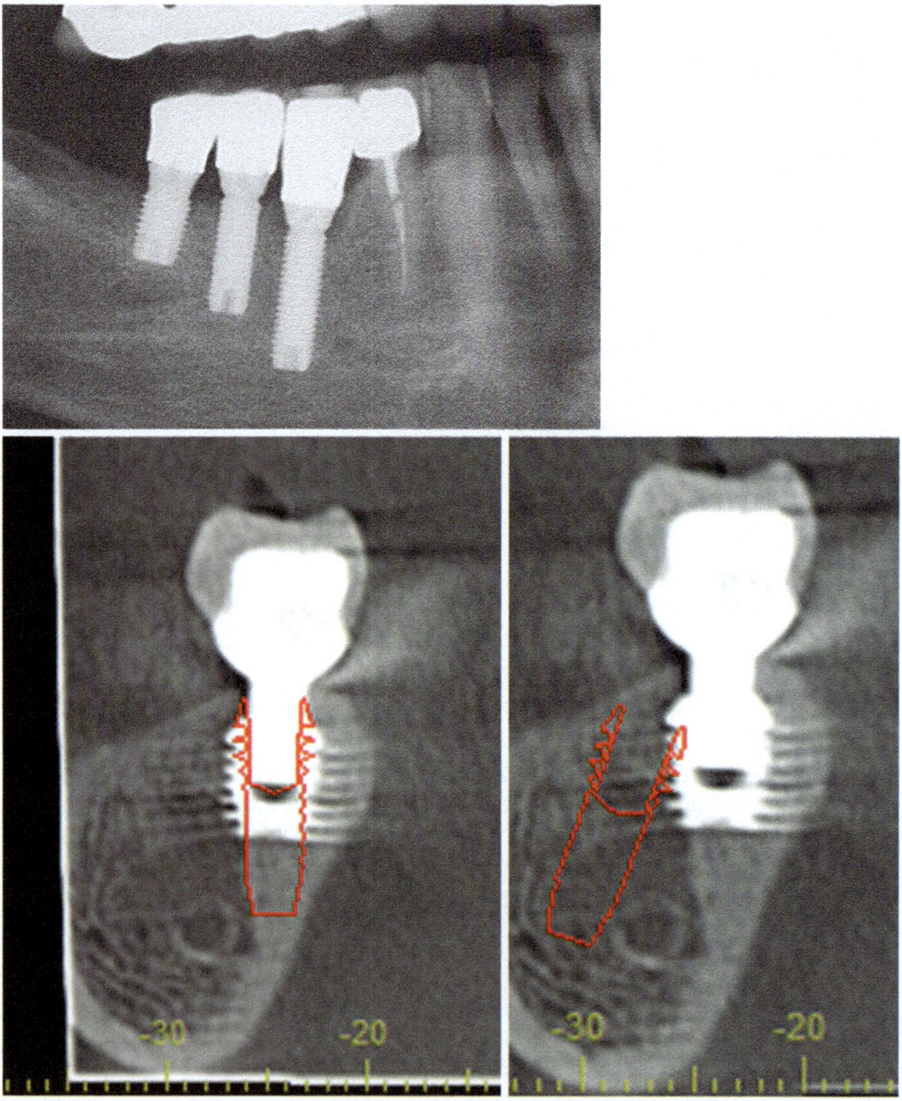

Fig. 8.1 Conventional restoring protocols advocate splinting shorter implants. Mandibular first and second molars were restored with splinted, premolar sized teeth presumably to protect the bone surrounding the shorter implants. A longer, single implant was used to restore the second premolar. Mandibular nerve paresthesia was caused during the surgery to place the long implant

The objective of this chapter is to question the validity of the above rationale and to present an alternative point of view. Our clinical and research experience with plateau root form implants restored with load-bearing implant abutment platforms support the hypothesis that any amount of bone loss is a sign of disease. That the bone surrounding a successful implant grows coronally or at the very least is stable overtime. That bone density and osseointegration surrounding functional implants is continually changing, it increases overtime and that masticatory forces have an anabolic effect in bone until the point of bone fracture. Since fracture of the implant-to-bone interface is uncommon, splinting implants to protect bone is unnecessary. It is clear to us that implants are splinted to achieve a restorative objective (to prevent screw/abutment loosening or fracture and/or to reduce the number of implants needed) but not necessary for biological reasons. The case presented in Figs. 8.2, 8.3, 8.4, 8.5, 8.6, 8.7, 8.8, and 8.9 illustrates, in the same patient shown on Fig. 8.1, the proposed rationale.

Since a *Long* implant has a larger endosteal surface when compared to a *Short* implant of similar width. It seems reasonable to question, will the implant with the longest bone support have the lengthiest survival? On the other hand, if the bone

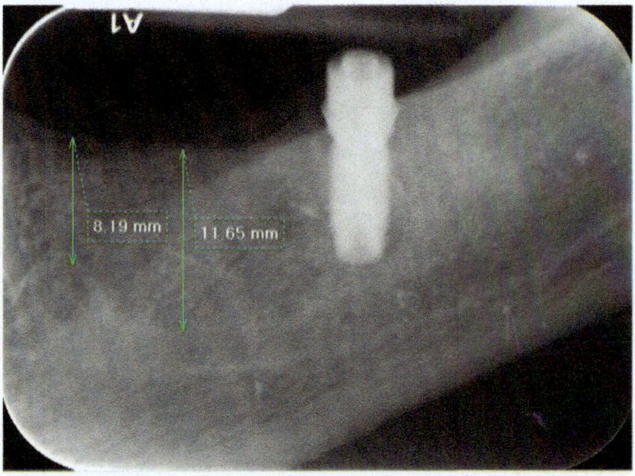

Fig. 8.2 Mandibular left posterior area of the same patient shown in Fig. 8.1. Limited bone length due to the location of the mandibular nerve

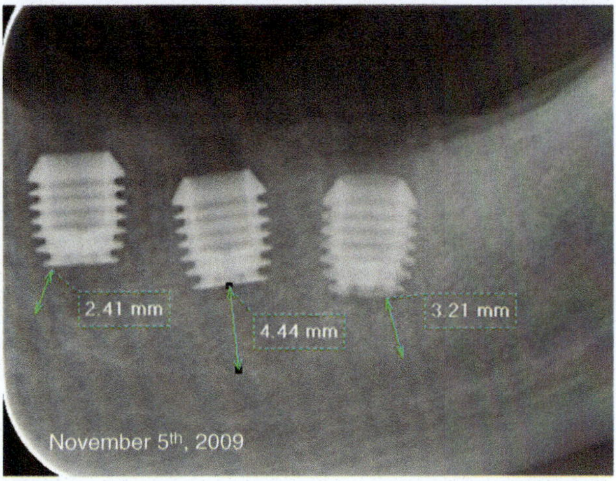

Fig. 8.3 Three ultrashort implants (5 mm wide by 6 mm long) were placed at a safe distance to the mandibular nerve. Implants placed Nov 5th, 2009

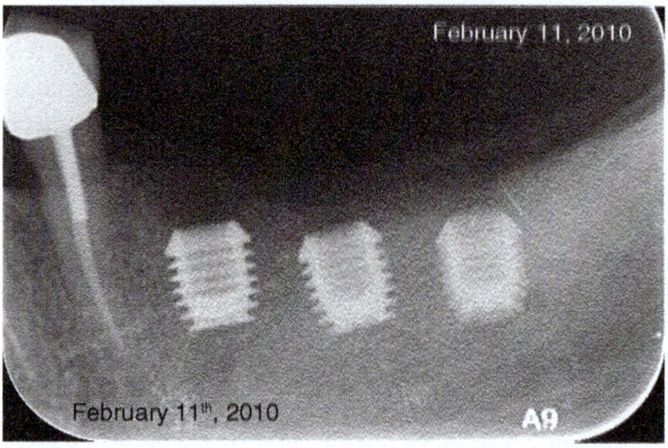

Fig. 8.4 Implants were uncovered after 3 months of healing, February 11, 2010

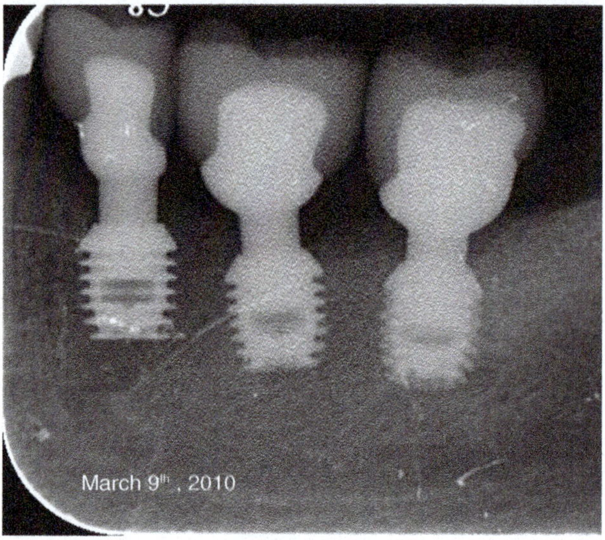

Fig. 8.5 Ultrashort implants were restored with single crowns/abutments, restorations were inserted March 9, 2010

surrounding a *Short* unsplinted implant is subjected to higher masticatory loads (due to its reduced endosteal surface and higher crown-to-implant ratio), would the bone strengthen or even grow around it overtime to the point of outliving a *Long* implant?

Figure 8.10 demonstrates in the same patient both the conventional restoring protocol and the proposed treatment approach. The bone response after 3 years of

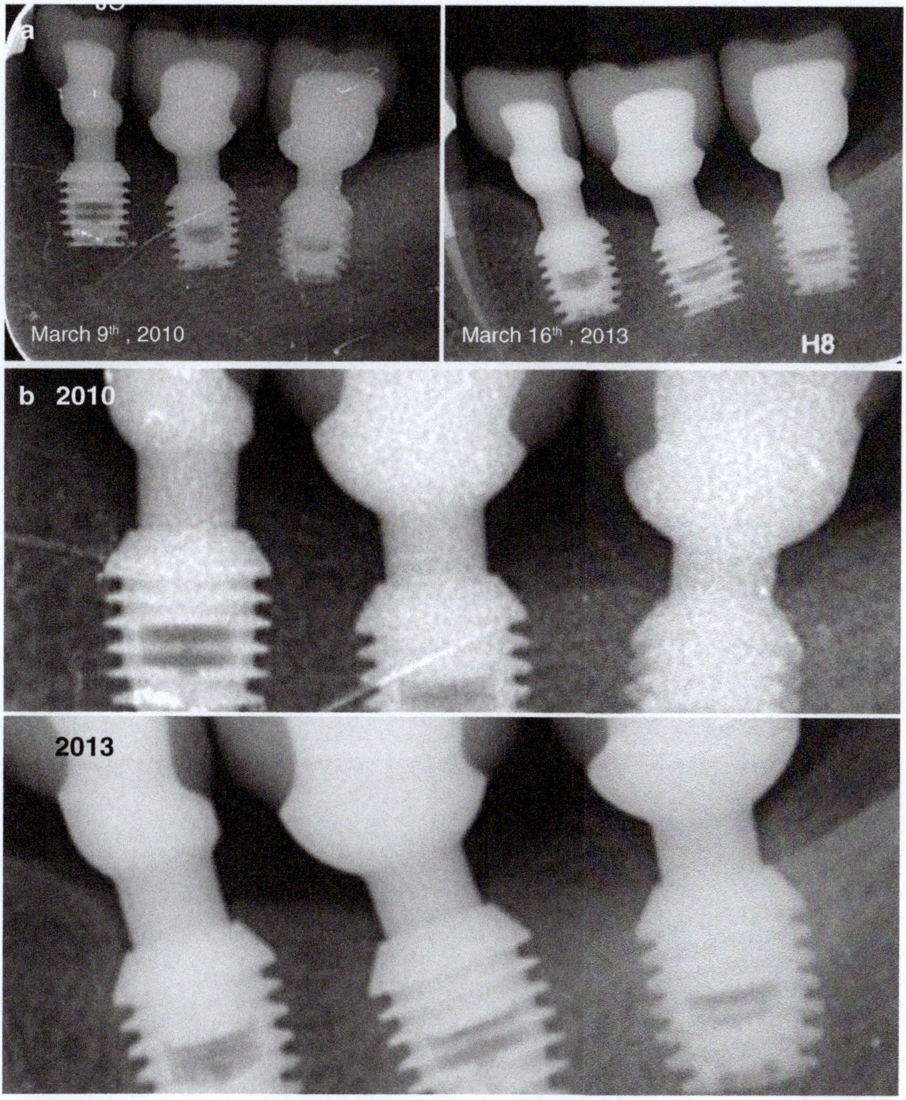

Fig. 8.6 (**a**) Periapical radiographs at crown/abutment insertion, (left) March 2010 and 3-year recall appointment, (right) May 2013. (**b**) Close up of the bone surrounding the implants, at crown insertion (above) and 3-year recall (below)

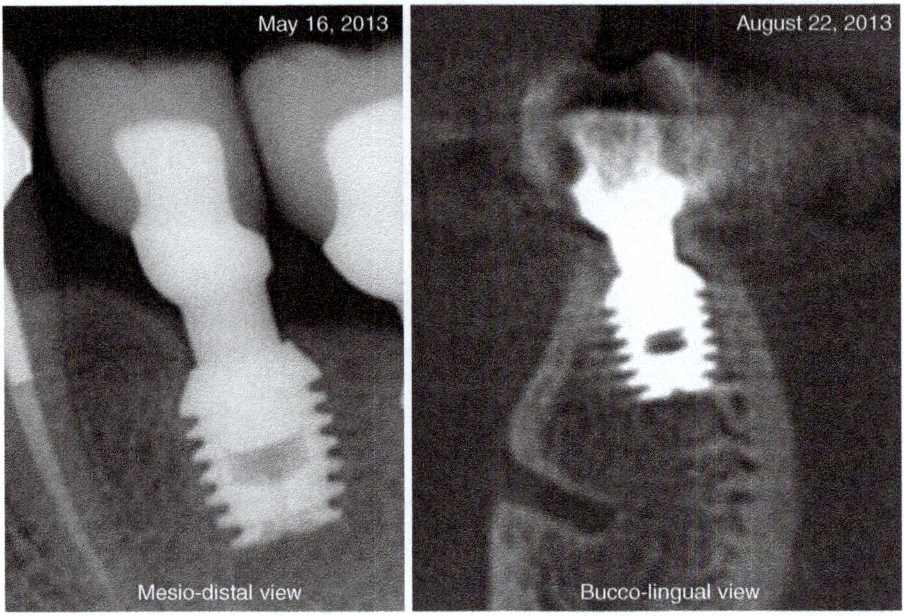

Fig. 8.7 Periapical radiograph (left) and CT-scan image (right) of the 5 × 6-mm implant restoring the mandibular left second premolar. Notice the healthy bone in both bucco-lingual and mesio-distal dimensions

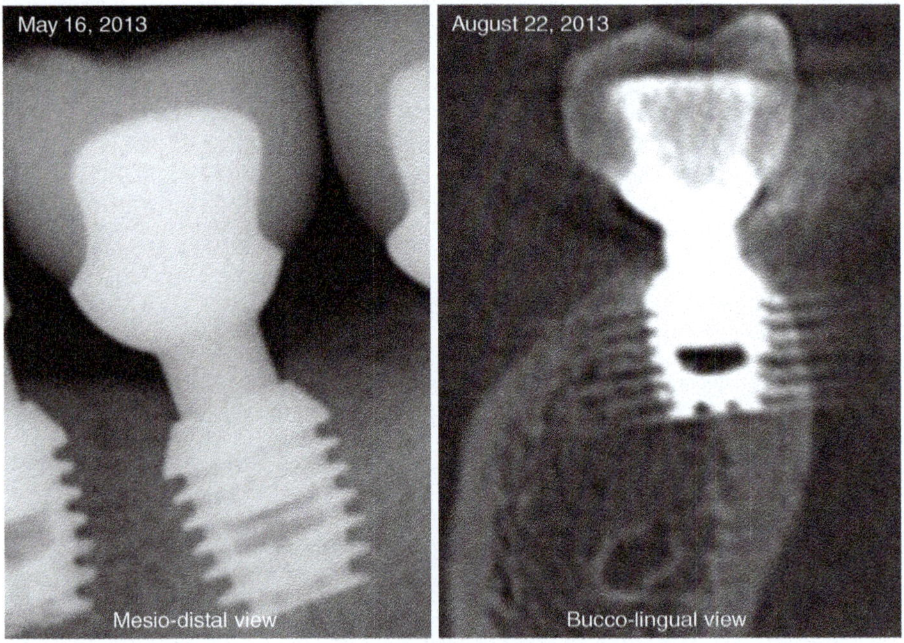

Fig. 8.8 Periapical radiograph (left) and CT-scan image (right) of the 5 × 6-mm implant restoring the mandibular left first molar. Notice the healthy bone in both bucco-lingual and mesio-distal dimensions

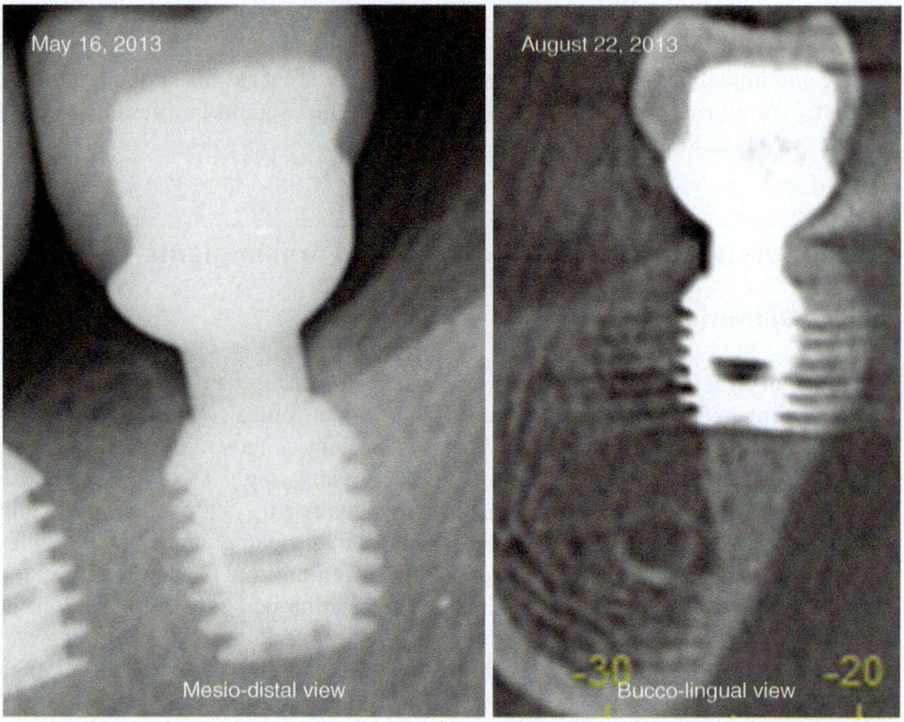

Fig. 8.9 Periapical radiograph (left) and CT-scan image (right) of the 5 × 6-mm implant restoring the mandibular left second molar. Notice the healthy bone in both bucco-lingual and mesio-distal dimensions, despite the fact that the implant was placed several mm apical to the crest of the bone

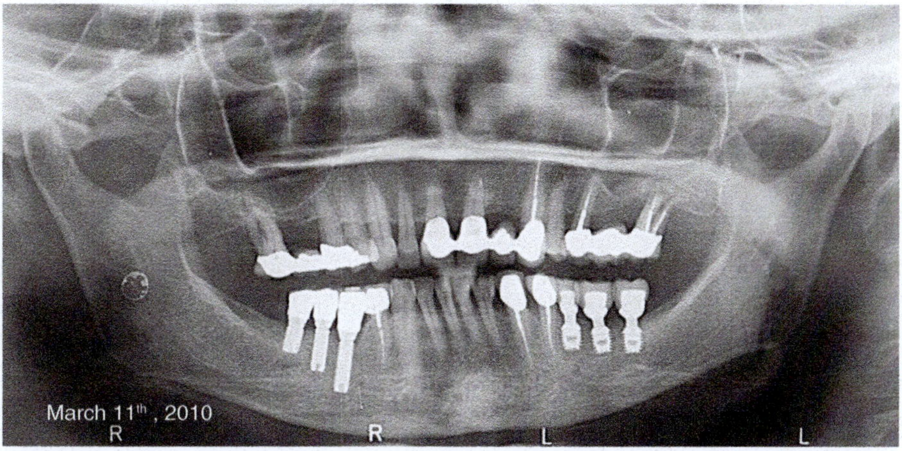

Fig. 8.10 Panoramic radiograph of the case presented in Figs. 8.1, 8.2, 8.3, 8.4, 8.5, 8.6, 8.7, and 8.9. The use of long implants led to mandibular nerve damage on the right side that could have been prevented with the use of short or ultrashort implants as in the left posterior area

loading surrounding the unsplinted *Ultrashort* implants restored with molar-sized crowns (Figs. 8.7, 8.8, and 8.9), as well as the limitations of splinting implants or using *Long* implants (impaired maintenance and increased surgical complications), suggest that the use of *Ultrashort* unsplinted implants should be presented to the patient as the ideal treatment plan.

8.2 Survival Studies on Plateau Root Form Implants

8.2.1 Definition

The term survival is defined by the Oxford dictionary as: the state or fact of continuing to live or exist, typically in spite of an accident, ordeal, or difficult circumstances. The dental implant literature reports as failures those implants that have been removed from the oral environment, assessing implant survival as those implants that remained in the mouth. When evaluating the survival of *Short* and *Ultrashort* implants, we need to distinguish between those implants that fail to integrate and those implants that fail after loading. Can an implant that fail to reach proper osseointegration and was not placed in function be considered a failure to survive in the oral environment? Perhaps, but only a failure to osseointegrate. Furthermore, the implants that failed after short periods of time, i.e., <6 months should be considered as well, osseointegration failures. Therefore, the term survival should include only those implants that "survived the oral environment" for more than 6 months, which can appropriately be classified as an ordeal. For the purpose of this book we are going to classify implant failures into three different categories:

Classification of implant failures	
Type I Failure to osseointegrate	Includes those implants that were removed prior, at the uncovering stage, and during the first 6 months of loading
Type II Failure to survive	Includes those implants that were removed after more than 6 months of loading
Type III Other failures	Includes those cases in which the implants were removed at the patients' request or were removed due to other reasons such as metal allergies, etc., but the implants were otherwise osseointegrated and were functioning properly

For dental implant practice, it is important to know which factors are associated with the failure to integrate as well as which factors may be involved in the failures observed after loading. In the studies done on survival of plateau root form (PRF) implants [1–10], the majority of implant failures occurred during the months of healing and/or within 6 months of function. Therefore, the clinical phenomenon being investigated in those studies was not necessarily "implant survival" but rather "failures to achieve osseointegration". This chapter will present scientific data on the factors associated with those implants that failed to achieve osseointegration or failed to survive for short periods of time. We will also present cases depicting the long-term survival of *Short* and *Ultrashort* PRF implants and what we have learned from them.

8.3 Statistical Models

When estimating the survival rates and risk factors affecting the behavior of an implant system in the oral environment, different statistical models may yield different results. Thus, it is important to utilize an appropriate model to analyze and interpret the data.

Before the year 2000, many studies analyzed the dental implant survival rate using the number of surviving implants divided by the number of total implants without considering the cluster effect of subjects. However, some subjects had multiple failed implants because of uncontrolled systemic disease, smoking history, poor bone quality, and other factors. It is reasonable to assume that implants in the same subject are submitted to similar conditions and therefore are "dependent" from one another while performing survival analysis. On the other hand, implants placed in different patients can be considered truly "independent" from each other.

Chuang et al. (2001) [1] utilized three different models to estimate the survival rate: (1) randomly selecting one implant per patient; (2) utilizing all implants, assuming independence among implants from the same subject; and (3) utilizing all implants, assuming dependence among implants from the same subject. It was found that patients at high risk for implant failure (smokers) manifested greater variation in the standard error estimates among the three models, 8.2%, 4.0%, and 5.6%, respectively even though these models had similar survival rates. The accumulative implant survival rates of all patients in the dependence model were 95.4, 93.8, 93.2, 91.8, and 91.2% in 1- to 5-year follow-up respectively. In smokers, the accumulative implant survival rates were 91.4, 84.5, 79.7, 79.7, and 79.9% in the same follow-up period. These results demonstrated that adjusting for dependence among clustered survival observations could explain the variability of survival rates and draw attention to the issue of clustered failures in some patients.

Chuang et al. (2005) [2], (2006) [3] also proposed a novel model, Cox proportional hazards model with frailty, to predict the survival rate of clustered implants in the same subject. This model could predict survival rate considering the dependence factor. Therefore, the statistical models utilized in the studies presented here adjusted for clustered observations.

8.4 Data Sample

The patient cohorts for the survival and risk factor analysis were composed of patients who had at least one PRF implant placed at the Dentistry Implant Dentistry Center at Faulkner Hospital (Boston, MA). Three different peer reviewed patient cohorts [1–10] were combined to form a master database. All implants in the master cohort were placed according to the recommended surgical protocols and restored by means of fixed or removable prostheses. There were 2944 implants placed in 969 patients (503 female). Between, 1 and 22 implants were placed per patient. One hundred and forty-eight implants failed (5%), 131 of them failed before loading (88.5%).

In terms of location, 1744 implants (59.2%) were placed in the maxilla and 2062 implants (70%) were placed in posterior areas. With regards to the timing of implant exposure and implant placement, 412 implants (14.0%) were placed using a one-stage surgical protocol, and 462 implants (15.7%) were placed immediately after tooth extraction. There were 1080 (36.7%) short implants and 1836 (62.4%) were narrow implants (3.5–4.0 mm wide). One thousand six hundred and fourteen implants (54.8%) had an HA coating, 655 were TPS coated and 418 uncoated with a sandblasted/acid etched treatment. The most commonly used implant sizes were: 4.0 × 11 mm (27.2%), 3.5 × 11 mm (24.3%), and 5.0 × 8.0 mm (19%).

8.5 Factors Associated with Failures of Osseointegration

Because 88.5% of the implant failures occurred before loading and the average follow-up time was relatively short, the factors evaluated here should be considered to be associated with Type I implant failures (fail to achieve osseointegration), rather than Type II failures (fail to survive after loading). The factors affecting implant survival after several years of loading still need to be determined by long-term studies.

To identify those factors associated with Type I failures, univariate and multivariate statistical models were developed. In the univariate model, the following variables were found to be associated with the failure of implants to osseointegrate (outcome):

1. Smoking, specifically in the maxilla and with a more pronounced effect in female patients and on TPS-coated implants.
2. Adjacent structures.
3. Maxillary location, specifically in molar areas.
4. One-stage surgical protocol in particular for those maxillary non-immediately placed implants and those implants placed immediately after the extraction of a mandibular tooth.
5. Surface coating, suggesting that TPS coatings affected osseointegration negatively and HA-coated implants being more likely to integrate.
6. Immediate placement, with an effect that seemed specific to those implants placed immediately after the extraction of a mandibular tooth.
7. Implant size/dimension:
   (a) Implant length, suggesting that 14-mm-long implants are more likely to integrate in posterior mandible.
   (b) Implant width suggesting that the narrowest implants (specifically 3.5 mm) and the widest implants (6.0 mm) are less likely to integrate.
   (c) Implant size: 3.5 × 8, 3.5 × 11, and 6 × 8 demonstrating lower rates of integration.

To further investigate those factors significantly associated with the failure of implants to osseointegrate, a multivariate statistical model was developed. The following variables remained statistically associated with Type I implant failures (P value <0.10) in the multivariate model.

Smoking in the maxilla ($P < 0.0001$), location, maxillary molar ($P = 0.0002$), implant length ($P = <0.0001$) one-stage surgical protocol ($P = 0.02$), placement of an implant immediately after the extraction of a mandibular tooth ($P = 0.0002$), well size ($P < 0.0001$), and implants sizes 3.5 × 8 ($P = 0.03$) and 3.5 × 11 ($P = 0.002$).

8.6 Smoking Impairs Osseointegration in the Maxilla

The data suggests that smoking's deleterious effect on implant survival seems to be more pronounced in the maxilla. Statistically significant higher failure rates were observed in maxillary implants (28 out of 178 implants failed, 15.7%) when compared to mandibular implants (7 out of 117 implant failed, 6%) in patients who smoke tobacco.

A maxillary implant is significantly more likely to fail if placed in a patient who smokes tobacco daily $P < 0.0001$ (hazard ratio: 5.1)

Whereas a mandibular implant was not statistically significantly more likely to fail if placed in a smoker $P = 0.77$ (hazard ratio: 1.173, statistics march 17, 2015)

The deleterious effect of smoking in the osseointegration of a maxillary implant seemed to be more pronounced on those implants placed in female patients (18 out of 77 implants failed, 23.4%) and those implants with a TPS coating (15 out of 51 implants failed, 29.4%) when compared to maxillary implants placed in male patients (10 out of 102 failed, 9.9%) and HA-coated implants (7 out of 112 implants failed, 6.25%). When TPS-coated maxillary implants were placed in female patients, a failure rate of 47.8% (11 out of 23 implants failed) was noted. As a comparison, 14.3% failure rate was documented on maxillary TPS-coated implants placed in male patients (4 out of 28 implants failed).

Surgical protocol was another factor that seems to hinder the survival of maxillary implants in patients who smoke tobacco. Higher failure rates were noted on maxillary implants placed in smokers when using a one-stage surgical protocol (10 out of 37 implants failed, 27%) as compared to implant placed using two-stage surgeries (18 out of 133 implants failed, 13.5%).

8.6.1 Clinical Recommendations Regarding Patients Who Smoke Tobacco

Based on the data evaluated and within its limitations, the following protocol is recommended for patients who smoke tobacco and are unwilling/unable to stop prior to implant placement:

Clinical recommendations when placing implants in patients who smoke tobacco
Use HA-coated implants and two-stage protocols
Avoid TPS coatings and one-stage surgeries
Particular attention given to female patients, the use of HA coatings is encouraged

8.7 One-Stage Surgical Protocol and Osseointegration

A higher number of one-stage implants failed to integrate (33 out of 412 implants failed, 8%) when compared to those implants placed using a two-stage surgical protocol (118 out of 2445 implant failed, 4.8%).

One-stage surgeries and Osseointegration
A plateau root form implant placed using a one-stage surgical protocol was significantly less likely to integrate, P = 0.02 (Hazard ratio: 2.0)

In the maxilla, one-stage surgical procedures seem to hinder the survival of TPS-coated implants but do not seem to have a significant effect on the survival of HA-coated implants. In the mandible, one-stage protocols do not appear to affect the survival of implants that have been placed in healed sites and rather its significance seems to be limited to those mandibular implants that have been placed immediately after the extraction of a tooth. For this discussion, failures in patients who smoke tobacco were excluded.

In patients who do not smoke tobacco, higher failure rates were documented on TPS maxillary implants placed using a one-stage surgical protocol (12 out of 120 implants failed, 10%) when compared to HA-coated maxillary one-staged implants (1 out of 99 implants failed, 1%).

It is interesting to note that when using two-stage surgical protocols in the maxilla in nonsmokers, TPS coatings (2 out of 205 implants failed, 1%) outperformed HA coatings (19 out of 454 implants failed, 4.18%).

One-stage surgeries in the maxilla
In the maxilla, one-stage surgical procedures were correlated with higher osseointegration failures on TPS-coated implants (P = 0.03, hazard ratio: 9.125)
Whereas an HA-coated implants were significantly more likely to osseointegrate that TPS-coated implants when using a one-stage surgical protocol (P = 0.03, hazard ratio: 0.110)

For implant placed in the mandible, we observed significant correlations between immediate implant placement and one-stage surgical protocols. The data suggests that in the absence of immediate placements, one-stage surgical procedures are not correlated with increased mandibular implant failures.

For implants placed immediately after the extraction of a tooth, we observed contrasting accounts in the maxilla and the mandible. In the maxilla, lower failure rates were observed when using of a one-stage protocol (1 out of 49 implant failed, 2%) as opposed to a two-stage surgical protocol (8 out of 97 implants failed, 8.2%).

The opposite was true in the mandible, higher failure rates were observed for immediately placed mandibular implants when a one-stage protocol was used (7 out of 18 implants failed, 38.9%) instead of a two-stage protocol (3 out of 45 implants failed, 6.7%).

One-stage surgeries and immediate placement in the mandible
For mandibular implants placed immediately after the extraction of a tooth, one-stage surgical protocols increase the risk for implant failures ($P = 0.0027$, hazard ratio: 24.547) when compared to two-stage surgeries

8.8 Immediate Implant Placement and Higher Failures in the Mandible

For patients who do not smoke tobacco, similar failure rates were observed on implants placed immediately after the extraction of a tooth (22 out of 410 implants failed, 5.3%) when compared to non-immediate implants (83 out of 1912 failed, 4.3%). However, the performance of immediately placed implants differ in the maxilla and the mandible and surface coatings seem to play a role as well.

When placing implants immediately after the extraction of a tooth In patients who do not smoke tobacco, higher failure rates were observed in the mandible (11 out of 138 implants failed, 7.97%) as compared to the maxilla (11 out of 272 implants failed, 4%).

Immediate implant placement and osseointegration
Implants placed immediately after the extraction of a tooth were significantly more likely to fail if placed in the mandible ($P = 0.02$, hazard ratio: 3.239)
Whereas maxillary location had a protective effect against failures of immediately placed implants ($P = 0.02$, hazard ratio: 0.309)

In fact, for the maxilla the failure rates of immediately placed (4%) and non-immediately placed implants (5.2%) were relatively similar. The deleterious effect of immediate placement in the mandible seems to further increase with the use of TPS-coated implants (6 out of 26 implants failed,23%) as opposed to HA-coated implants (5 out of 100, failed, 5%). TPS-coated implants performed significantly better when placed immediately after the extraction of a maxillary tooth (only 1 out of 62 implants failed, 1.6%).

8.8.1 Clinical Recommendations

Based on the data evaluated and within its limitations, the following may be concluded:

There is an increased risk of failure when implants are placed immediately after the extraction of a mandibular tooth but there is not an increased risk of failure for immediately placed maxillary implants.

Clinical recommendations with regards to the placement of implants immediately after the extraction of a *Mandibular* tooth
For implants placed in previously healed sites, one- and two-stage surgical protocols and different surface coatings lead to comparable survival rates
When placing implants immediately after the extraction of a tooth, there is an increased risk for mandibular failures. In these cases, avoid one-stage procedures and choose HA coatings

8.9 Implant Size and Osseointegration

The multivariate statistical model depicted in Table II revealed that longer implants are significantly more likely to integrate.

Implant length and Osseointegration
Longer implants are significantly more likely to osseointegrate, P = <0.0001 (Hazard ratio: 0.74)

When each implant length was evaluated individually, only one implant length was statistically significant correlated to implant failure, 14-mm-long implants were significantly more likely to integrate, $P = 0.02$.

However, when implant lengths were classified as either being *Short* (5–8 mm) or *Long* (11 and 14 mm). There was no statistically significant difference between the failures of *Short* when compared to Long implants, $P = 0.16$.

Furthermore, the beneficial effect of implant length in osseointegration is limited to the mandible. A long implant was significantly more likely to integrate in the mandible, $P = 0.003$ but not more likely to integrate in the maxilla, $P = 0.56$.

Implant length and Osseointegration
Long implants were significantly more likely to osseointegrate in the mandible, P = 0.0002 (Hazard ratio: 0.74). This effect was specific to 14-mm-long implants

There were 15 different implant sizes evaluated, two of which were significantly associated to implant failures. Both 3.5 × 8 and 3.5 × 11 implants were significantly less likely to osseointegrate. These findings suggest that very narrow implants (3.5 mm) of shorter lengths (8 mm and 11 mm) are less likely to osseointegrate and that increasing implant width to 4.0 mm or increasing implant length to 14 mm may help reduce this risk. Implant length seems particularly important in the osseointegration of very narrow implants (3.5 mm wide).

Implant size and Osseointegration
3.5 × 8 implants (P = 0.03, hazard ratio:2.5) and 3.5 × 11 (P = 0.002, hazard ratio:2.0) were significantly less likely to osseointegrate

The statistical models revealed that 2-mm-welled implants are less likely to integrate when compared to 3-mm-welled implants. Since both 3.5 × 8 and

3.5 × 11 implants have 2 mm wells, it is possible that the correlation between implant failure and well size may be due to the association between 2 mm well and 3.5 width.

Does the fact that 14-mm-long implant were more likely to integrate in the mandible mean that we should use 14-mm-long implants when restoring missing teeth in the mandible? Of course not. Failure to osseointegrate is not the most severe complication that can be encountered when placing a mandibular implant. Damage to the inferior alveolar nerve/paresthesia and perforation of lingual plate/submandibular bleeding are severe complications with may lead irreversibly to patient impairment.

It is obvious that the longer the implant, the more likely it is to encroach into important anatomical boundaries and lead to severe complications. The increased risk of a reversible complication, such as implant failure, should never take precedence over the increased risk for irreversible damage to a patient.

Clinical relevance of Implant length and osseointegration
The higher rate of osseointegration of 14-mm-long implants cannot justify their use when the risk of severe complications, however uncommon or remote, exists

8.10 Failure to Survive after Loading

Our clinical experience over the last 20 years has taught us that implant length has no clinical relevance long term. The following cases are examples that clearly demonstrate that short implants not only have similar survival rates but in some instances, outlast longer implants.

Why would a short implant outlast a larger implant? Because a short implant distributes a larger masticatory load over a smaller surface area. Since it is well known that bone changes its configuration in response to loads and larger loads are particularly osteogenic, bone around a shorter implant should be expected to be denser that bone surrounding a longer one of similar width.

The following cases demonstrate the long-term performance of plateau root form implants of difference lengths. We believe that cases present a clearer picture, than words.

The case depicted in Figs. 8.11, 8.12, 8.13, and 8.14 taught us that bone, unlike metal, is a living tissue that responds to masticatory loads. In this environment it is not only possible but reasonable to expect that a shorter implant with less anchorage in bone can survive a longer one.

Longer angled implants vs. Short "straight" implants
The use of longer angled implants in posterior mandible, with the obvious increased risk for severe complications, such as damage to the inferior alveolar nerve or perforation of the lingual plate cannot longer be justified since shorter implants are available

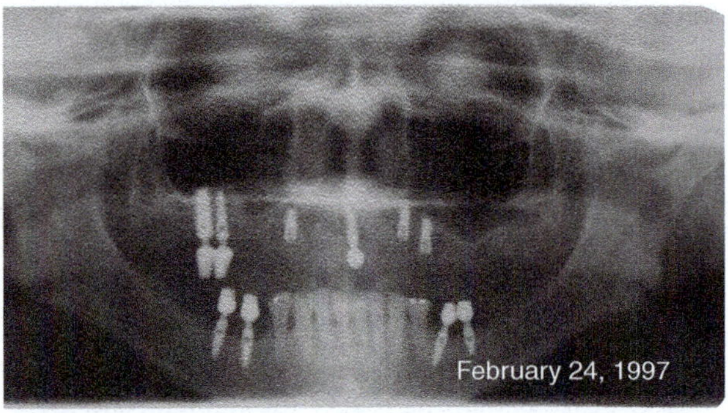

Fig. 8.11 Panoramic radiograph of mandibular implants in posterior areas on the day of implant uncovering, February 24, 1997. A 3.5 × 8-mm implant was placed in the area of the mandibular left first molar and 3.5 × 11-mm implants were placed to restore the mandibular right second premolar and first molar

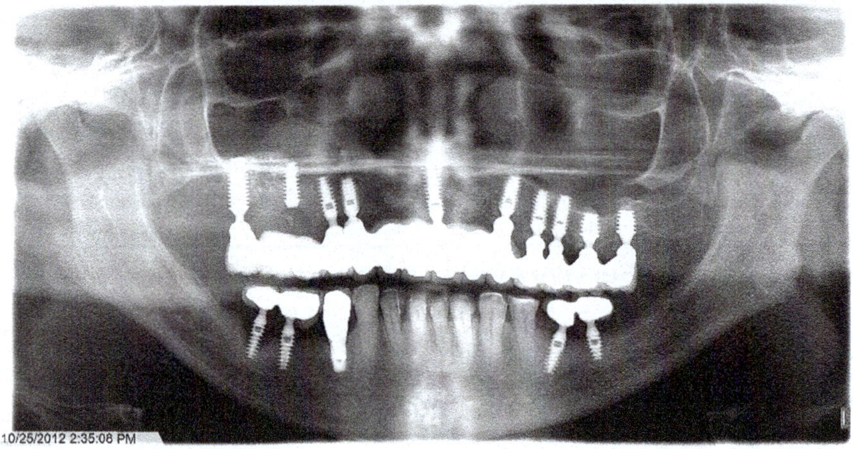

Fig. 8.12 Panoramic radiograph of mandibular implants in posterior areas on a recall appointment, October 2012. Notice crestal bone stability in the shorter, 3.5 × 8-mm implant restoring the mandibular left first molar and the bone loss in the longer, 3.5 × 11-mm implant placed to restore the mandibular right first molar. In this case, the longer implant (11 mm) did not prove to have better long-term survival when compared to the shorter implant (8 mm)

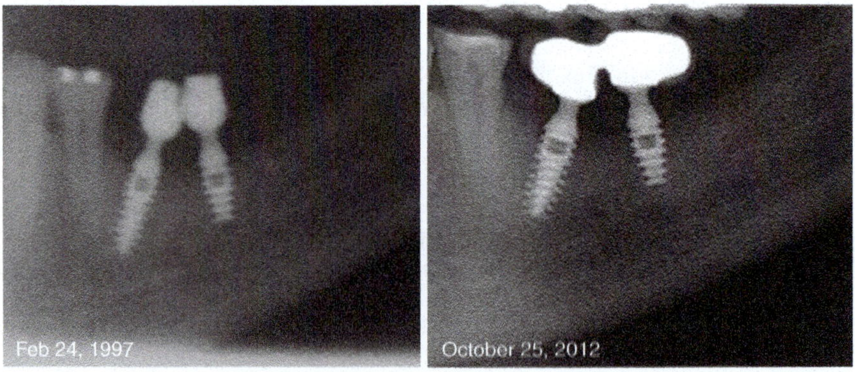

Fig. 8.13 Radiographs of mandibular left posterior implants at uncovering (left, Feb 1997) and at recall appointment (right, Oct 2012). Note peri-implant bone stability after 15 years of loading surrounding the 3.5 × 8-mm implant

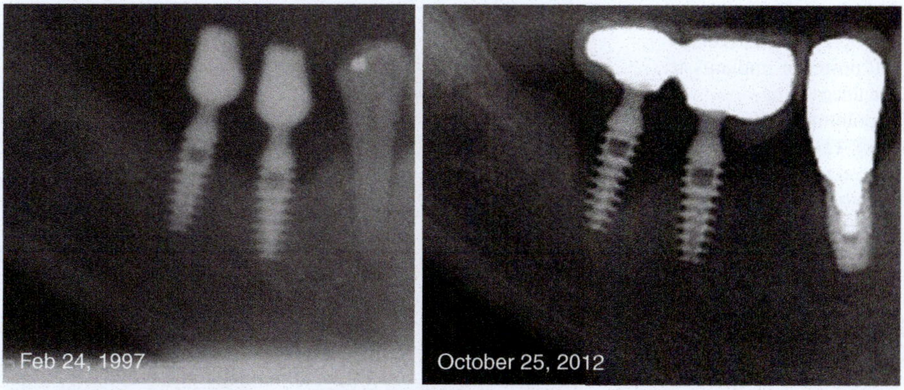

Fig. 8.14 Radiographs of mandibular right posterior implants at uncovering (left, Feb 1997) and at recall appointment (right, Oct 2012). Note peri-implant bone loss in the 3.5 × 11-mm implant placed to restore the first molar

8.11 Long-Term Performance of Ultrashort Implants in Posterior Maxilla

We have reported that for PRF implants, the short-term survival of ultrashort wide implants is similar to the survival of longer implants. We have also reported that the short-term survival of 5- and 6-mm-long implants is similar to that of 8-mm-long implants [10].

It has been suggested that a 6-mm-long implant is insufficient to support a maxillary molar. Conventional restoring protocols call for longer implants which often require large grafting procedures when restoring posterior maxilla. This rationale is based on the belief that the surface provided by an ultrashort implant will offer insufficient contact between the poorly mineralized maxillary bone and the implant to withstand masticatory forces. This rationale seems to come from the fact that the torqueing forces necessary to restore screw-type implant systems is often capable of fracturing the bone-to-implant connection in cases with limited maxillary bone height. It is possible that 5 and 6 mm length is not sufficient for predictable implant treatments using screw-type implants and consequently, they should not be recommended in these types of cases.

On the other hand, the use of 5- and 6-mm-long single-tooth plateau-type implants in posterior maxilla has proved to be a successful long-term treatment approach in our clinical practice. The cases shown in Figs. 8.15, 8.16, 8.17, 8.18, 8.19, 8.20, 8.21, 8.22, 8.23, 8.24, 8.25, and 8.26 are examples of long-term survival of Bicon implants restoring maxillary posterior areas.

Longer implants and larger grafting vs. Short implants with minimal grafts
The use of longer implants and larger grafts can no longer be justified when short plateau root form implants with limited-to-no grafting can be used

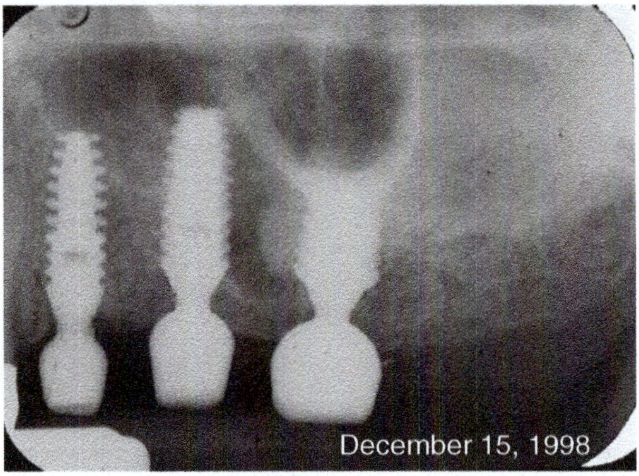

Fig. 8.15 Periapical radiograph of maxillary left posterior implants at the uncovering appointment, Dec 1998. A 3.5 × 11-mm implant was placed in the second premolar area, a 4 × 11-mm was placed in the first molar area and a 5 × 8-mm placed to restore the second molar

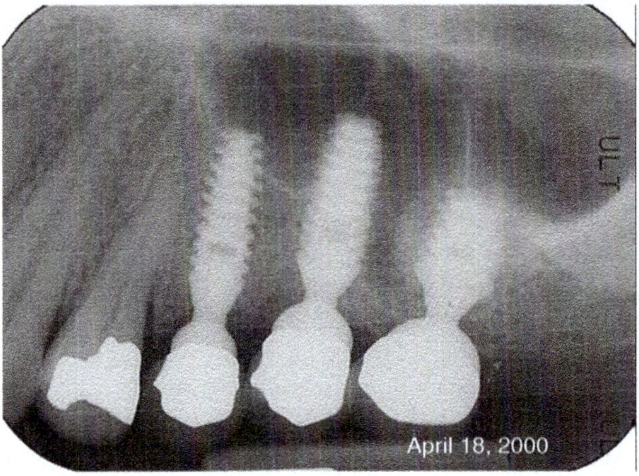

Fig. 8.16 Periapical radiograph of maxillary left posterior implants restored with single PFM crowns at a recall appointment, April 2000

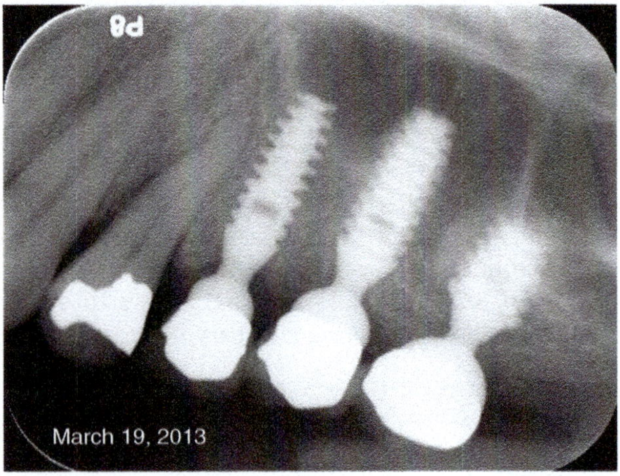

Fig. 8.17 Periapical radiograph of maxillary left posterior implants at the 15-year recall appointment, March 2013. A 3.5 × 11-mm implant was placed in the second premolar area, a 4 × 11-mm was placed in the first molar area, and a 5 × 8-mm placed to restore the second molar. Notice the peri-implant bone stability surrounding all the implants. It seems clear that short 8-mm-long implants can survive as well as the 11-mm-long ones, so they should be considered the standard of care

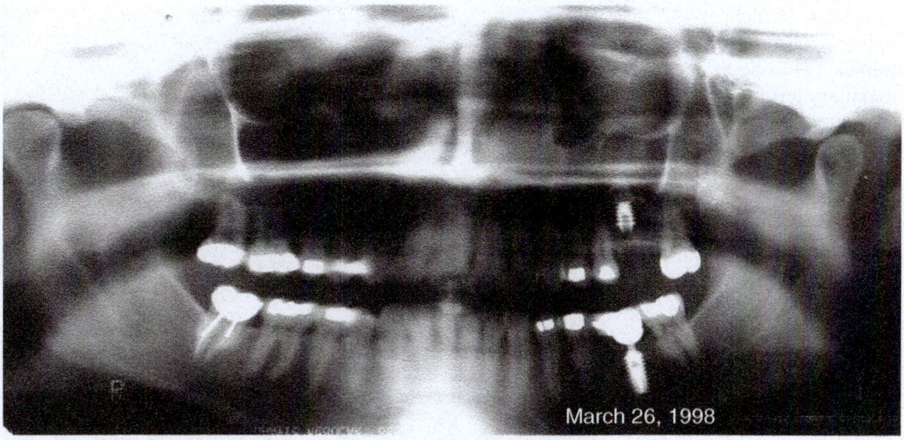

Fig. 8.18 Panoramic radiograph of a short implant placed in the maxillary left first molar area at uncovering March 1998

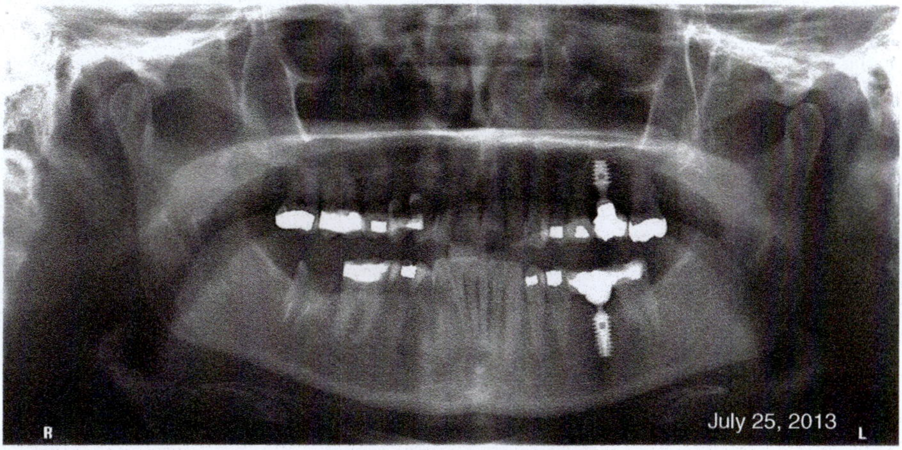

Fig. 8.19 Panoramic radiograph of a short implant restoring a maxillary left first molar area after 15 years of loading, July 2013

8.12 Long-Term Performance of Ultrashort Implants in Posterior Mandible

The use of ultrashort implants in posterior mandible has not been challenged as often as in the maxilla due to the increased density of mandibular bone. When we place long implants to restore posterior mandibular teeth we assume that the patient is going to be able to keep them for the rest of their lives. The longer the implants, the longer their function, right? The case presented in Figs. 8.27 and 8.28 presents a more realistic view of the oral environment.

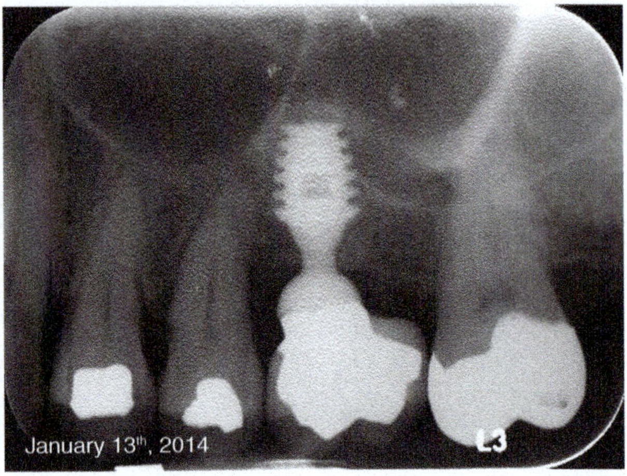

Fig. 8.20 Periapical radiograph of a short implant restoring a maxillary left first molar area after 16 years of loading, July 2013. Note peri-implant bone stability

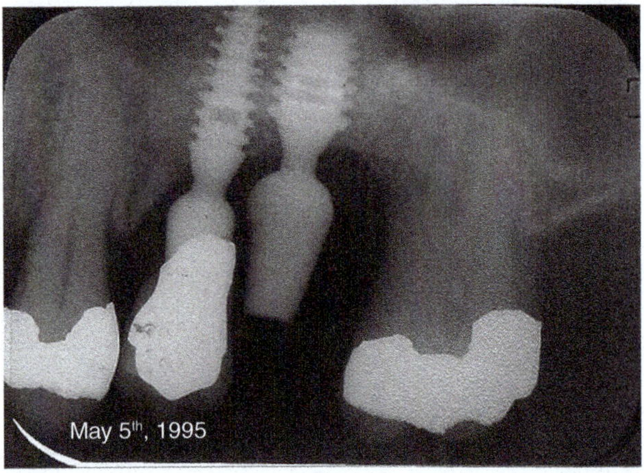

Fig. 8.21 Periapical radiograph of a short implant placed to restore the maxillary left first molar at uncovering appointment, May 1995

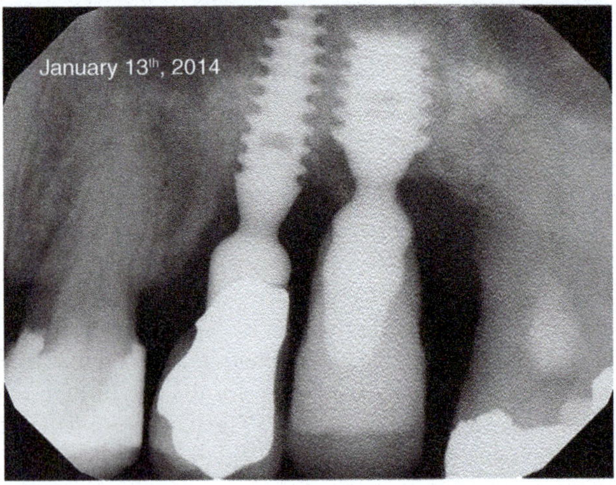

Fig. 8.22 Periapical radiograph of a short implant placed to restore the maxillary left first molar at uncovering appointment, January 2014. Note peri-implant bone stability after 19 years of loading

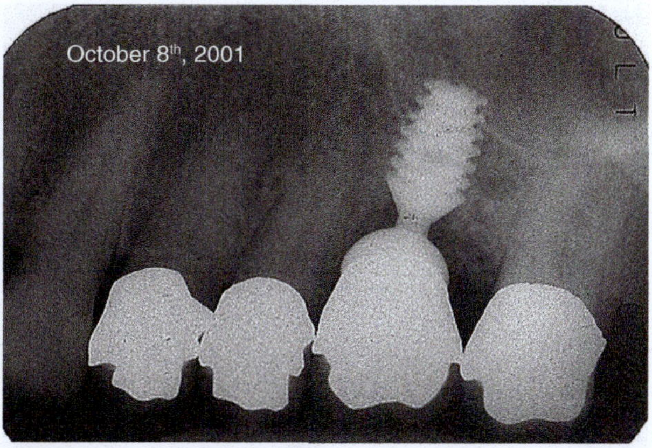

Fig. 8.23 Periapical radiograph of a short implant placed to restore a maxillary left first molar at crown insertion appointment, Oct 2001

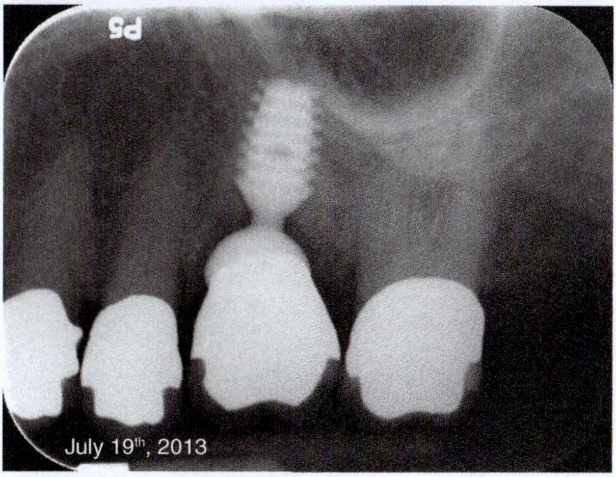

Fig. 8.24 Periapical radiograph of a short implant placed to restore the maxillary left first molar at recall appointment, July 2013. Notice long term, peri-implant bone stability (12 years)

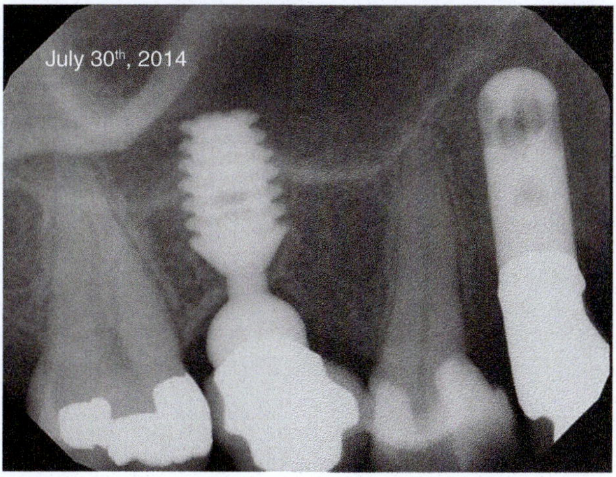

Fig. 8.25 Periapical radiograph of a short implant placed restoring a maxillary right first molar at a recall appointment (July 30, 2014) after 17 years of loading (implant was placed June 26, 1997)

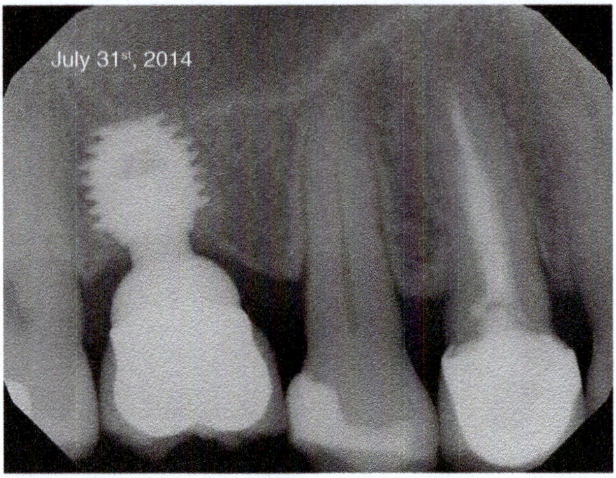

Fig. 8.26 Periapical radiograph of an ultrashort 6 × 6-mm implant placed restoring a maxillary right first molar at a recall appointment (July 31, 2014) after more than 10 years of loading

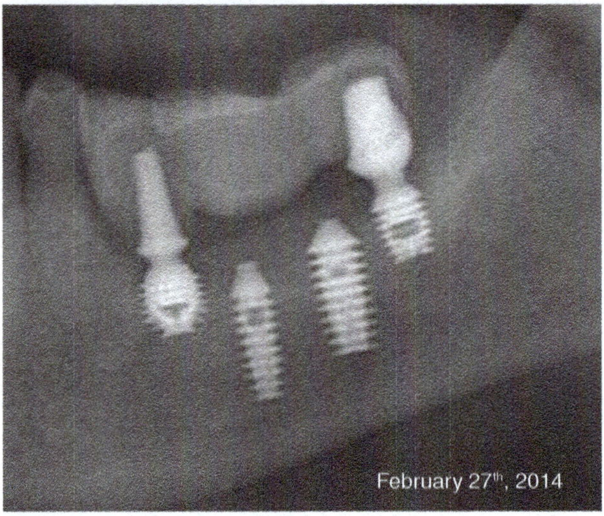

Fig. 8.27 Periapical radiograph of mandibular left posterior implants. A fixed partial denture is supported by two ultrashort implants, a 5 × 6-mm implant was placed in the second molar area and a 6 × 6 in the second premolar area. The ultrashort implants replaced longer implants that failed due to abutment fractures. This case depicts the changes in our clinical practice over the years. The shorter/wider implants with wider/stronger components are preferred over longer/thinner implants that can fracture in posterior areas

The cases showed in Figs. 8.27, 8.28, 8.29, 8.30, 8.31, 8.32, 8.33, 8.34, 8.35, 8.36, 8.37, 8.38, 8.39, 8.40, 8.41, 8.42, 8.43, 8.44, 8.45, 8.46, and 8.47 support the rationale that ultrashort implants should be presented to the patient as the ideal treatment option when restoring posterior mandible.

The use of Ultrashort implants in posterior mandible

Permanent damage to the inferior alveolar nerve and/or perforation of the lingual plate are serious complications that in most cases can be avoided with the use of short implants. Is the use of long implants in posterior mandible still indicated?

As shown in Fig. 8.27, shorter and wider implants have replaced longer and thinner implants in our clinical practice. The use of wider implants with larger

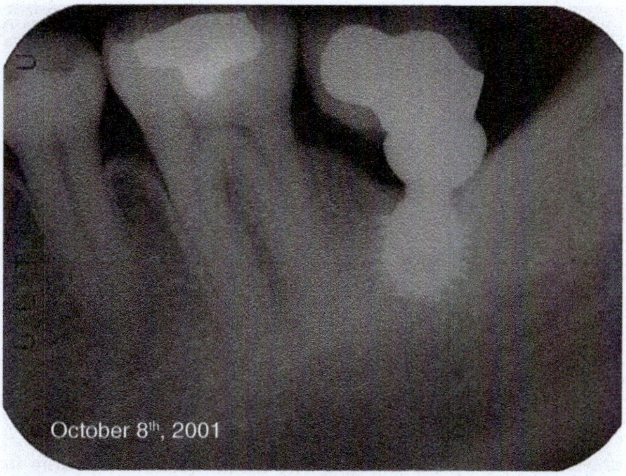

Fig. 8.28 Periapical radiograph of an ultrashort 6 × 6-mm implant placed in the area of a mandibular left second molar, at crown insertion 2001

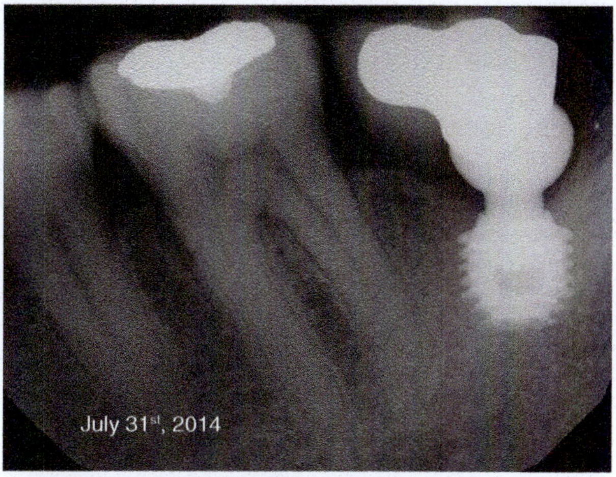

Fig. 8.29 Periapical radiograph of an ultrashort 6 × 6-mm implant placed in the area of a mandibular left second molar, at recall appointment 2014. Note the long-term crestal bone stability despite the less than ideal implant angle

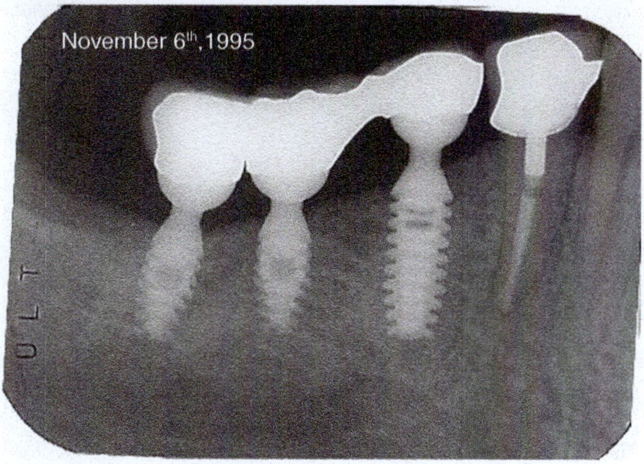

Fig. 8.30 Periapical radiograph of dental implants restoring mandibular right posterior teeth, at crown insertion 1995. 8-mm-long implants were placed in the first and second molar areas and 11-m-long ones in the second premolar

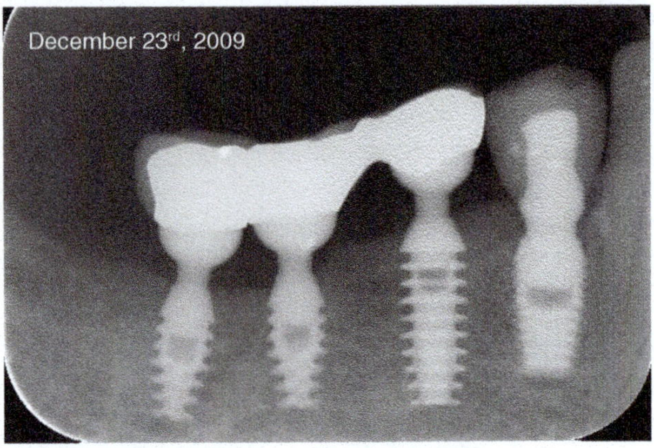

Fig. 8.31 Periapical radiograph of dental implants restoring mandibular right posterior teeth, at recall appointment 2009. Note the crestal bone stability of both the 8 mm long implants restoring the first and second molar areas and the longer, 11-mm-long implant placed in the second premolar. The increased risk of complications (such as paresthesia) when using longer implants can no longer be justified since shorter implants have similar clinical performance

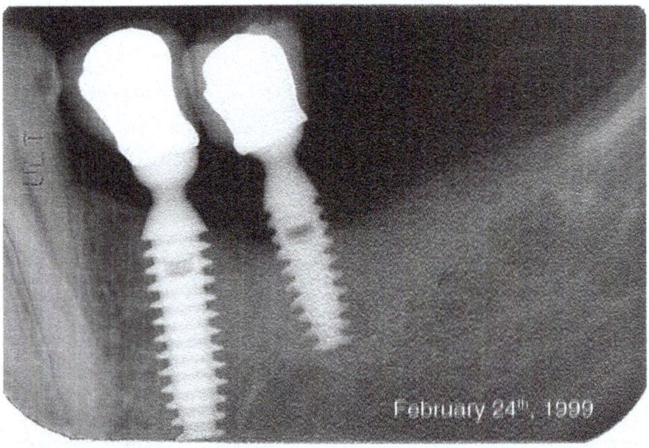

Fig. 8.32 Periapical radiographs of a 3.5 × 11-mm implant placed to restore a mandibular left second premolar. Shown here at a recall appointment Feb 1999. Implant was placed January 1997. Note that endosteal implant height is only 8 mm (only 8 of the 11 mm are in bone)

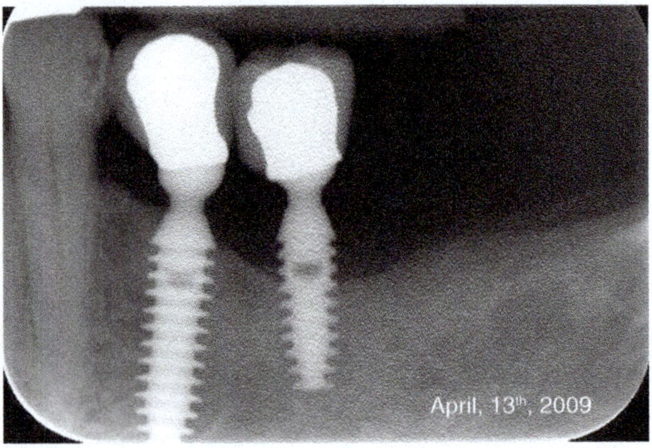

Fig. 8.33 Periapical radiographs of a 3.5 × 11-mm implant placed to restore a mandibular left second premolar. Shown here at a recall appointment April 2009. Crestal bone stability noted after more than 10 years in function, 8 mm endosteal implant height seems to be enough to withstand masticatory forces long term

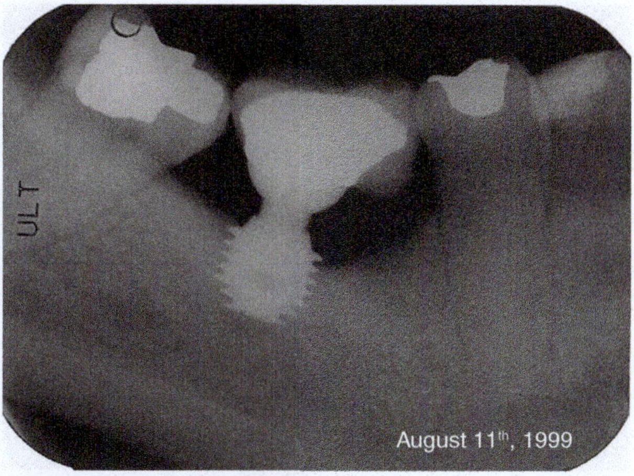

Fig. 8.34 Periapical radiograph of an ultrashort 6 × 6-mm implant restoring a mandibular first molar area at crown insertion 1999

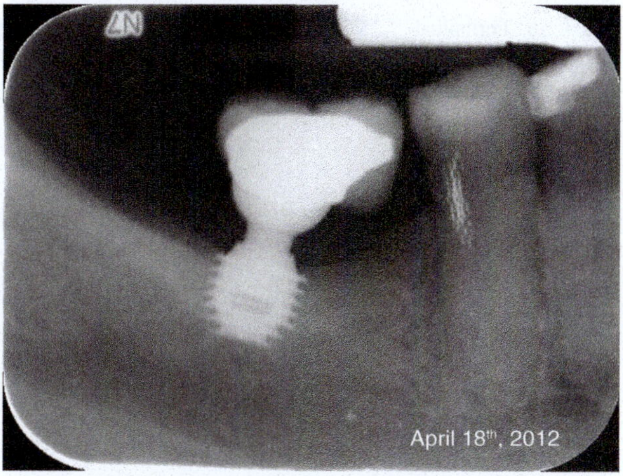

Fig. 8.35 Periapical radiograph of an ultrashort 6 × 6-mm implant restoring a mandibular first molar area at recall appointment 2012. Notice crestal bone stability after more than 10 years of loading, the radiograph suggests crestal bone growth on the mesial side when compared to the crown insertion radiograph

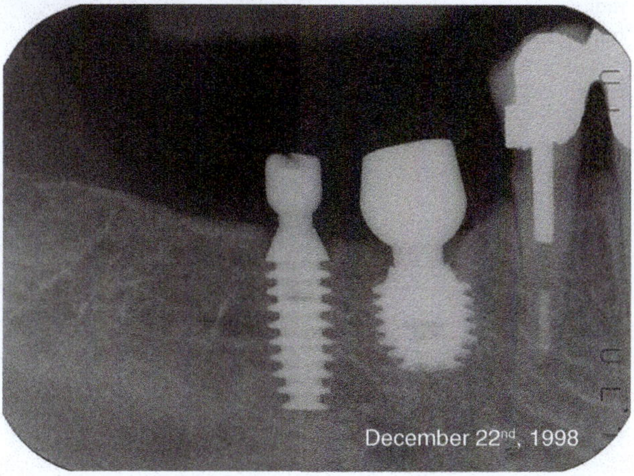

Fig. 8.36 Periapical radiograph of implants placed in mandibular right posterior area. A 6 × 6-mm was placed in the first molar and a 3.5 × 11-mm was placed in the second molar area. Shown here at crown insertion 1998

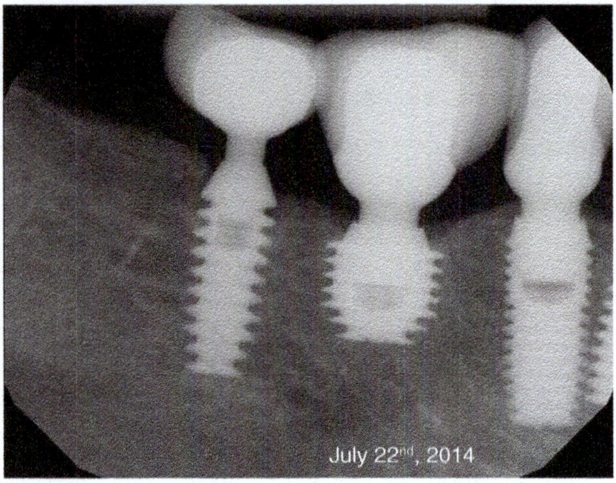

Fig. 8.37 Periapical radiograph of implants placed in mandibular right posterior area. Shown here at a recall appointment 2014. Note crestal bone stability surrounding both ultrashort and long implants after more than 15 years of loading

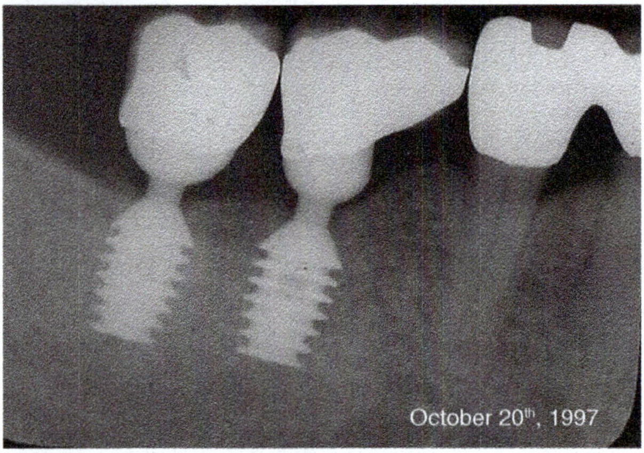

Fig. 8.38 Periapical radiograph of two short implants restoring mandibular right molars shown at crown insertion Oct 1997

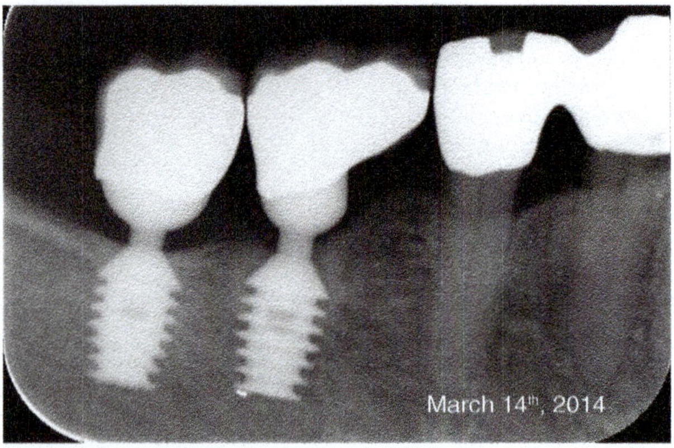

Fig. 8.39 Periapical radiograph of two short implants restoring mandibular right molars shown at recall appointment March 2014. Notice crestal bone stability after more than 15 years of loading

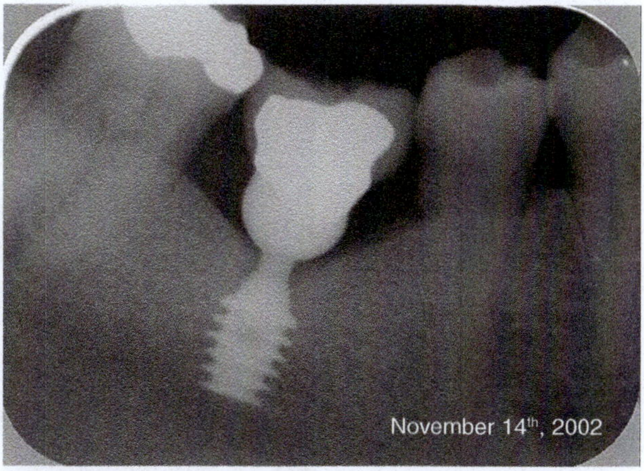

Fig. 8.40 Periapical radiograph of a mandibular right first molar restored with an implant supported restoration shown here 4 years after implant placement, Nov 2002 (implant was placed in 1998)

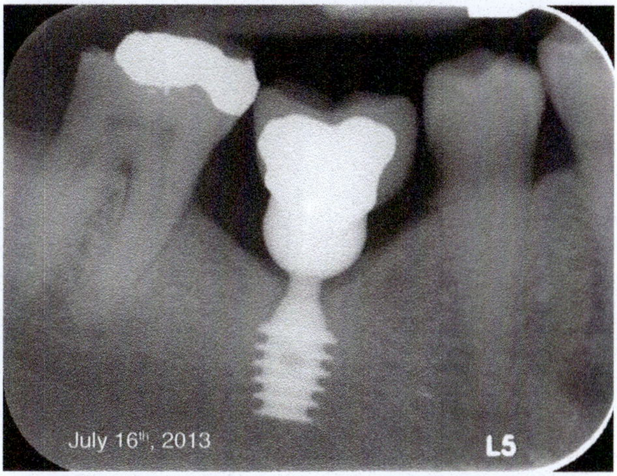

Fig. 8.41 Periapical radiograph of a mandibular right first molar restored with an implant supported restoration shown here 15 years after implant placement, July 2013

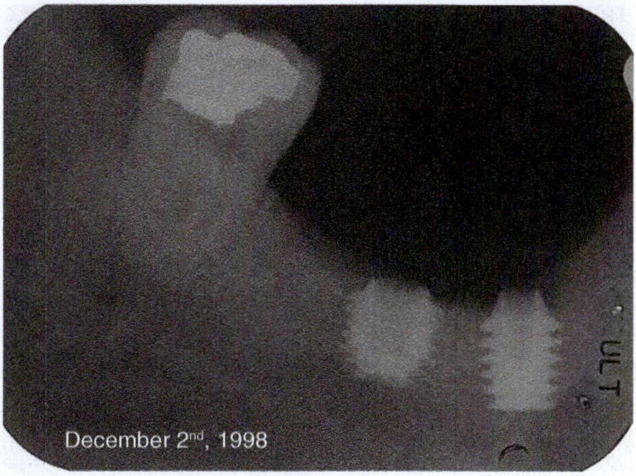

Fig. 8.42 Periapical radiographs of ultrashort implants restoring mandibular right molars. A 6 × 6-mm was placed in the area of the second molar and a 5 × 8-mm (shortened by the surgeon to about 7 mm, to avoid nerve trauma). Shown here at uncovering appointment, Dec 1998

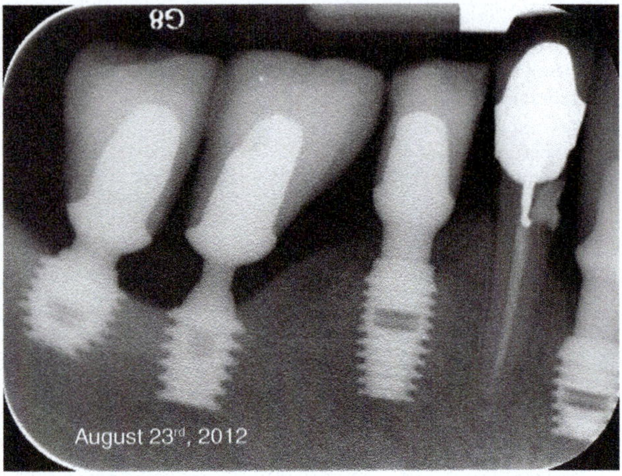

Fig. 8.43 Periapical radiographs of ultrashort implants restoring mandibular right molars. Note crestal bone stability more than 10 years at implant placement. Shown here at recall appointment, August 2012

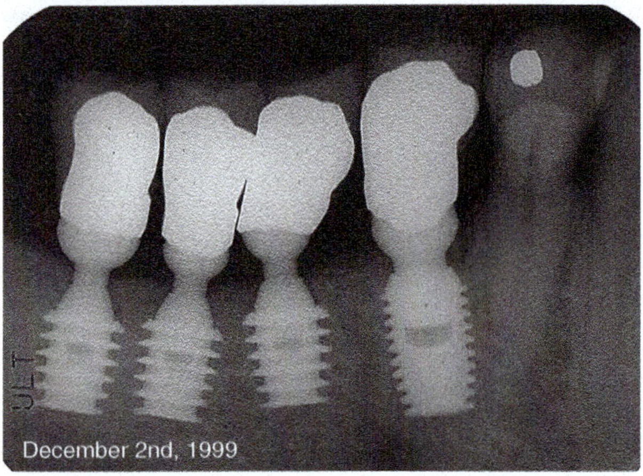

Fig. 8.44 Periapical Radiographs of four implants restoring mandibular right posterior teeth. A 5 × 8-mm with a 3 mm abutment post was placed to restore the first premolar. Three 5 × 8-mm (2 mm abutments post) implants were adjusted by the surgeon (reduced in length to approx. 6.5 mm) before being inserted in the 1990s. Shown here at crown insertion Dec 1999

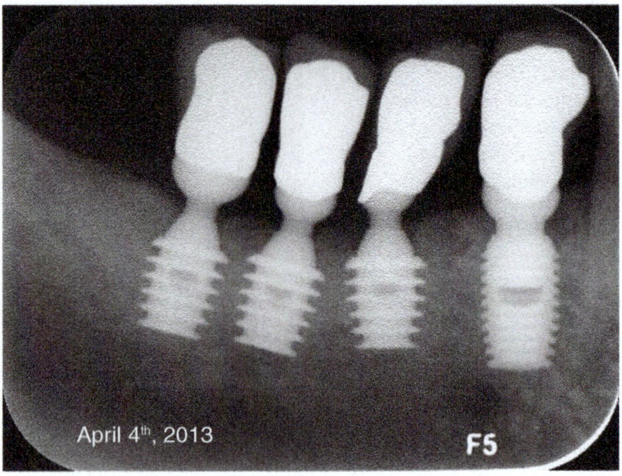

Fig. 8.45 Periapical Radiographs of four implants restoring mandibular right posterior teeth. A 5 × 8-mm with a 3 mm abutment post was placed to restore the first premolar. Three 5 × 8-mm (2 mm abutments post) implants were adjusted by the surgeon (reduced in length to approx. 6.5 mm) before being inserted in the 1990s. Shown here at a recall appointment April 2013. Note crestal bone stability after more than 10 years of loading

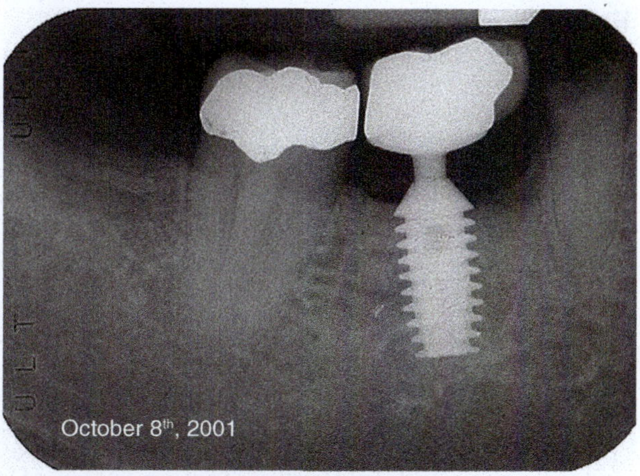

Fig. 8.46 Periapical radiograph of a 5 × 11-mm implant placed to restore a mandibular right first molar. Shown here at a recall appointment in Oct 2001, 6 years after implant placement (1995)

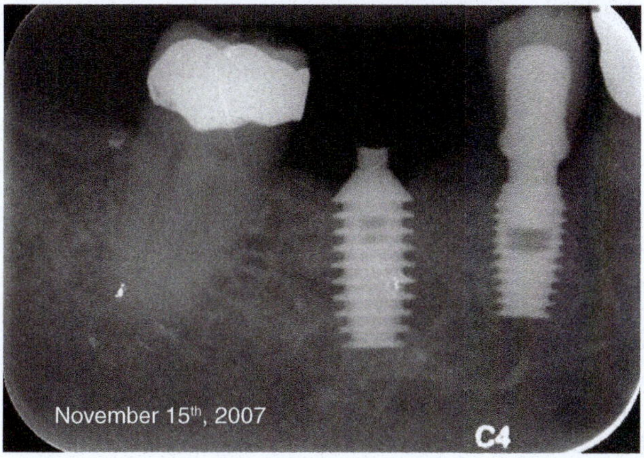

Fig. 8.47 Periapical radiograph of a 5 × 11-mm implant restoring a mandibular right first molar. Shown here at an emergency visit in Nov 2007 due to the fracture of the abutment, 12 years after implant placement (1995). Shorter implants with wider restorative components (i.e., 3 mm abutment posts vs. 2 mm posts) like the 4.5 × 8-mm restoring the second premolar are preferred over longer implants with thinner components when restoring posterior areas

components, i.e., 3-mm-wide abutments vs. 2-mm-wide abutments has shown better survival and a lesser risk of prosthetic complications, such as abutment post fracture, under long-term function. Therefore, the use of implants with 3 mm abutments (≥4.5 mm implant width) is preferred in posterior areas.

Ultrashort ≥4.5 mm wide implants in posterior areas
3 mm abutment posts have shown better long-term performance, i.e., less fractures when compared to 2-mm-wide posts which have shown to be more prone to fracture under long-term function

References

1. Urdaneta RA, Rodriguez S, McNeill DC, Weed M, Chuang SK. The effect of increased crown-to-implant ratio on single-tooth locking-taper implants. Int J Oral Maxillofac Implants. 2010;25:729–43.
2. Urdaneta RA, Leary J, Lubelski W, Emanuel K, Chuang SK. The effect of implant size 5 9 8 on crestal bone levels around single-tooth implants. J Periodontology. 2012;83:1235–44.
3. Urdaneta, RA, Daher S, Leary J, Emanuel K, Chuang SK. Factors associated with crestal bone gain on single-tooth locking-taper implants: The effect of nonsteroidal anti-inflammatory drugs. Int J Oral Maxillofacial Implants. 2011;26:1063–78.
4. Urdaneta RA, Leary J, Panetta KM, Chuang S-K. The effect of opposing structures, natural teeth vs. implants on crestal bone levels surrounding single-tooth implants. Clin. Oral Impl. Res. 2014;25:e179–e188. https://doi.org/10.1111/clr.12087.
5. Urdaneta RA, Leary J, Lubelski W, Emanuel KM, Chuang SK. The effect of implant size 5 x 8 mm on crestal bone levels around single-tooth implants. J Periodontol. 2012;83:1235–44.
6. Urdaneta RA, Daher S, Leary J, Emanuel KM, Chuang SK. The survival of ultrashort locking taper implants. Int J Oral Maxillofac Implants. 2012;27:644–54.
7. Urdaneta RA, Seemann R, Dragan IF, Lubelski W, Leary J, Chuang SK. A retrospective radiographic study on the effect of natural tooth-implant proximity and an introduction to the concept of a bone loading platform switch. Int J Oral Maxillofac Implants. 2014;29:1412–24.
8. Chuang SK, Wei LJ, Douglas CW. Risk factors for dental implant failure: A strategy for the analysis of clustered failure-time observations. J Dent Res. 2002;81:572–77.
9. Chuang SK, Cai T, Douglass CW, Wei LJ, Dobson TB. Frailty Approach for the analysis of clustered failure-time observations in dental research. J Dent Res. 2005;84:54–58.
10. Chuang SK, Cai T. Predicting clustered dental implant survival using frailty methods. J Dent Res. 2006;85:1147–51.

Short Implant in Cleft Cases

9

Dusan Poruban, Rastislav Slavik, and Adam Stebel

Contents

9.1 Dental Implants Overview 130
9.2 Summary 131
References 142

Cleft cases represent an extremely broad interdisciplinary issue in oral and maxillofacial rehabilitation. They have a great impact not only on the function which is the main point of interest but also on the facial esthetics [1]. In terms of oral and maxillofacial treatment, the planned result can be accomplished by controlled long-term therapy consisting of orthodontics, cranio-maxillofacial surgery and/or oral surgery, restorative dentistry, and long-term follow-up [2].

D. Poruban (✉)
Department of Maxillofacial Surgery, F.D. Roosevelt University Hospital, Banska Bystrica, Slovakia

Dental and Oro-Maxillofacial Surgery Office StomEst, Bratislava, Slovakia
e-mail: dporuban@stomest.sk; d.poruban@chello.sk

R. Slavik · A. Stebel
Department of Maxillofacial Surgery, F.D. Roosevelt University Hospital, Banska Bystrica, Slovakia

Medical Faculty of Comenius' University, Bratislava, Slovakia

B. J. Tomasetti, R. Ewers (eds.), *Short Implants*,
https://doi.org/10.1007/978-3-030-44199-9_9

The goals and outlines of treatment steps are essentially as follows:

1. Orthodontics—the goal: the size and the position of the jaw and dental arch along with proper tooth position regardless of the opposite jaw/arch. In cases of cranio-maxillofacial procedures, it is essential to adhere to the postoperative sequential therapy.
2. Cranio-maxillofacial surgery—the goal: the correction of the intermaxillary relation usually by bimaxillary orthographic procedures after growth is finished. Figures 9.1, 9.2, 9.3, 9.4, 9.5, 9.6, 9.7, and 9.8 show the functional and

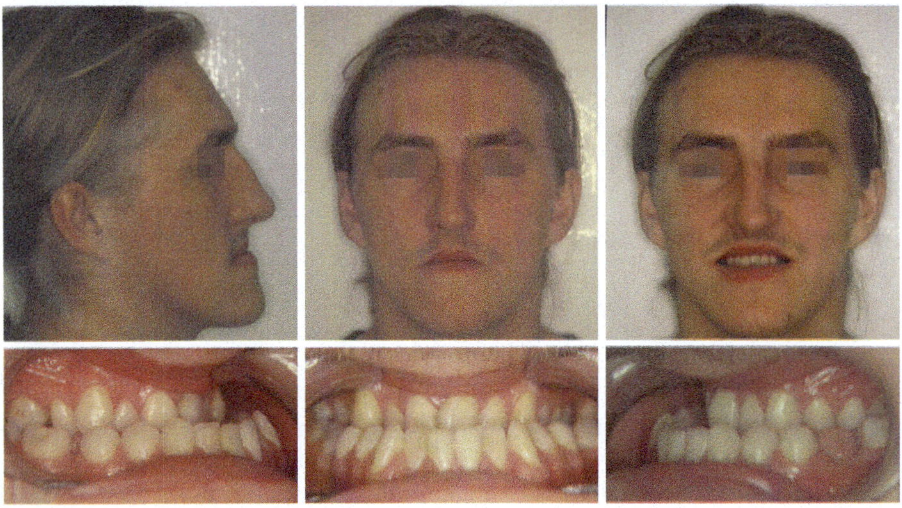

Fig. 9.1 Before the complex treatment

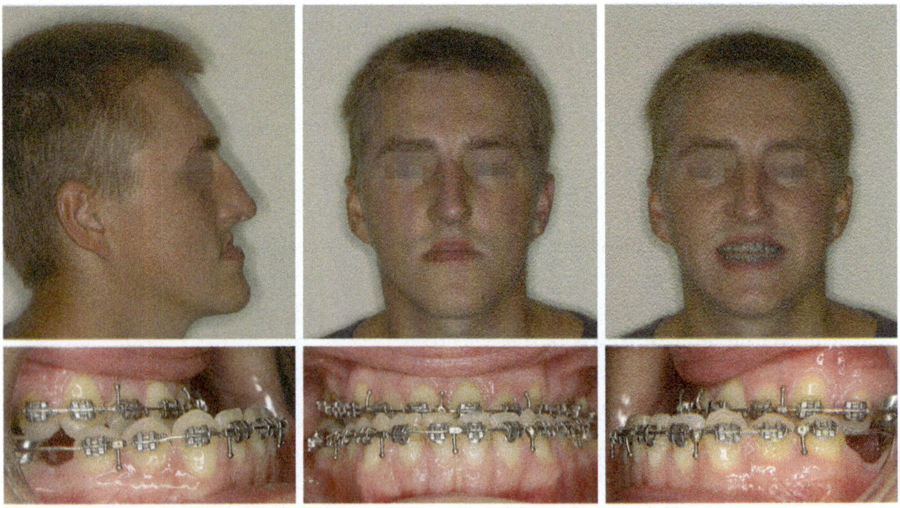

Fig. 9.2 The decompensation after orthodontic therapy and before surgery

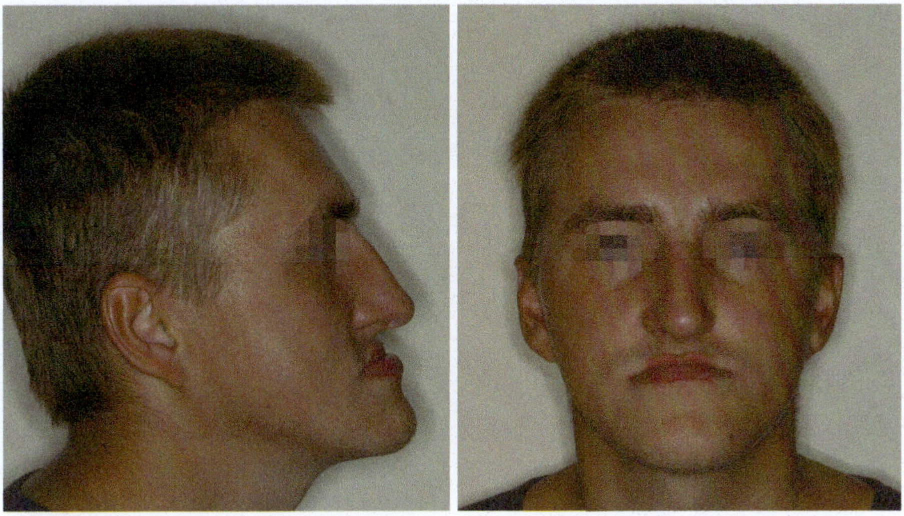

Fig. 9.3 Esthetics in central occlusion before surgery without the splint

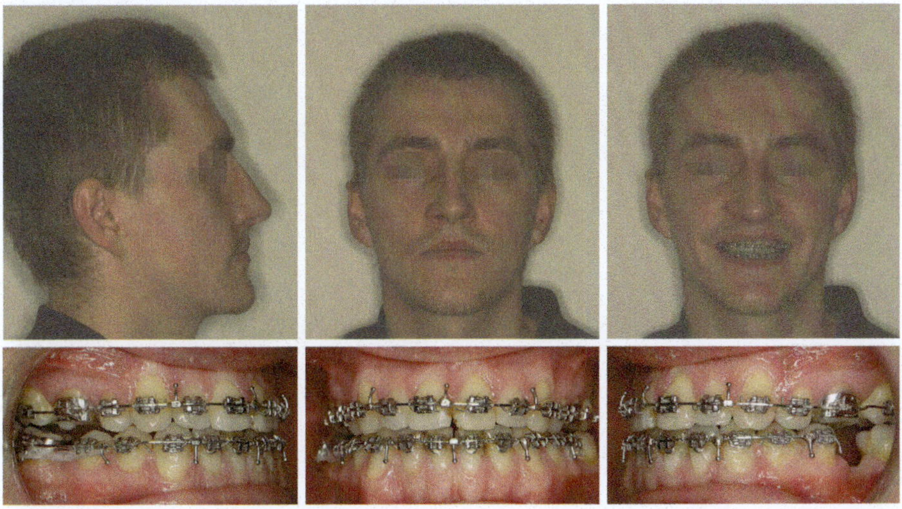

Fig. 9.4 After the bi-maxillary surgery

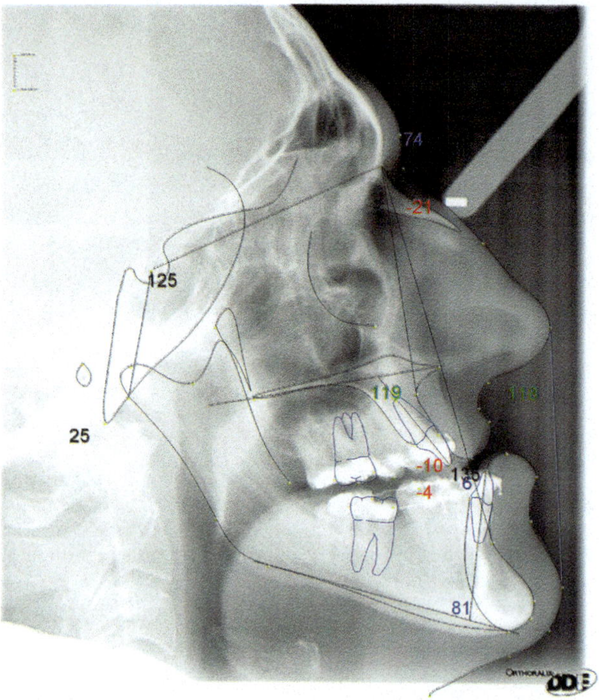

Fig. 9.5 The pre-surgery lateral cephalogram

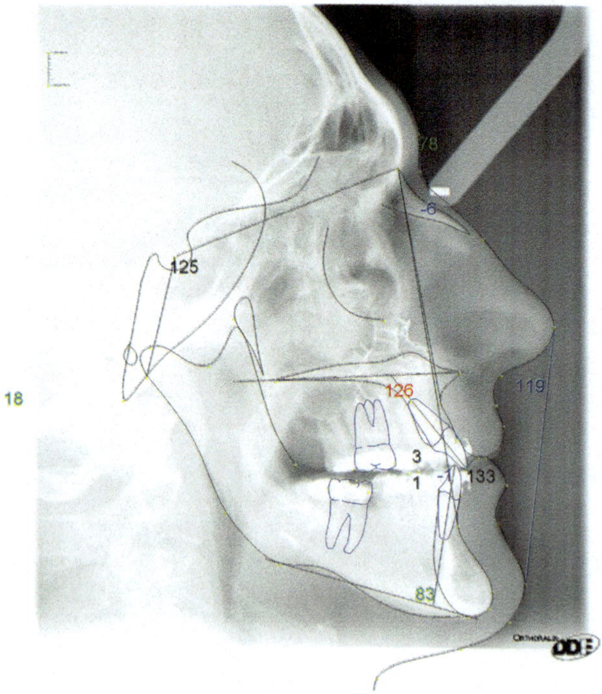

Fig. 9.6 The post-surgery lateral cephalogram

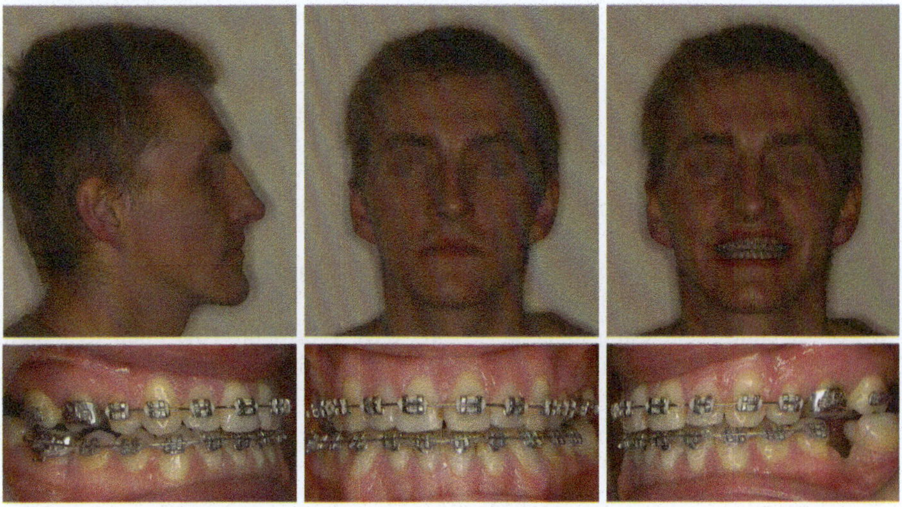

Fig. 9.7 Final result after finishing post-surgery orthodontic

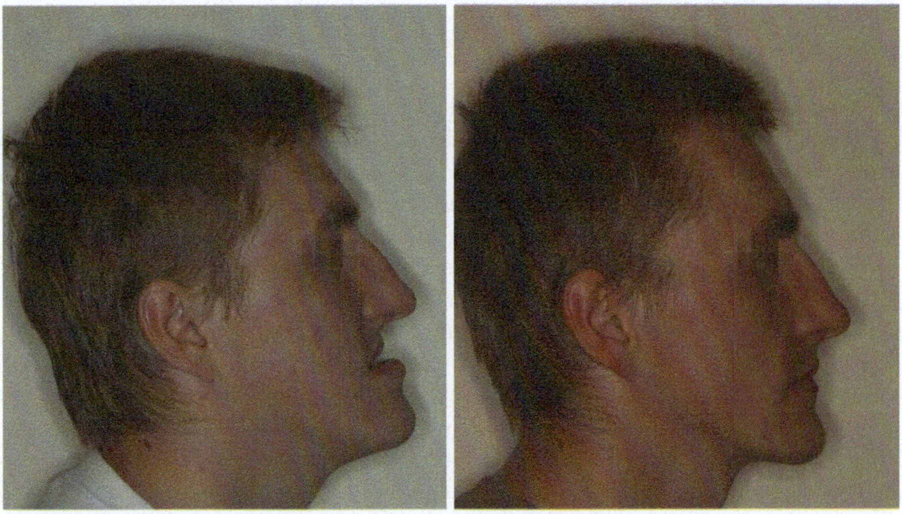

Fig. 9.8 Profile comparison before and after the complex therapy

aesthetic results of a patient with similar combined intermaxillary and aesthetic discrepancies. Oro-nasal fistulas can be closed in the age range of 10–14 years [3].
3. Oral surgery—the goal: the reconstruction of the alveolar ridge within the cleft along with soft tissue coverage (by means of GTR—guided tissue regeneration techniques) [4, 5], followed by dental implant placement and dental restorations. Steps 2 and 3 can be accomplished in the same session or in the reverse order.
4. Prosthodontics—the goal: the prosthetic reconstruction of the dental arches including the use of dental implants.
5. All specialties including dentistry—long-term follow-up—the goal: to sustain the treatment results and prevent any possible complications.

9.1 Dental Implants Overview

Missing teeth are a major problem in cleft patients. Cleft lip, alveolus, and palate patients require specialized prosthetic management including dental implants. The long-term prognosis of the dental implants, successful bone grafting in cleft areas and the optimal date for implant placement are essential for a good long term result. Unfortunately, biological and morphological conditions are often compromised by both the origin of the cleft and by previous treatment. As a result, the bone and soft tissue regeneration are much more negatively affected in comparison with the usual implant cases.

With respect to dental implants the final result depends on various factors. The most important factor is the bone quantity/quality at cleft site and the position of adjacent teeth. Thus, bone grafting represents one of critical steps in the therapy and it can in diffrent individual extent help to achieve the best possible final dental result along with other benefits (e.g. support of alar cartilage). Implant placement itself along with the period from the placement to successful osseointegration can be critical in compromised tissue cases. Complete or partial bone continuity loss and bone stress is proportional to the size and length of the implant used and the extent of primary stability. When considering most common screw implants the general recommendation has been to use implants with a length greater than 10 mm along with a diameter of at least 4 mm. The primary stability is achieved by threading the implant into position with a final torque of 40 Ncm. The implant to abutment connection is important for long-term prognosis and minimal alveolar bone resorption. Any movements (even minimal) of this connection caused by flexibility of material when loaded, may result in bone resorption beginning in proximity of the connection. In this case, bone gain is not possible. Standard dental implant therapy has traditionally been limited by the patient's age due to the fact that it was difficult to follow multidimensional growth changes. This resulted in implants rarely being placed before the age of 16–18 years of age.

The extensive bone grafting procedures and soft tissue flaps used along with previous treatment history represent complex treatment at a young age and a general anesthetic with intubation is the standard option [6].

9.2 Summary

In cleft patients, traditional dental implant treatment does not solve many potential problems in those cases with severely compromised tissues. An example is the case of a bilateral cleft with alveolar clefts and mucoperiosteal oro-nasal micro-fistulas. This often results in a mobile premaxilla which has been stabilized by an orthodontic appliance and space maintainer. There is often very little bone covering and supporting the teeth along the cleft margins. As well, we see an unsatisfactory result of bone-grafting procedures that were done at an early age. The treating surgeon now must contend with:

- Inadequate alveolar height for any traditional implant of 10 mm or more in length.
- Risk of repeated oro-nasal perforation.
- Risk of adjacent tooth root injury.
- Risk of a premaxilla disunion.
- Restricted prognosis counting on time-related marginal bone resorption.
- Compromised esthetics and the need for secondary mucogingival surgery.

9.2.1 Short and Ultrashort Implants

Short and ultrashort dental implants are generally indicated to be those with a length up to 8 mm and 6 mm respectively. It does not, however, specify anything about design, function, and prognosis. Traditional dental implants when shortened often keep their original pros and cons. Recently, increasing data are collected using dental implants of this category with different attributes of design and function (Bicon System) [7]:

- Plateaued and tapered macrogeometry—fast secondary stability/osseointegration.
- Sloping shoulder—extended vitality for marginal alveolar bone and gingiva regeneration.
- Bacterial seal—perfect implant-abutment connection prevents bacterial colonization of the implant surface.
- Short length—minimally invasive thus allowing limited augmentation or no augmentation at all.
- Narrow width—minimally invasive often requiring no augmentation or orthodontic movement.
- Slow drilling—minimally invasive and preserves the vitality of adjacent tissues while allowing bone to be collected.
- Spherical biomechanics—gives support for bone gain induction through load transfer.
- The locking-taper implant to abutment connection—secure abutment in place without the use of internal screws. It simply avoids the additional concern of technical failure of the screw.

- Precise and delicate osteotomy—allows intramembranous-like healing/osseointegration.
- Osteotomy technique (especially hand reamers) —allows complete collection of autologous bone chips for additional immediate alveolar bone augmentation.
- Age limitation—compensation of 3D skeletal changes in adolescent group of patients with help of step-by-step abutments and/or prosthetic suprastructures modification instead of the implant replantations.

Figures 9.9, 9.10, 9.11, 9.12, and 9.13 demonstrates the long-term result of typical implant case and Figs. 9.14, 9.15, 9.16, 9.17, 9.18, 9.19, 9.20, 9.21, 9.22, and 9.23 shows the case of bilateral cleft patient with compromised tissue conditions as mentioned above. Bony and soft tissue regeneration is significant along with the interdental papilla formation.

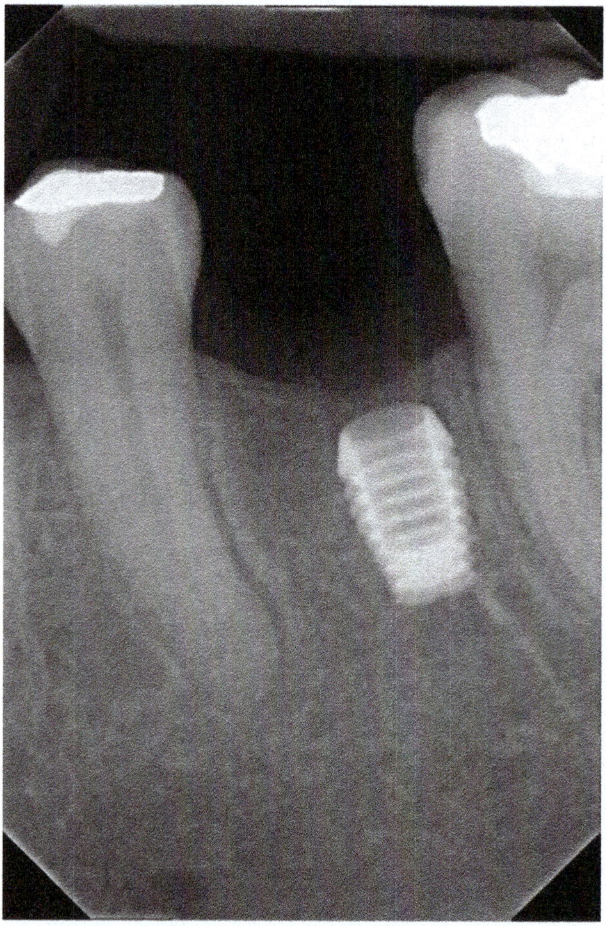

Fig. 9.9 Post-setting time X-ray Bicon 4 × 6 × 2.5 mm into the site 35

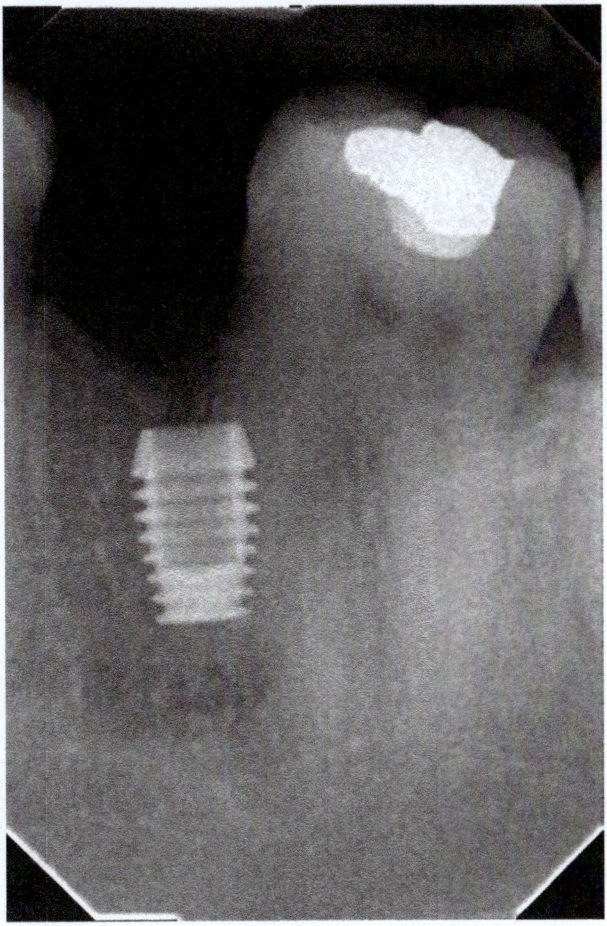

Fig. 9.10 Three-months post-implantation 35

While there is a slightly higher implant failure in all cleft patients with compromised tissue conditions, this should not prevent the use of short and ultrashort implants early in the complex cleft patient's therapy. The extension and time consumption of three-wall bone regeneration techniques with short and ultrashort implants often results in the same or better functional and aesthetic result in comparison to traditional "long" dental implants.

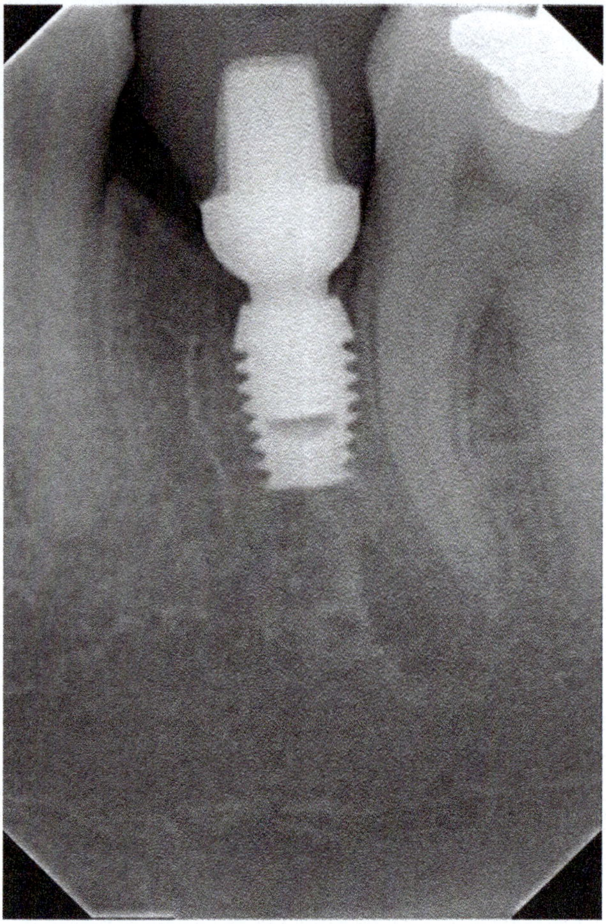

Fig. 9.11 Four-months after integrated crown abutment (IAC) setting

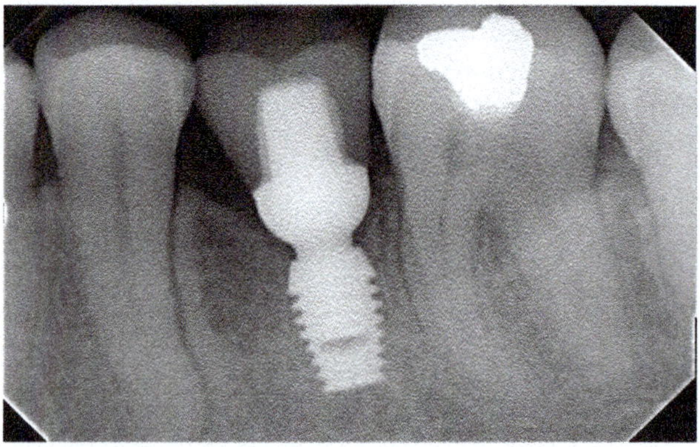

Fig. 9.12 Five-weeks after IAC setting

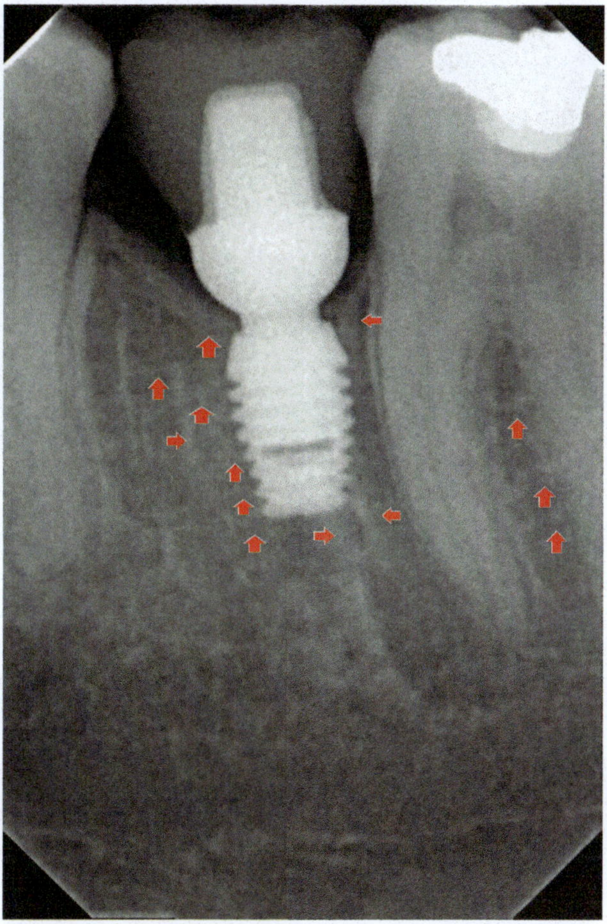

Fig. 9.13 Seven-months after IAC setting, arrows show the functional bony trabecular structure remodeling

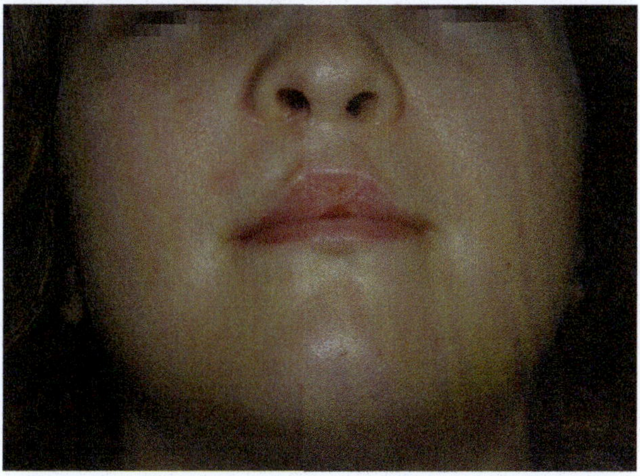

Fig. 9.14 Lip contour with scars in bilateral complete cleft patient

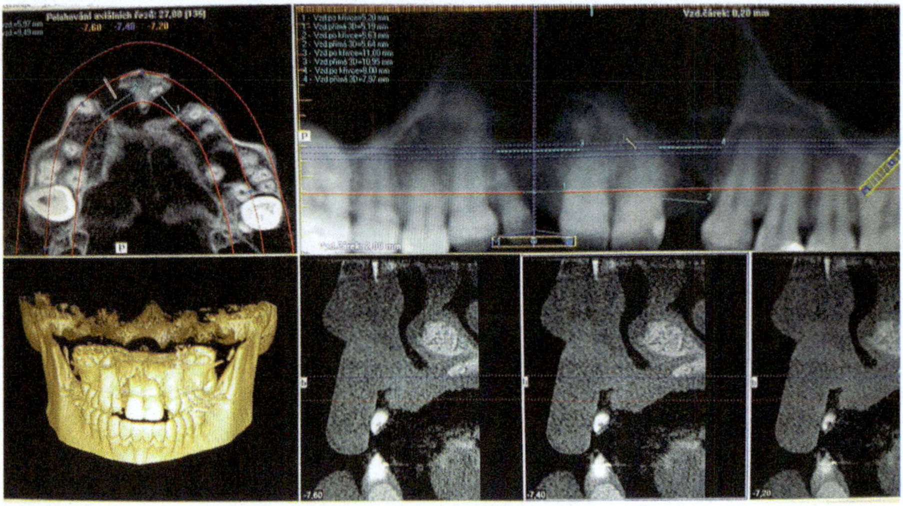

Fig. 9.15 CBCT before the autologous bone graft (mental region) placement and bilateral transpositional extended gingival plasty to restore soft tissue cover

Fig. 9.16 Immediate postoperative view

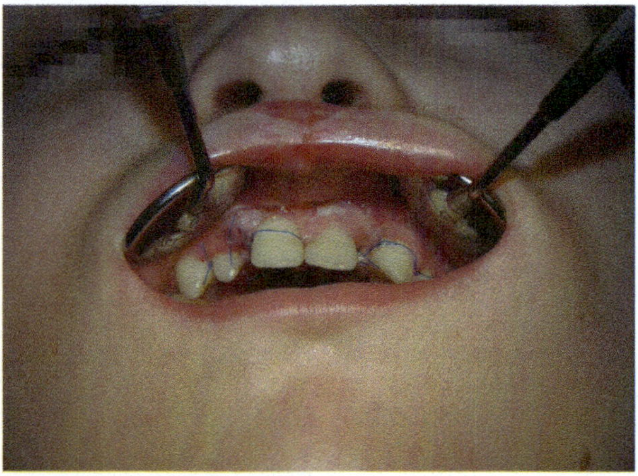

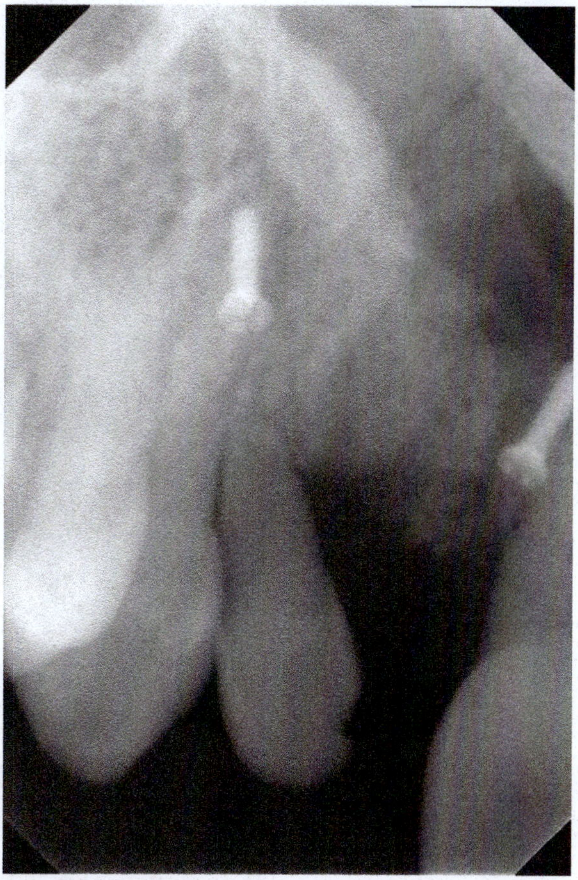

Fig. 9.17 The site 12; 2-months after the surgery

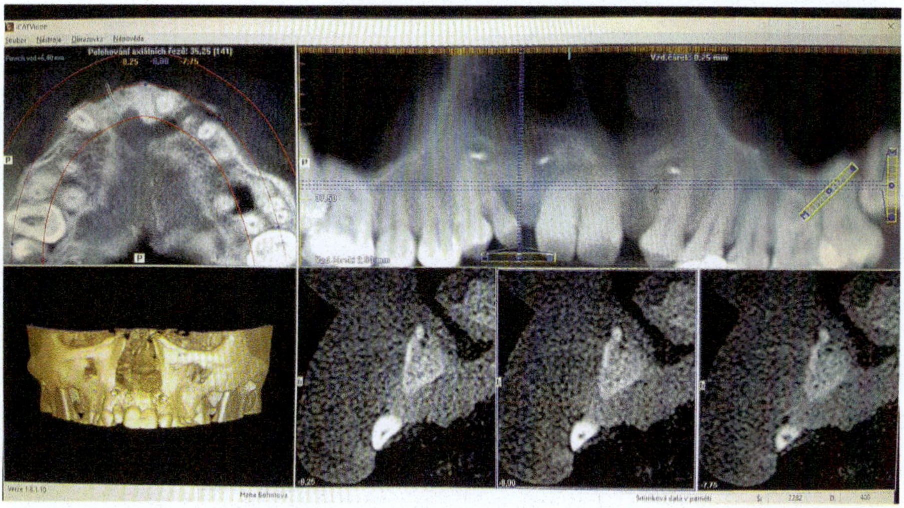

Fig. 9.18 CBCT 3-months after the mental free bone graft surgery

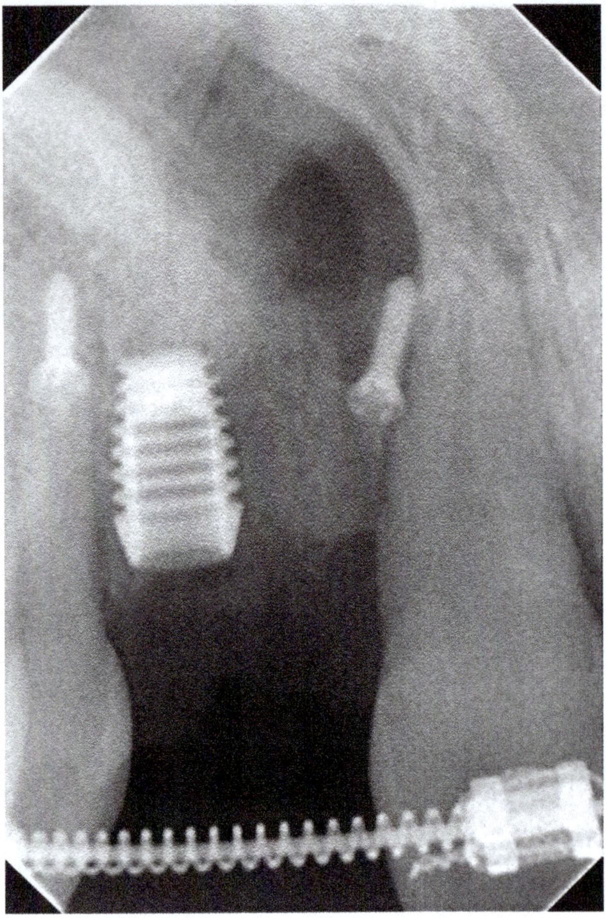

Fig. 9.19 Dental implant Bicon 4 × 6 × 2.5 mm in position of 12 after the implantation

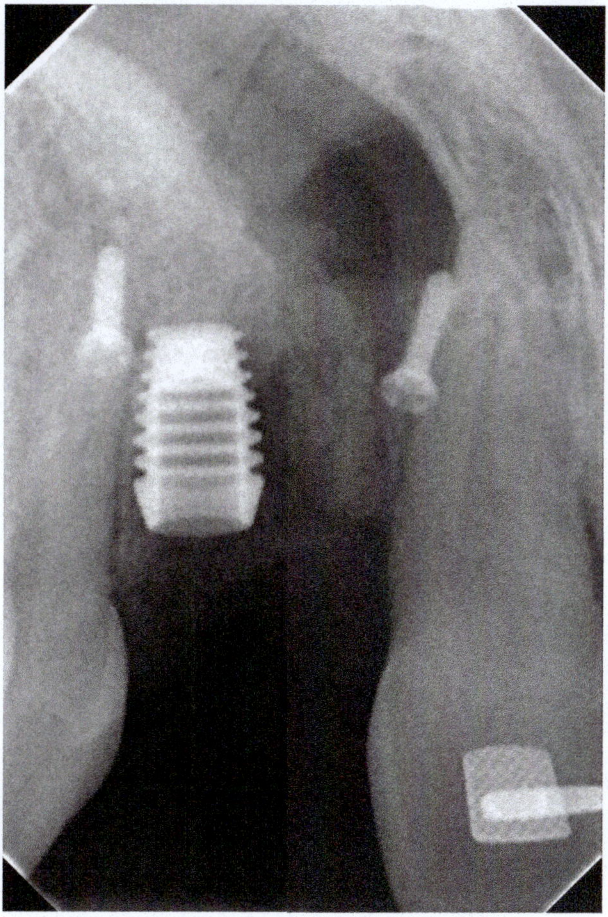

Fig. 9.20 Dental implant 12 3-months post-insertion

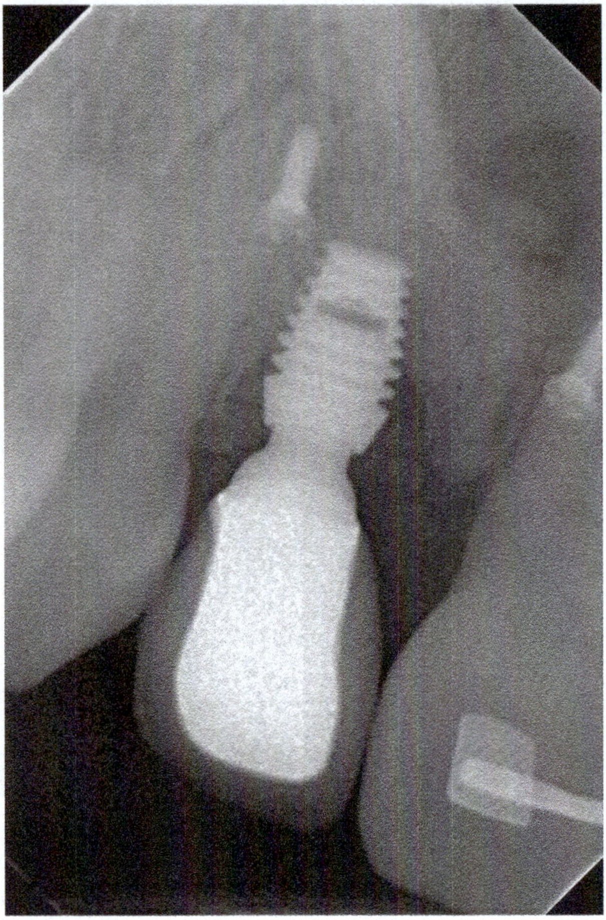

Fig. 9.21 Dental implant 12 with IAC 3-months in function

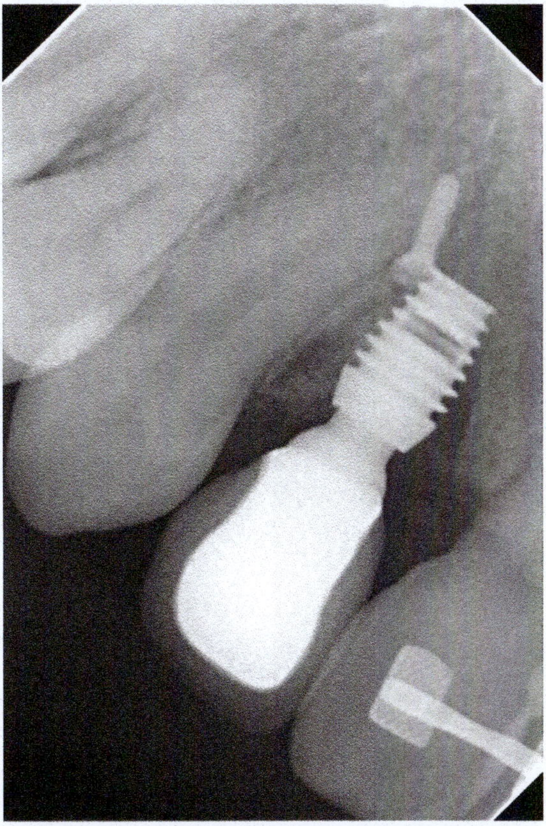

Fig. 9.22 Dental implant 12 with IAC 9-months in function

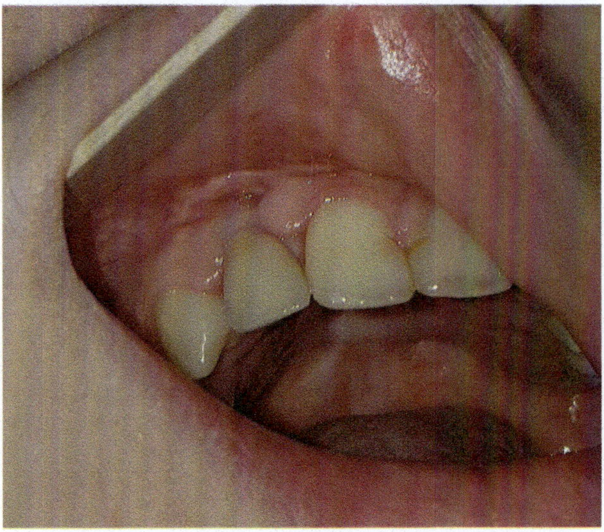

Fig. 9.23 Intraoral view after 9 months

References

1. Obwegeser HL. Pioneer steps in correcting secondary cleft lip and palate deformities: my philosophy and procedures. JCMFS. 2014;42:1023–47.
2. Arnett GW, McLaughlin RP. Facial and dental planning for orthodontists and oral surgeons. London: Mosby; 2004. 314pp, ISBN 0 7234 3320 8.
3. Stanko P, Mracna J, Stebel A, Vojtassak J. Letter to the editor BMJ—contribution to long-term functional results in cleft patients. Bratisl Lek Listy. 2013;114(3):177.
4. Poruban D, Bakos D, Danisovic L, Böhmer D, Blasko M, Vojtassak J. In vitro prepared autologous graft from buccal mucosa—clinical application. Case Rep Clin Pract Rev. 2005;6:107–12. http://www.crcpr-online.com/pdf/vol_6/6726.pdf.
5. Greenlagh DG. The role of growth factors in wound healing. J Trauma. 1996;41:159–67.
6. Holly D, Mracna J. Využitie augmentačných techník v chirurgickej terapii parodontopatií (Augmentation techniques in periodontal surgery). Aktuality súčasného biomedicínskeho výskumu I. (Spotlights of biomedical research I.), Asklepios, Bratislava; 2007, p. 34–8.
7. Morgan VJ. The Bicon short implant. Quintessence, USA; 2017. 326pp, ISBN 9780867157284.

Rehabilitation of Tumour Patients with Ultra-Short Implants and TRINIA Bridges

10

Rolf Ewers and Rudolf Seemann

Contents

10.1 Epidemiology and Aetiology of Oral Squamous Cell Carcinomas 144
10.2 Multimodal Therapy of the OSCC 144
10.3 Implant Rehabilitation of Tumour Patients 144
10.4 Discussion 158
References 159

A variety of head and neck tumours manifest in the jaws. The range extends from rare benign odontomas to semi-malignant tumours such as keratocystic odontogenic tumours or ameloblastomas. Especially, the most frequent malignant tumour, the squamous cell carcinoma, requires a combination of therapies, each with serious side effects. The therapy often comprises tumour resection, lymphadenectomy of the neck, radiotherapy, chemotherapy, reconstruction with microvascular re-anastomosed flaps, and finally rehabilitation with implants and fixed full arch prosthesis.

R. Ewers (✉)
CMF Institute Vienna, Vienna, Austria
e-mail: rolf@cmf-vienna.com

R. Seemann
Department of Otorhinolaryngology, Institute of Head and Neck Diseases, Evangelical Hospital, Vienna, Austria

R. Ewers, B. J. Tomasetti (eds.), *Short Implants*,
https://doi.org/10.1007/978-3-030-44199-9_10

10.1 Epidemiology and Aetiology of Oral Squamous Cell Carcinomas

The high incidence of the oral squamous cell carcinoma (OSCC) finds its etiologic factors in heavy abuse of nicotine and alcohol. Bosetti et al. demonstrated that cessation of smoking halves the cumulative risk of upper aerodigestive cancer even in the age of 50 in comparison to lifetime smokers aged 75 [1]. Unfortunately, a single pathway of OSCC genesis is not identifiable. The effect of tobacco is partly explained by its ability to mutate the tumour suppressor gene p53 [2]. Besides the nuclear factor kappa B, NFKB1 or NFKBIA gene polymorphisms are one of the several other pathogenic pathways [3].

10.2 Multimodal Therapy of the OSCC

Without a profound knowledge of all therapeutic steps, the complexity of implant rehabilitation cannot be understood. Two main concepts of multimodal tumour therapy have to be distinguished by the order of radio-chemotherapy and surgery. If the therapy is started with the tumour resection and followed by a radio-chemotherapy, an adjuvant therapy was chosen. In case of primary radio-chemotherapy followed by tumour resection, we speak of neo-adjuvant therapy. After surgical removal of the OSCC, the defect is frequently reconstructed with a microvascular re-anastomosed flap. The main difference between both concepts is that neo-adjuvant therapy irradiates the tumour and finally leaves a non-irradiated flap whilst during adjuvant therapy the tumour is first removed and then the peri-tumorous tissues as well as the flap is irradiated. On the other side, flap transfer to an irradiated transplant bed is by far more complicated and prone to complication and flap failure. A direct comparison of both concepts shows significant better cumulative survival rates especially in patients with metastatic lymphatic spread [4]. Especially in tumours invading neighbouring tissues (TNM stage T4N2) showed significantly better 5-year survival rates (37.3% vs. 9.7%). Depending of the resection defect, a graft composed of different tissues is required. Bony defects may be reconstructed with a limited number of flaps. The workhorses are the free fibula, the iliac crest, and the scapula transplants [5].

10.3 Implant Rehabilitation of Tumour Patients

The potential risk of radio-osteonecrosis after irradiation, the reduced dimensions of microvascular bone transplants comparable to atrophic jaws and mouth opening, and last but not least the confirmed smoker are the principal challenges of implant rehabilitation in tumour patients. In a systematic review, the time of implantation and radiotherapy in adjuvant therapy was investigated by Nooh [6]. Preimplantation radiation showed smaller overall implant survival rates (88.9%) when compared to post-implantation radiation (92.2%). This suggests that the early osseointegration process is more disturbed by radiation than the late osseointegration. In the conventional preimplantation radiation group, the overall survival rates of implants depended on the location with lowest survival in non-vascularized bone grafts (81.7%), 89.3% in vascularized free flaps, 78.9% in the maxilla, and 93.3% in the mandible. Focused on fibula-reconstructed mandibles Parbo et al. reported an implant survival rate of 96% [7]. In another study, 5-year CSR was reported to be 97.0% and 10-year CSR 79.9% [8]. Compared to non-irradiated healthy individuals a slightly higher implant loss rate has to be expected in tumour patients.

We present a 69-year-old female patient, nonsmoker since 40 years who showed first a white lesion in the left mandibular alveolar part, which confirmed histologically to be a fibrotic metaplasia without any signs of leucoplakia. Four years later, she came again with an ulcerating, reddish lesion in the same region (Fig. 10.1). The biopsy confirmed an invasive squamous cell carcinoma. The patient received neoadjuvant radio-chemotherapy according to the therapeutic scheme at our institution comprising Mitomycin C (15 mg/m^2, bolus on the first day), 5-Fluoruracil (750 mg/m^2 from day 1 to 5), and irradiation (25 sessions of 2 Gy each, a total dosage of 50 Gy) over a time span of 6 weeks. After a recovery period of 11 weeks after

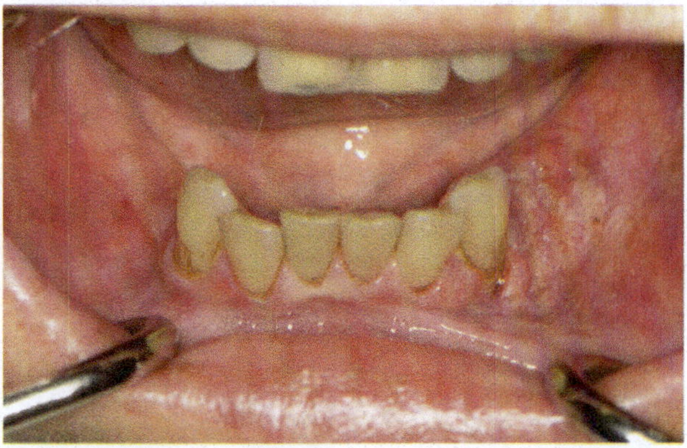

Fig. 10.1 Oral squamous cell carcinoma spreading from the left canine to the second molar region (further stages shown in Figs. 10.2, 10.3, 10.4, 10.5, 10.6, 10.7, 10.8, 10.9, 10.10, 10.11, 10.12, 10.13, 10.14, 10.15, 10.16, 10.17, 10.18, 10.19, 10.20, 10.21, 10.22, 10.23, 10.24, 10.25, 10.26, 10.27, 10.28, 10.29, 10.30, 10.31, 10.32, 10.33, 10.34, 10.35, 10.36, and 10.37)

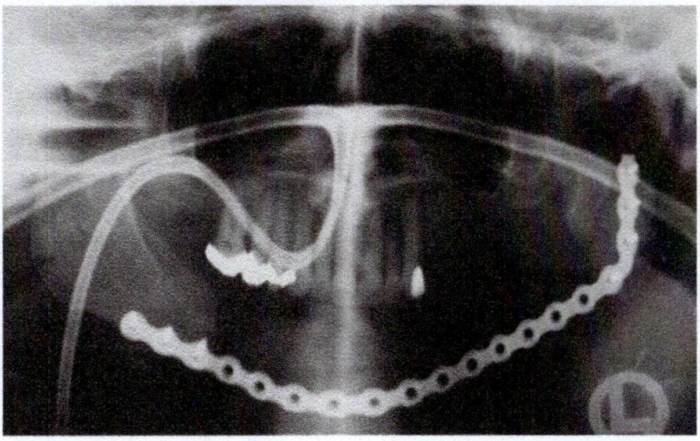

Fig. 10.2 Panoramic radiograph after extensive resection of the mandible from the left angle to the right molar region and stabilizing the mandible by means of osteosynthesis plate and screws

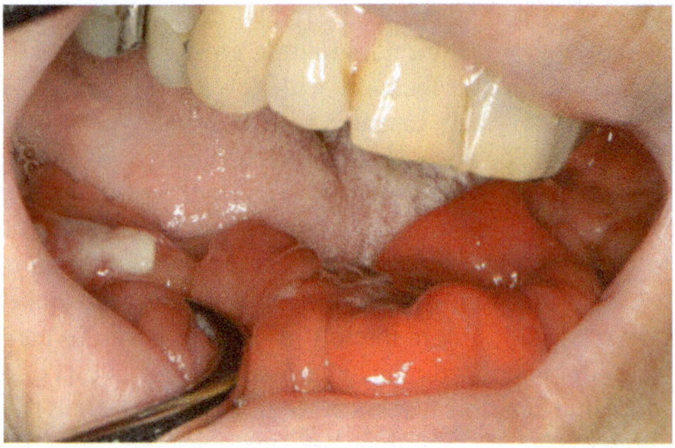

Fig. 10.3 Intraoral view postoperatively of the microvascular re-anastomosed jejunal free flap which was transplanted to cover the huge mucosa defect after tumour resection

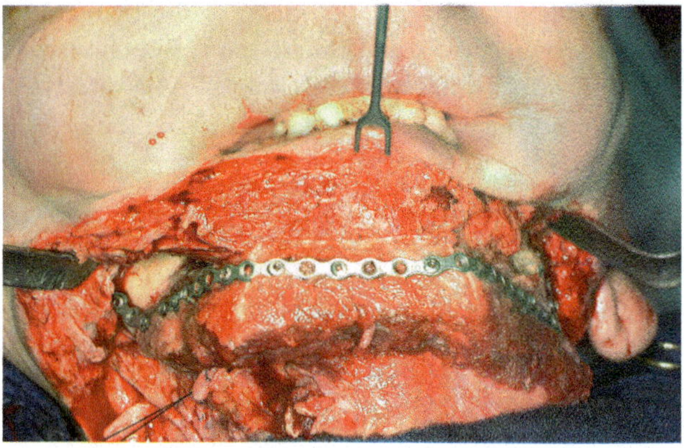

Fig. 10.4 Frontal clinical photograph after secondary reconstruction with microvascular re-anastomosed fibula free flap partially osteotomized to be precisely pressed under the osteosynthesis plate in between the mandibular stumps

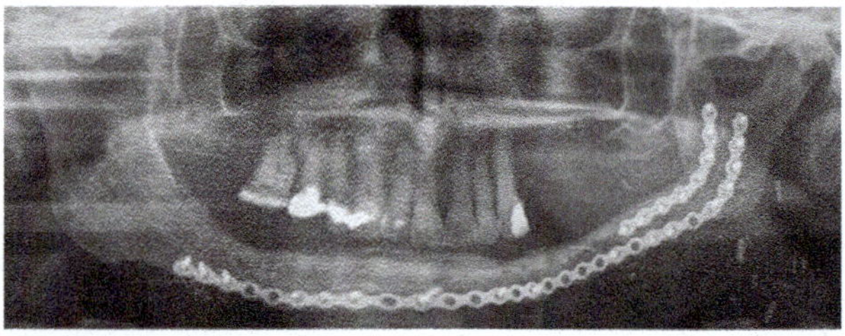

Fig. 10.5 Panoramic radiograph 3 years after primary reconstruction with jejunal graft and 6 month after secondary reconstruction with fibular transplant

irradiation, the tumour was resected; a selective neck dissection on the left side, stabilisation of the mandible by means of a stale osteosynthesis plate and a reconstruction with a microvascular re-anastomosed jejunum flap was performed (Figs. 10.2 and 10.3). As the patient did not show any signs of tumour recurrence 3 years later, the bony defect was finally reconstructed with a microvascular re-anastomosed fibula transplant (Figs. 10.4, 10.5, 10.6, 10.7, and 10.8). One year later, the patient received four 4.0 × 5.0 mm Bicon CP implants (Figs. 10.9, 10.10, 10.11, 10.12, 10.13, and 10.14). After 4 months, we uncovered the four Bicon implants and

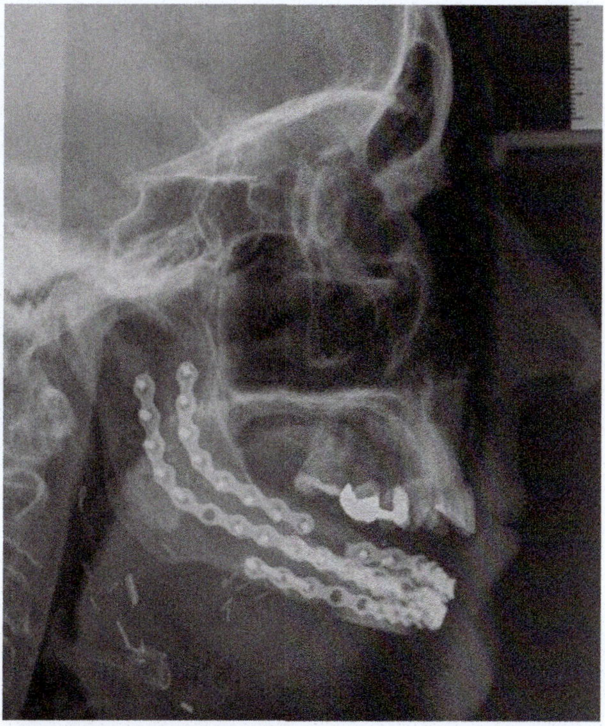

Fig. 10.6 Lateral cephalometric radiograph 3 years after primary reconstruction with jejunal graft and 6 month after secondary reconstruction with fibular transplant

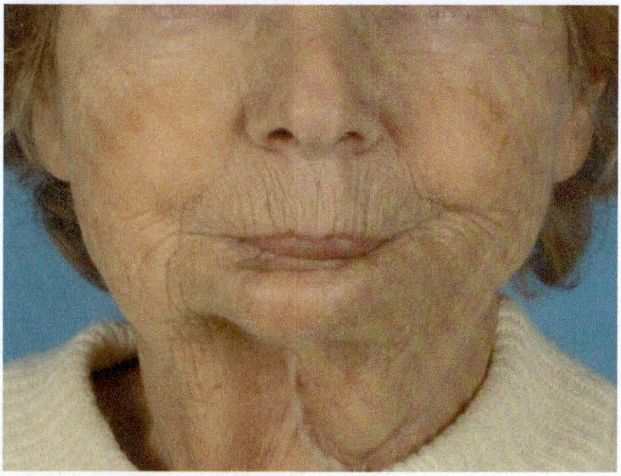

Fig. 10.7 Frontal view 3 years after primary reconstruction with jejunal graft and 6 month after secondary reconstruction with fibular transplant

took in the same session a full arch implant-level transfer impression (Figs. 10.15 and 10.16). After 10 days, we tested the TRINIA™ base, produced by the Perpetuini laboratory in Cisterna di Latina/Italy for their fit on the screw abutments (Fig. 10.17) and 10 days later we had a special wax try-in session (Fig. 10.18). Finally, 30 days later, the implants were loaded with a metal-free resin reinforced TRINIA™ full

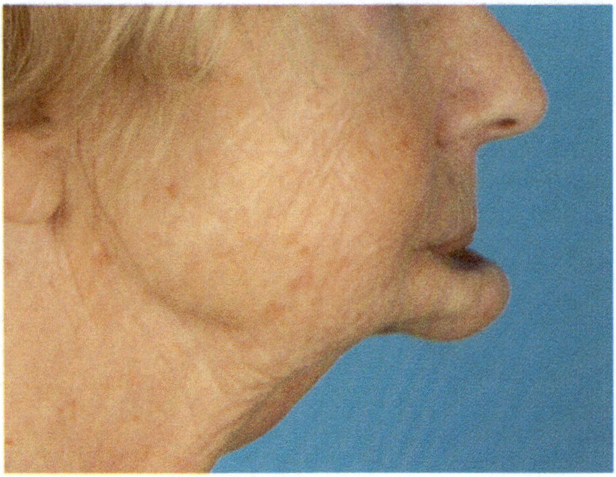

Fig. 10.8 Lateral view 3 years after primary reconstruction with jejunal graft and 6 month after secondary reconstruction with fibular transplant

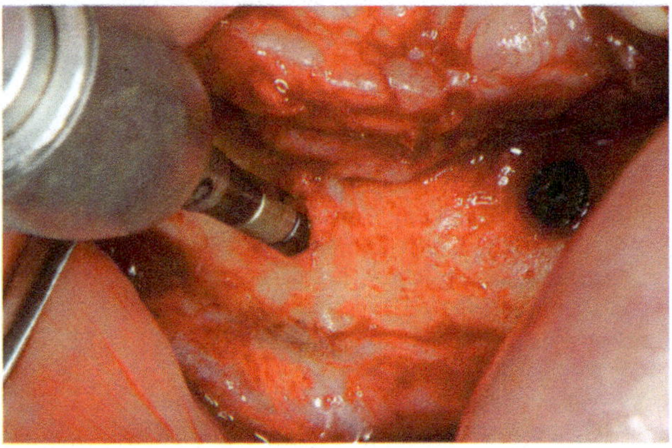

Fig. 10.9 Consecutive steps of implant placement 1 year after reconstruction with a microvascular re-anastomosed fibula transplant. Osteotomising the implant socket on the right side with a 2.5 mm latch reamer as second step after using the pilot drill

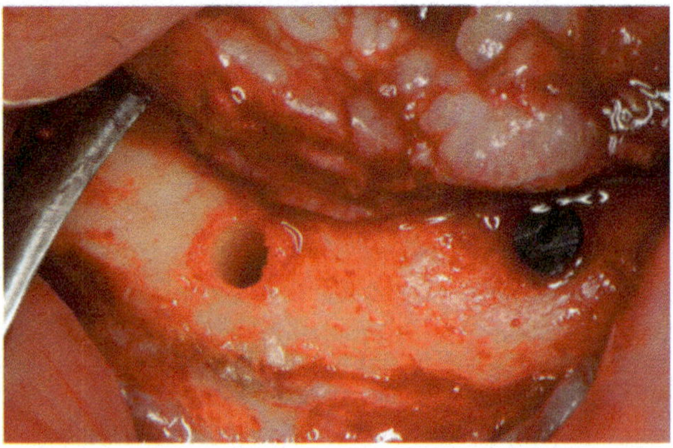

Fig. 10.10 Finalised 4 mm wide osteotomy on the right side

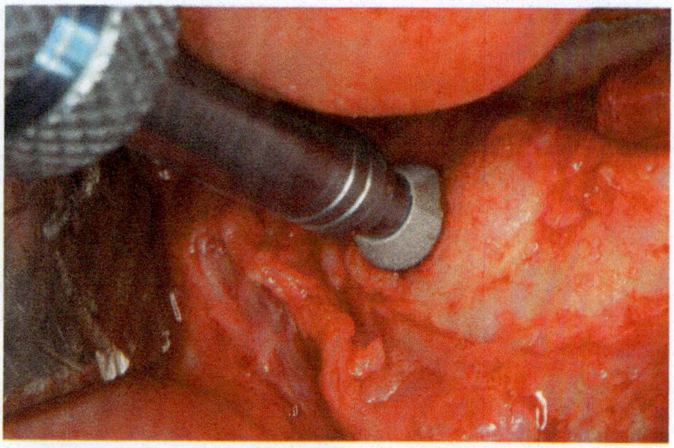

Fig. 10.11 Inserting the 4.0 × 5.0 mm Bicon implant

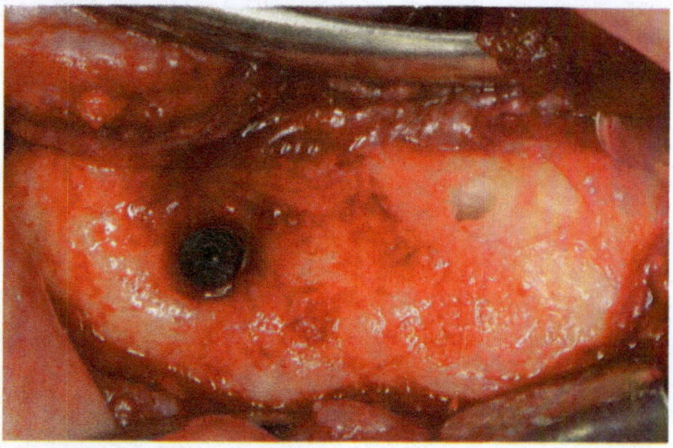

Fig. 10.12 After inserting the cut polyethylene healing plug into the 2.5 mm well of the Bicon implant

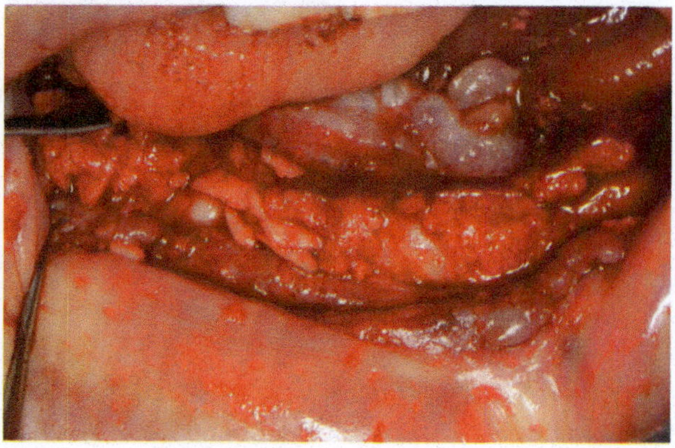

Fig. 10.13 After placing over the shoulders of the four 4.0 × 5.0 mm Bicon implants the harvested bone

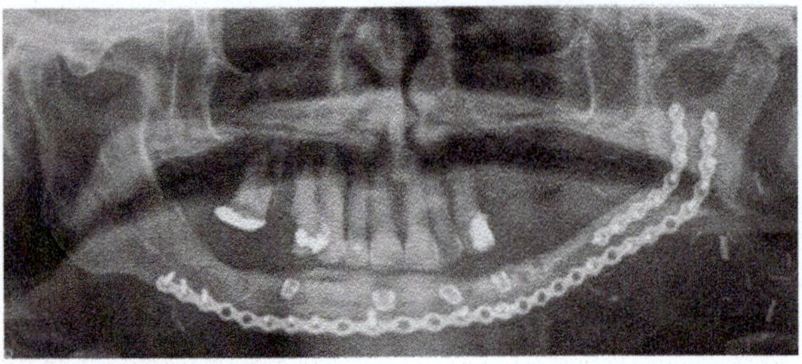

Fig. 10.14 Postoperative panoramic radiograph with four 4.0 × 5.0 mm Bicon implants in good position in the fibula transplanted neo mandible

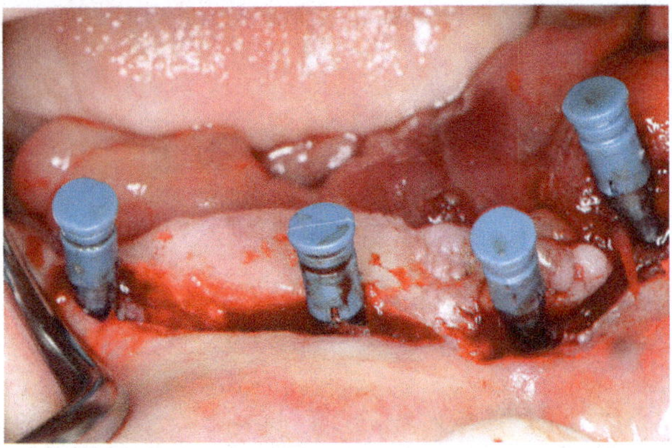

Fig. 10.15 After uncovering the Bicon implants 4 months later, inserting the blue 2.5 mm titanium impression posts with their corresponding blue acrylic sleeves for making of a full arch implant level impression

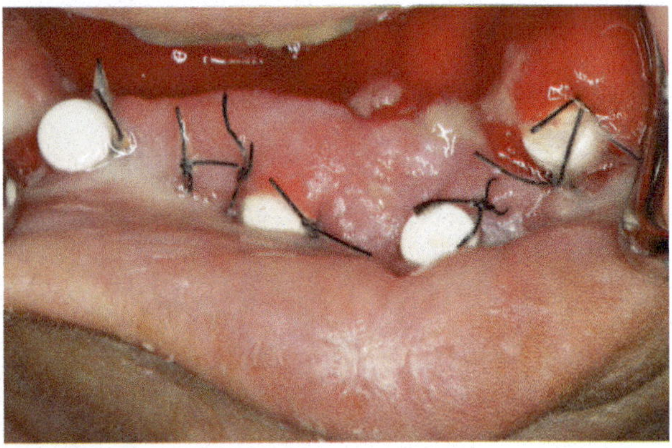

Fig. 10.16 View of the four white PEEK healing abutments seated in the wells of their implants after suturing

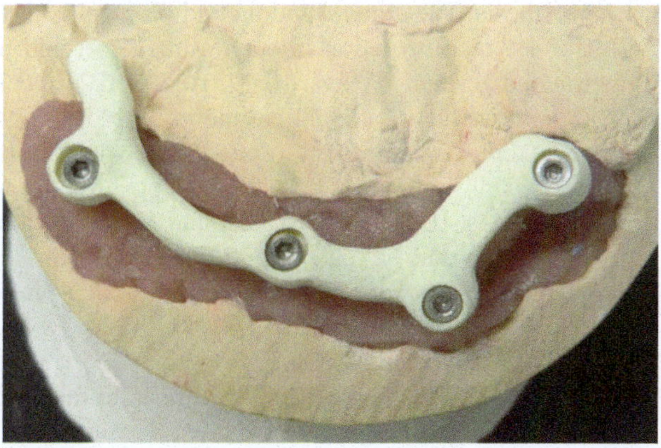

Fig. 10.17 Fiber-reinforced 3 D CAD/CAM milled TRINIA™ scaffold fixed on screw abutments in stone model

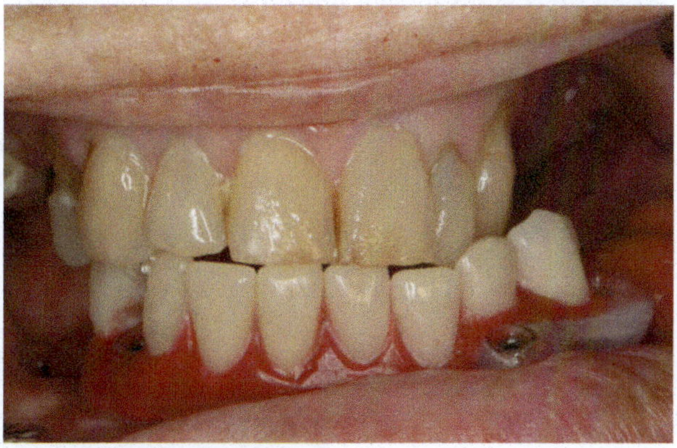

Fig. 10.18 Wax try-in with the TRINIA™ base and teeth fixed in wax to check the occlusion

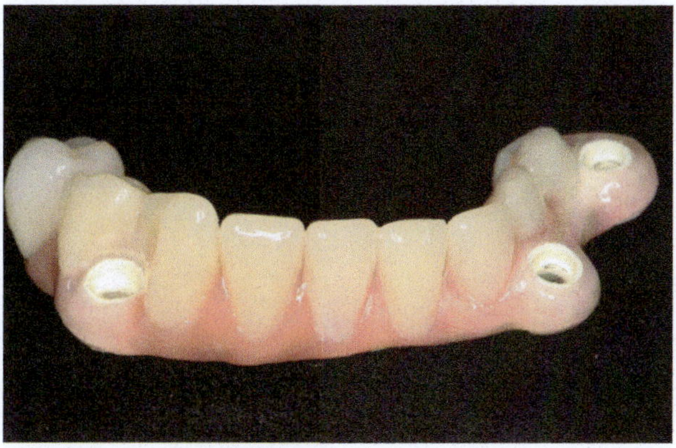

Fig. 10.19 Frontal view of the metal free resin reinforced TRINIA™ full arch prosthesis

arch prosthesis. The clinical and the radiological control showed a very satisfactory result of the reconstruction of such a huge soft and hard tissue defect with good function and aesthetics (Figs. 10.19, 10.20, 10.21, 10.22, 10.23, 10.24, and 10.25). The patient was very satisfied but the left middle implant bothered her closing the lip so we kept it sleeping and removed the socket for the screw in the TRINIA™ prosthesis. This implant was in this labial position due to the wide curve in the fibula transplant (Figs. 10.26, 10.27, 10.28, and 10.29). At the last follow-up (5 years after primary loading and 11 years after tumour resection), the CT scan did not show any tumour recurrence of lymphatic spread. Clinical photographs and radiograms are shown in Figs. 10.30, 10.31, 10.32, 10.33, 10.34, 10.35, and 10.36. Interesting is the comparison of the panoramic radiographs short after loading and 5 years later. According to Wolff's law [9] and the threshold theory of Frost [10], we recognise a bone level change and gain on the crest between the two-loaded left and the right Bicon implants (Fig. 10.37), as reported by Urdaneta et al. 2011 [11]. It is especially interesting as this is a microvascular re-anastomosed fibula transplant with a 4- to 5-mm-thick cortical bone structure.

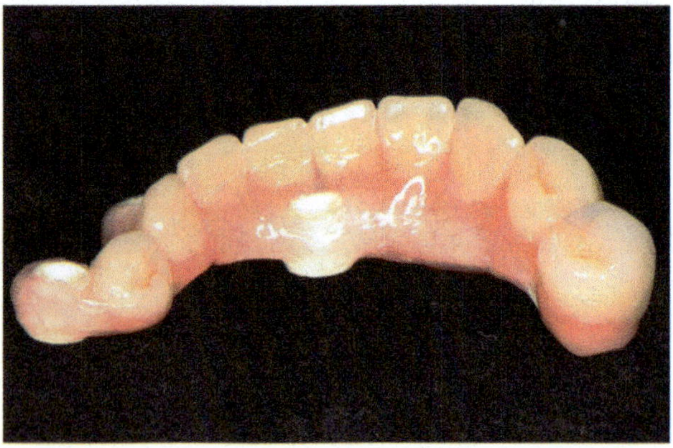

Fig. 10.20 Lingual view of the metal free resin reinforced TRINIA™ full arch prosthesis

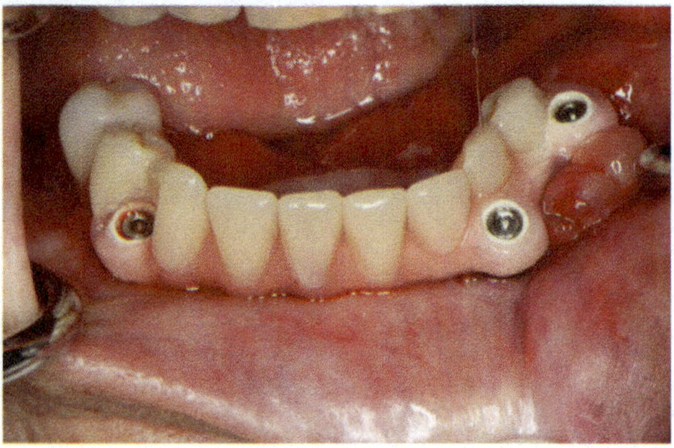

Fig. 10.21 Enoral view after loading

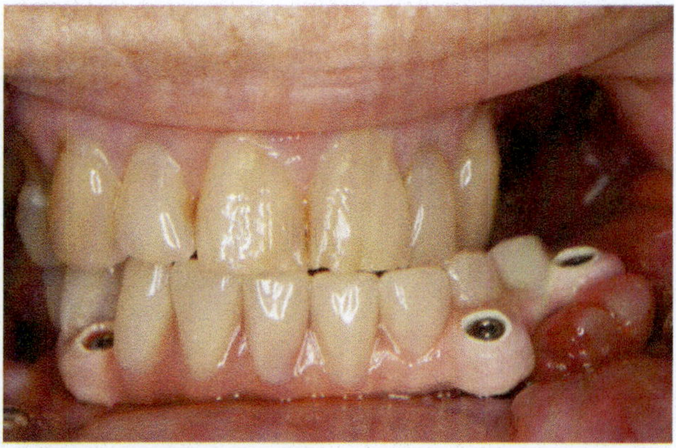

Fig. 10.22 Enoral view of the new lower prosthesis in cross bite occlusion with patients natural maxillary teeth

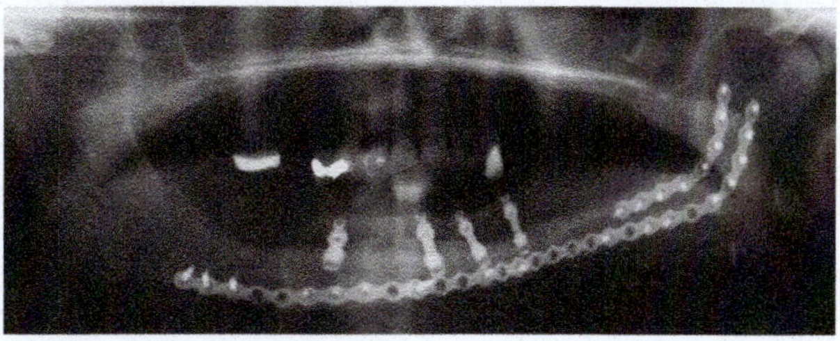

Fig. 10.23 Panoramic radiograph after starting to load

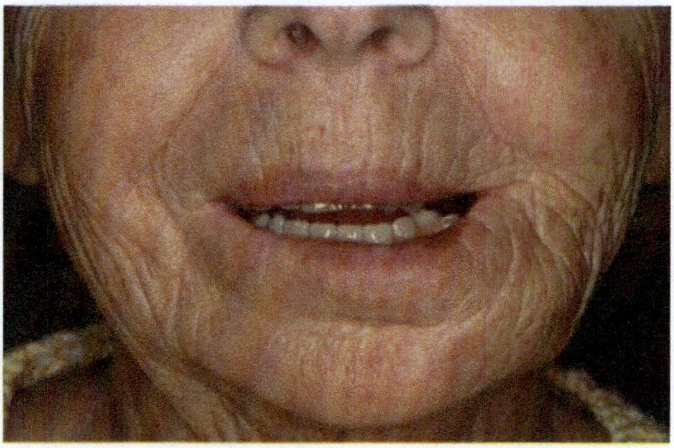

Fig. 10.24 Frontal view after incorporation of the mandibular prosthesis

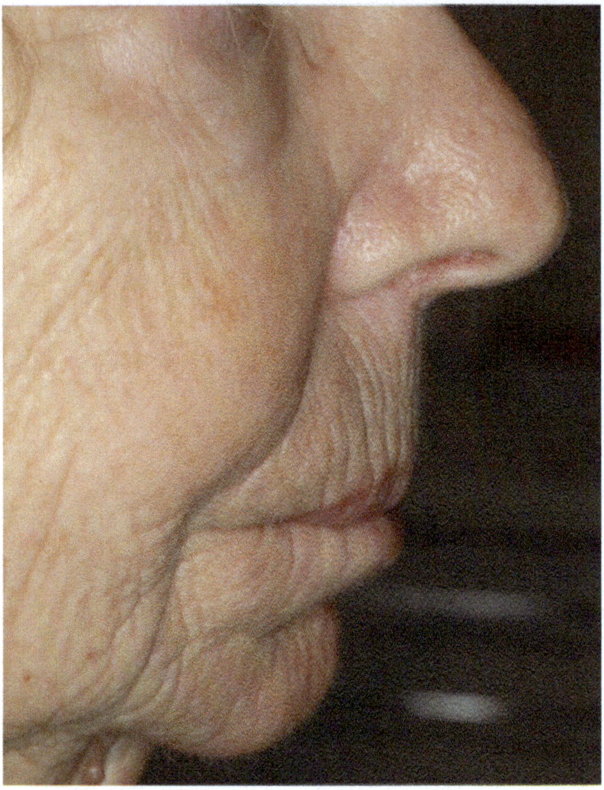

Fig. 10.25 Lateral view after incorporation of the mandibular prosthesis

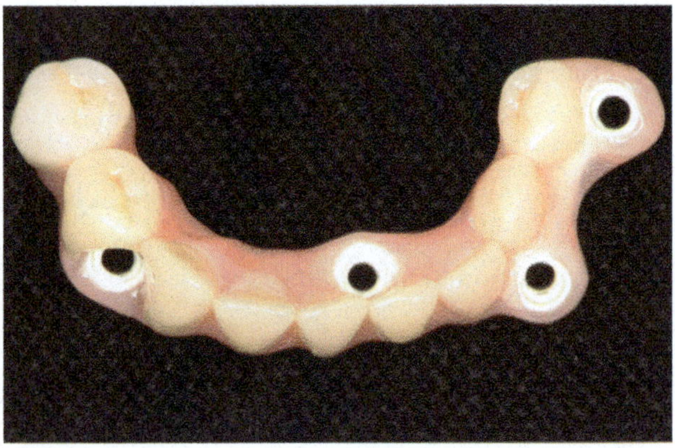

Fig. 10.26 Axial view of the TRINIA™ full arch prosthesis. The middle left implant is positioned far too lingual

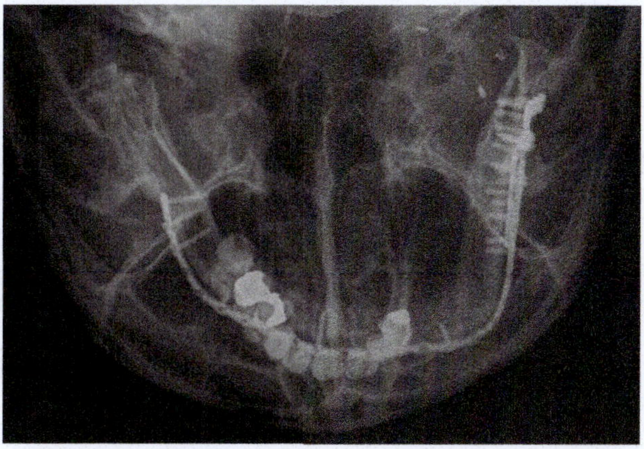

Fig. 10.27 The axial radiograph shows the incongruent arch of the reconstructed mandible

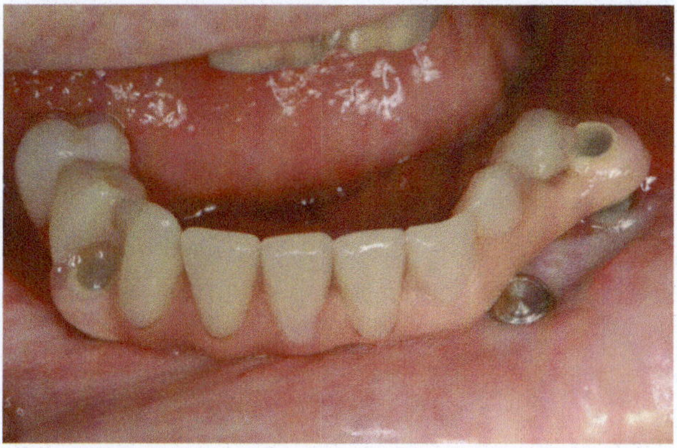

Fig. 10.28 Enoral view after putting the middle left implant to sleep and removing the abutment socket out of the TRINIA™ full arch prosthesis

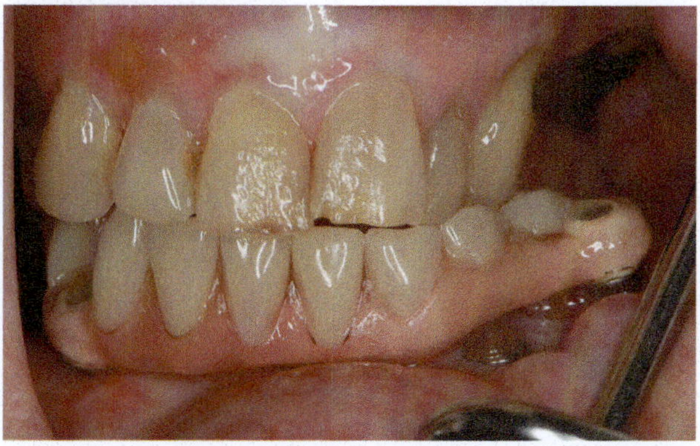

Fig. 10.29 Enoral view of the new lower prosthesis in cross bite occlusion with patients natural maxillary teeth after putting the middle left implant to sleep and removing the abutment socket

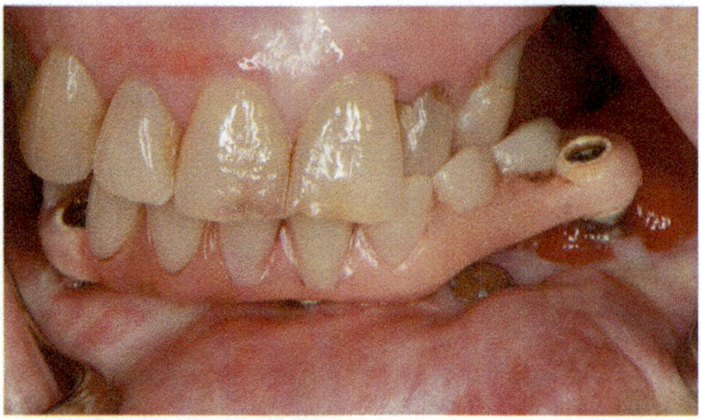

Fig. 10.30 Frontal view of mandibular prosthesis in occlusion 5 years after primary loading and 11 years after tumour resection

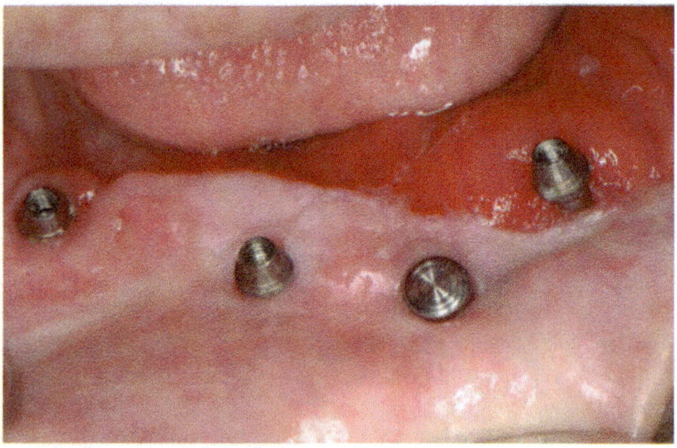

Fig. 10.31 Intraoral view of three screw abutments one gingiva former 5 years after primary loading and 11 years after tumour resection. Note the infect free mucosa also around the jejunal graft mucosa

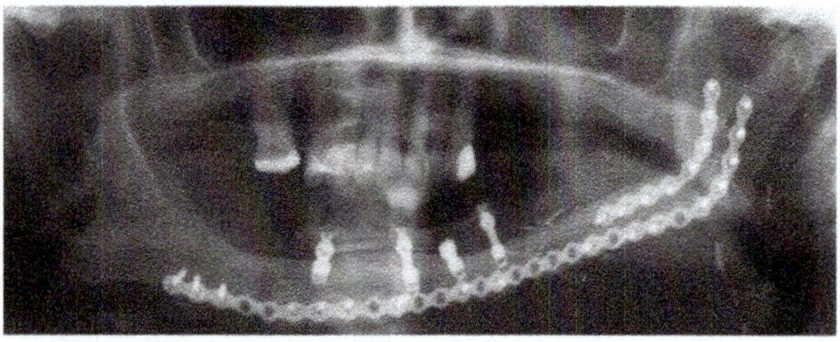

Fig. 10.32 Panoramic radiograph 5 years after primary loading and 11 years after tumour resection

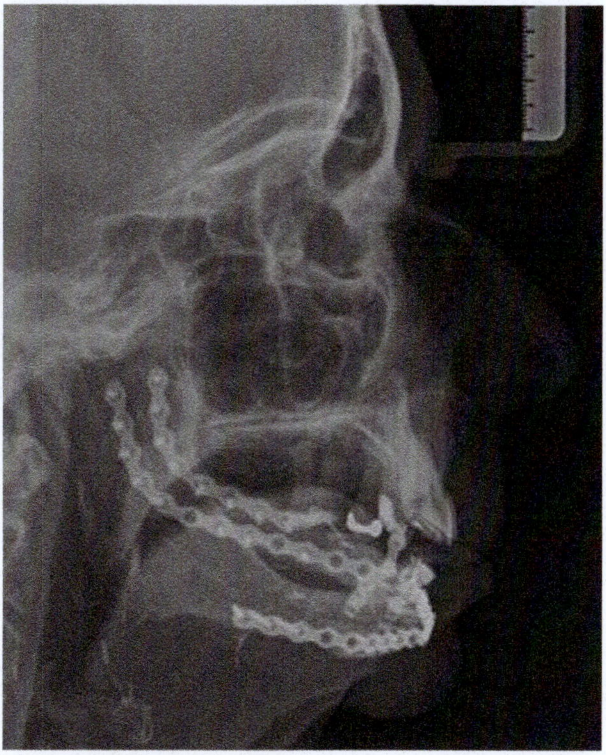

Fig. 10.33 Lateral cephalometric radiograph 5 years after primary loading and 11 years after tumour resection

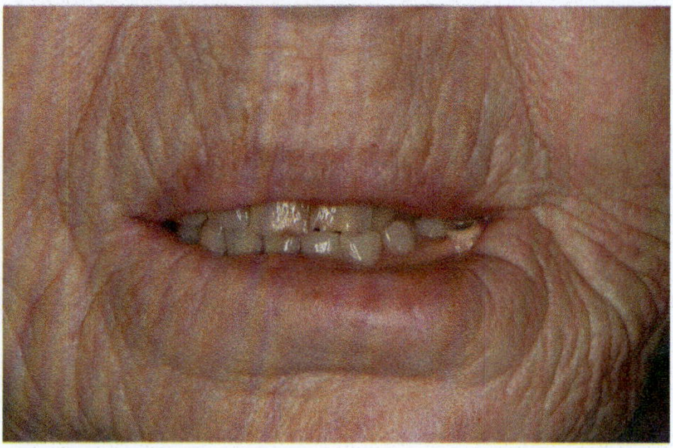

Fig. 10.34 Frontal view in occlusion 5 years after primary loading and 11 years after tumour resection

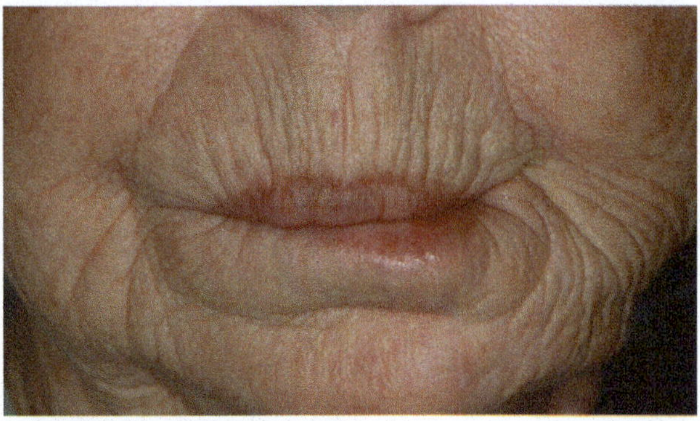

Fig. 10.35 Frontal view in occlusion with closed lips 5 years after primary loading and 11 years after tumour resection

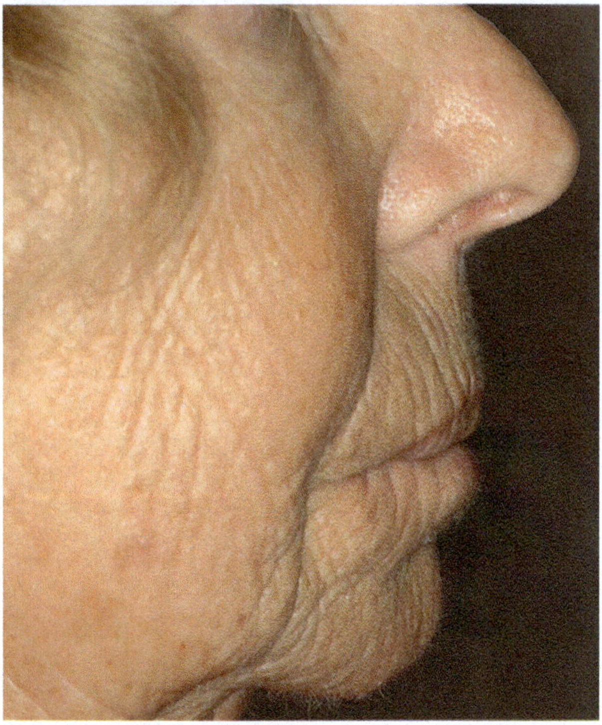

Fig. 10.36 Lateral view 5 years after primary loading and 11 years after tumour resection

10.4 Discussion

As described we do have with our multimodal therapy approach excellent results and are able to report about very long lasting good results with our free fibula flap reconstruction. Since more than 5 years by now we have reconstructed ten of these patients with four 4.0 × 5.0 mm Bicon implants and a TRINIA full arch prosthesis with very satisfactory stable results. In addition to these good results we could

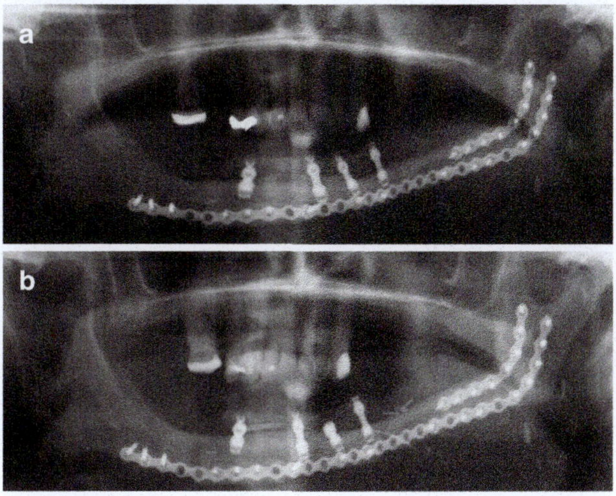

Fig. 10.37 Panoramic radiographs. Top: short after starting to load. Bottom: 5 years after loading. According to Wolff's law [9] and Frost's threshold theory [10] we recognize a bone level change and gain on the crest between the two-loaded left and the right Bicon implants as reported by Urdaneta et al. 2011 [11]

observe bone gain around the implant neck and a functional adaptation of the cortical bone between and around the implants as described by Wolff [9]. Finally, we found a solution to reconstruct also our tumour patients in the full scope of Oral & Maxillofacial Surgery and Dentistry of today.

References

1. Bosetti C, Gallus S, Peto R, Negri E, Talamini R, Tavani A, et al. Tobacco smoking, smoking cessation, and cumulative risk of upper aerodigestive tract cancers. Am J Epidemiol. 2008;167(4):468–73.
2. Braakhuis B, Rietbergen M, Buijze M, Snijders P, Bloemena E, Brakenhoff R, et al. TP53 mutation and human papilloma virus status of oral squamous cell carcinomas in young adult patients. Oral Dis. 2014;20(6):602–8.
3. Lin C-W, Hsieh Y-S, Hsin C-H, Su C-W, Lin C-H, Wei L-H, et al. Effects of NFKB1 and NFKBIA gene polymorphisms on susceptibility to environmental factors and the clinicopathologic development of oral cancer. PLoS One. 2012;7(4):e35078.
4. Kreppel M, Eich H-T, Brüggenolte C, Dreiseidler T, Rothamel D, Drebber U, et al. Preoperative vs. postoperative radiochemotherapy in patients with N2 squamous cell carcinoma of the oral cavity. Oral Oncol. 2012;48(10):1019–24.
5. Lutz BS, Wei F-C. Microsurgical workhorse flaps in head and neck reconstruction. Clin Plast Surg. 2005;32(3):421.. -30–vii
6. Nooh N. Dental implant survival in irradiated oral cancer patients: a systematic review of the literature. Int J Oral Maxillofac Implants. 2013;28(5):1233–42.
7. Parbo N, Murra NT, Andersen K, Buhl J, Kiil B, Nørholt SE. Outcome of partial mandibular reconstruction with fibula grafts and implant-supported prostheses. Int J Oral Maxillofac Surg. 2013;42(11):1403–8.
8. Teoh KH, Huryn JM, Patel S, Halpern J, Tunick S, Wong HB, et al. Implant prosthodontic rehabilitation of fibula free-flap reconstructed mandibles: a Memorial Sloan-Kettering Cancer Center review of prognostic factors and implant outcomes. Int J Oral Maxillofac Implants. 2005;20(5):738–46.

9. Wolff J. Das Gesetz der Transformation der Knochen. Berlin: Verlag von August Hirschwald, 1892.
10. Frost HM. Wolff's law and bone's structural adaptations to mechanical usage: an overview for clinicians. Angle Orthod. 1994;64(3):175–88.
11. Urdaneta RA, Daher S, Leary J, Kimberly E, Chuang SK. Factors associated with crestal bone gain on single-tooth locking taper implants: the effect of nonsteroidal anti-inflammatory drugs. Int J Oral Maxillofac Implants. 2011;26:1063–78.

Minimally Invasive Sinus Lift Using Short Implants

11

Mauro Marincola, Rolf Ewers, and Boyd J. Tomasetti

Content

References.. 175

The premature loss of maxillary molars usually leads to pronounced atrophy of the posterior maxillary alveolar ridge and pneumatization of the maxillary sinus [1]. The original sinus lift was performed via a lateral approach by Tatum in 1974—no graft material was used. Tatum presented his findings in 1976 at the Alabama Implant Congress [2]. In 1980, Boyne and James published about sinus grafting using autogenous bone, again using a lateral approach [3]. The lateral approach maxillary sinus lift soon become the standard and the graft materials used began to shift away from autogenous bone [4, 5] (Fig. 11.1).

In 2005, Ewers published one of the seminal papers describing the long-term success of the lateral approach to sinus grafting [6]. Prior to this, the American Association of Oral and Maxillofacial Surgeons and the Academy of Osseointegration

M. Marincola
University of Cartagena, School of Dentistry, Bolívar, Colombia

R. Ewers (✉)
CMF Institute Vienna, Vienna, Austria
e-mail: rolf@cmf-vienna.com

B. J. Tomasetti
Department of Oral and Maxillofacial Surgery, Denver Health and Hospitals, Denver, CO, USA

Tomasetti and McLain Oral and Maxillofacial Surgery, Littleton, CO, USA

B. J. Tomasetti, R. Ewers (eds.), *Short Implants*,
https://doi.org/10.1007/978-3-030-44199-9_11

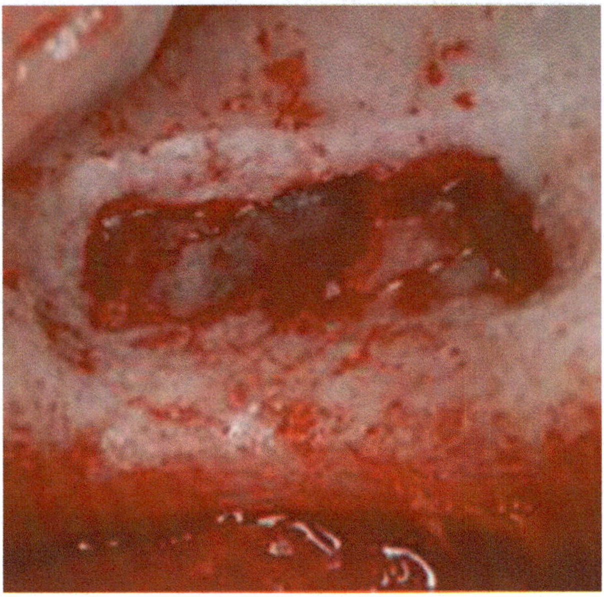

Fig. 11.1 Lateral sinus lift

had held Consensus Conferences on Sinus grafting and published their results. Both organizations concluded that the lateral approach to maxillary sinus grafting with an appropriate graft material was successful in restoring the severely atrophic maxilla [7–9].

As surgeons became more comfortable with sinus augmentation procedures, they began to look for ways to perform less-invasive procedures. One such method was to eliminate the lateral approach and its "sinus window" in favor of performing the lift procedure and subsequent grafting by going through the implant crestal osteotomy. This indirect sinus lift procedure using the crestal approach was initially described by Summers in 1994 [10, 11]. The indirect sinus lift proved to be both less invasive and less time consuming. This resulted in less patient discomfort and minimal complications. As more experience has been gained, the methods used have become more minimally invasive [12, 13].

In order to address clinical-related sinus pneumatization issues, two main surgical approaches have been suggested—internal and lateral sinus lift techniques. The minimally invasive internal sinus lift approach is indicated whenever there is residual bone height of 3–7 mm. The procedure involves using an osteotome inserted through the implant osteotomy site to perform a comminuted fracture of the very thin cortical bone of the sinus floor (Fig. 11.2).

Implant placements into grafted sinuses were historically done with traditional length implants—over 10 mm in length. The thought process was "the longer, the better." This was certainly the case with the lateral sinus approach. In many cases, restorative dentists found it necessary to splint the restorations together. Even with a minimal crestal sinus lift, the traditional length implant was deemed to be necessary. One of the concerns with any sinus lift procedure has always been sinus membrane perforation. When using the lateral approach, the membrane is easily

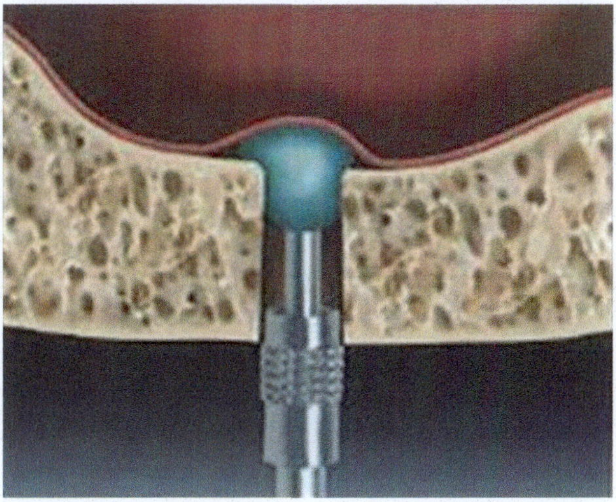

Fig. 11.2 Minimal sinus lift using an osteotome

visualized and any perforations can be repaired. With the crestal approach, visualization is almost nonexistent and perforations can be frequent [14]. The crestal approach, compared to the lateral approach, has a lower amount of vertical gain.

The short implant presents a unique opportunity to combine a minimally invasive crestal approach sinus lift with an implant that can be accommodated within the limited amount of vertical gain. The use of short implants is recognized as a standard of care for treatment in the atrophied posterior maxilla. Recent papers have shown that short implants can also be used in combination with a minimally invasive crestal sinus lift [15].

Marincola et al. [16] described a classification which determined the type of sinus graft based upon the residual bone height. At this time the implants being used were all traditional length—usually 10 mm or longer. Their classification based on Cawood and Howell's original work [17] was (Fig. 11.3):

- Less than 1 mm of residual bone height—A horizontal horseshoe Le Fort I osteotomy with an interpositional iliac crest bone graft.
- 1–5 mm of residual bone height—Staged procedures with lateral approach sinus lift and graft followed by implant placement approximately 6 months later.
- 5–8 mm of residual bone height—Lateral approach sinus lift with simultaneous implant placement.
- 8 mm or more of residual bone height—A sinus floor intrusion through the implant osteotomy along with simultaneous implant placement.

When short and ultrashort implants are used the indications change dramatically:

- Less than 1 mm of residual bone height—A horizontal horseshoe Le Fort I osteotomy with an interpositional iliac crest bone graft. One can also consider a lateral sinus lift and graft or a crestal sinus lift/graft.

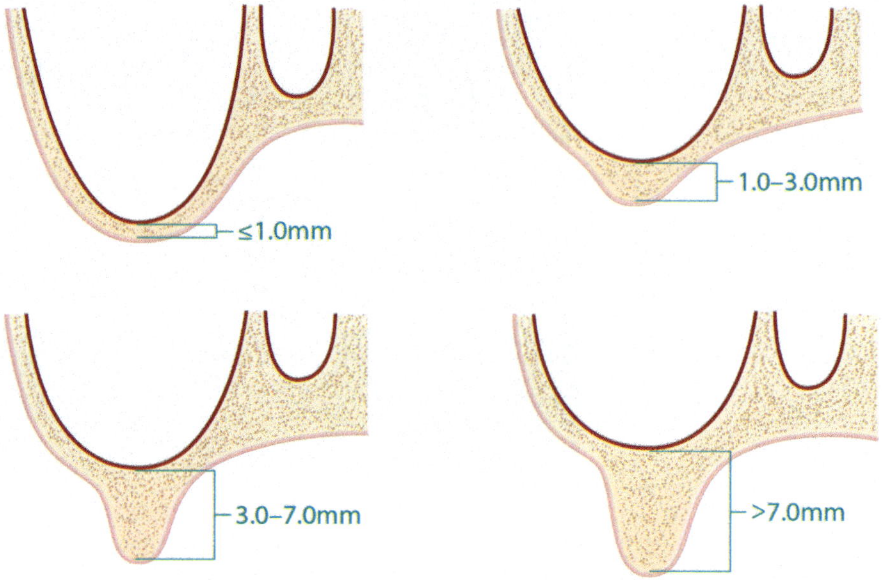

Fig. 11.3 Procedures are dictated by alveolar crest height or residual bone height—the **RBH**

- Less than 3 mm of residual bone height—Either a lateral sinus lift/graft or a crestal lift/graft.
- 3–7 mm of residual bone height—A sinus floor intrusion through the implant osteotomy with immediate placement of a short or ultrashort implant.
- 7 mm or more of residual bone height—A normal implant placement using short or ultrashort implants.

As mentioned earlier, Summers introduced the internal sinus lift (ISL) in 1994. Osteotomes are used to lift the sinus floor by going through the implant osteotomy. An additional approach is via a crestal sinus lift in which an osteotomy is made on the ridge crest and the bone is tapped upwards using osteotomes—graft material is then placed and covered with a membrane. The ISL technique has been shown to be less invasive, takes less time, and has less postoperative discomfort than a lateral approach.

The ISL is indicated when there is a residual bone height of 3–7 mm and short and ultrashort implants will be used. There has been increasing debate as to whether or not a graft needs to be done at the time of sinus lift. Of interest is that Tatum's original work was done without any graft material being used. Summer's original work recommended using autogenous, allogenic, or xenogenic graft materials. Recently Nedir et al. [18] showed no difference between ISL procedures performed with or without graft material being placed. Rammelsberg et al. [19] did a retrospective study of 66 patients who had an ISL without graft material and implants placed.

They noted some small bone gain and subsequently stated that implants done with an ISL without graft material would have bone gain.

While there is still no consensus on whether to use or not use graft material in performing an ISL, it is our opinion that using graft material is the better option. This is particularly so when using short and ultrashort implants because of the benefits observed with respect to maintaining a good bone level around the implant. Maintenance of crestal bone is the most critical issue for long-term implant survival [20]. This is achieved by placing the implant subcrestal. The bone level is further maintained by the sloping implant shoulder and allowing platform switching.

Platform switching allows an increase in residual crestal bone around the implant neck [21]. It also results in a papilla that is repositioned to a more esthetic level and reduces the mechanical stress in the crestal bone area. The reduction of mechanical stress also enhances the vascular supply to both hard and soft tissue. These qualities become more important with short and ultrashort implants particularly when placed in sites in conjunction with an ISL.

The figures below demonstrate a minimally invasive sinus lift procedure using a 4.5 × 6 mm Bicon implant. The patient is a 58-year-old healthy ASA I female missing teeth in her posterior maxilla. Radiographs showed 4 mm of residual alveolar bone height (Figs. 11.4 and 11.5).

Figure 11.6 shows the complete edentulous area of the bicuspids and first molar. Surgery is performed through a crestal incision and initially blood is collected for use with the graft material (Fig. 11.7). The implant osteotomy is performed after first using a pilot drill to perforate the cortical bone (Fig. 11.8).

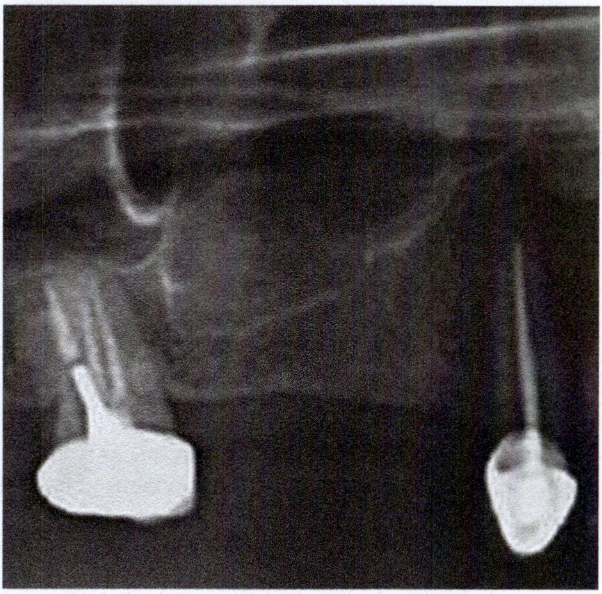

Fig. 11.4 Pre-op radiograph

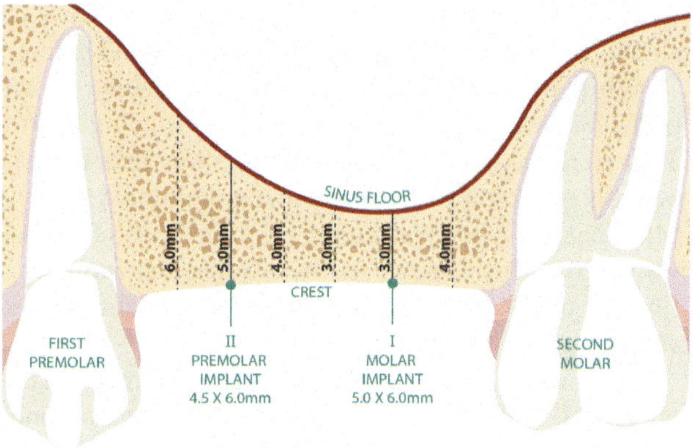

Fig. 11.5 Schematic showing RBH

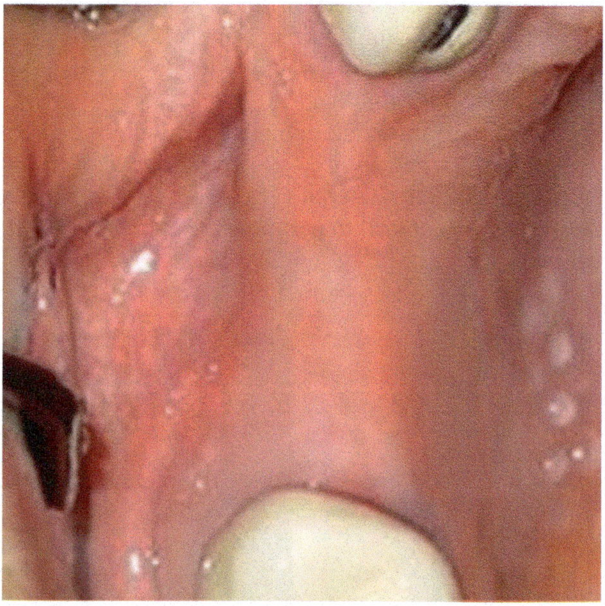

Fig. 11.6 Pre-op view

Once the pilot drilling has been completed, the osteotomy is widened using a series of latch reamers **without** irrigation. This allows the surgeon to collect bone from the osteotomy site. This bone will be used in combination with the previously collected blood and graft material for insertion into the graft site—the ISL. It is recommended that a radiograph of the site be taken with the 2.5 mm latch reamer in place in order to determine the final drilling length (Fig. 11.9).

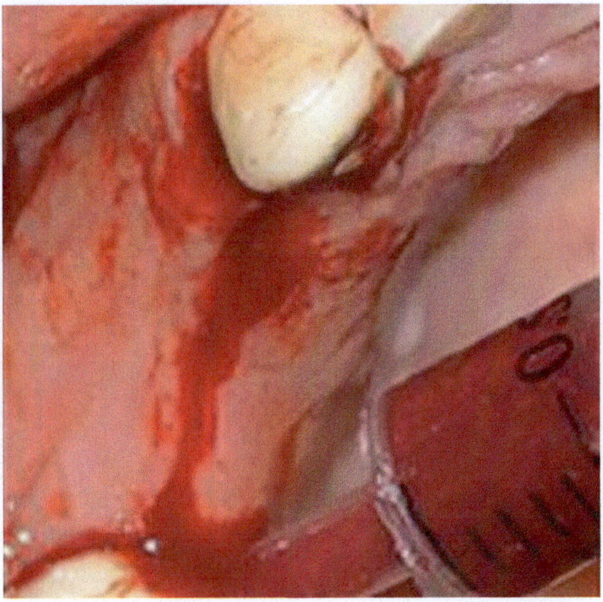

Fig. 11.7 Crestal incision and collecting blood for use with the graft material

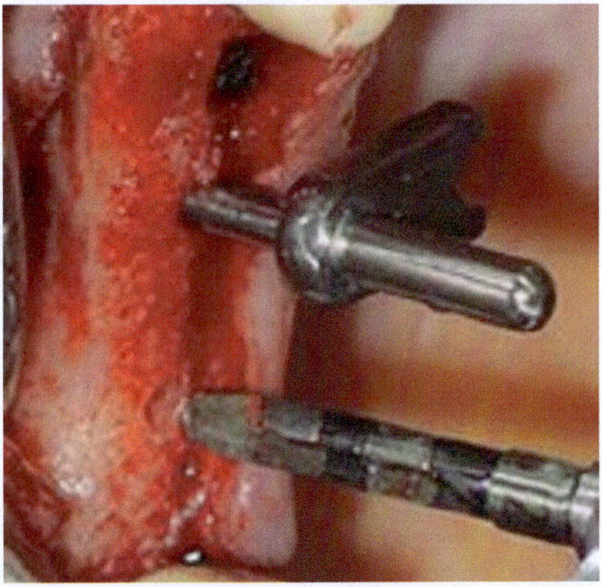

Fig. 11.8 The pilot osteotomy is made 1–2 mm less than the residual bone height

The osteotomy is gradually widened to the desired size using 0.5 mm increasing latch reamers and hand reamers.

When the desired diameter is reached, a hand reamer is used to perform a comminuted fracture of the cortical bone of the sinus floor. In this case a 3.5 mm reamer that has a single vertical cutting edge and a knife edge at its apex is used. Using a

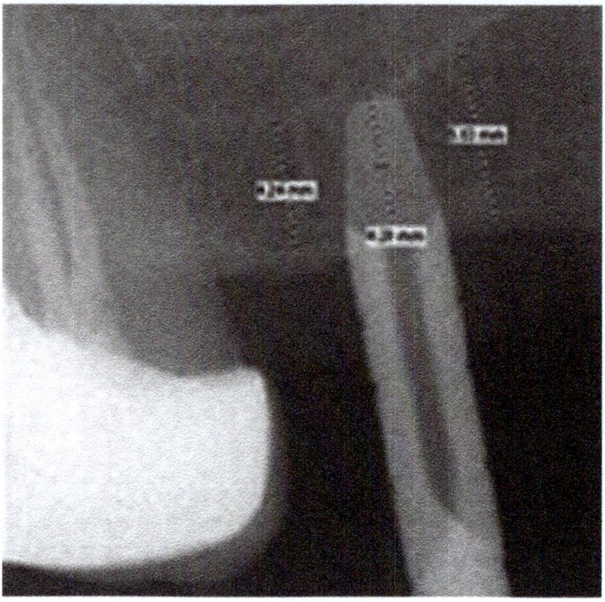

Fig. 11.9 Radiograph showing reamer but just short of sinus floor

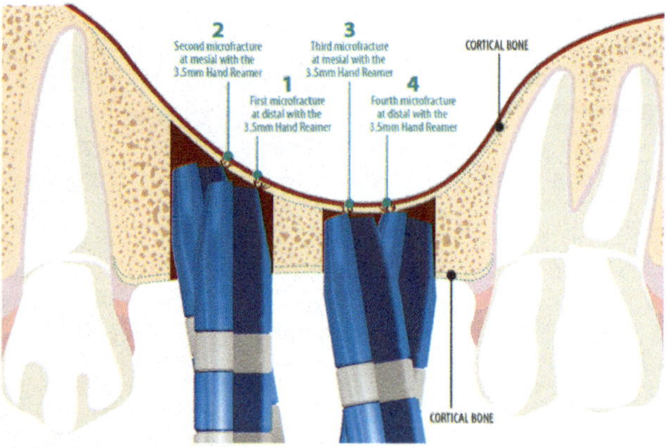

Fig. 11.10 Schematic showing microfracture points along sinus floor

reamer with a smaller diameter than the osteotomy site allows the sharp tip of the reamer to be placed at four different points at the apex of the site (Fig. 11.10).

The reamer is gently tapped to fracture the thin cortical layer of the sinus floor at the distal aspect of the osteotomy site and then the buccal and mesial areas followed by the palatal area. The second and fourth fracture points are always the buccal and palatal because of the higher sinus pneumatization in these areas (Fig. 11.11a, b).

The sinus floor fracture is completed using an osteotome slightly smaller in size than the implant being placed—in this case a 4.5 mm implant. The synthetic graft

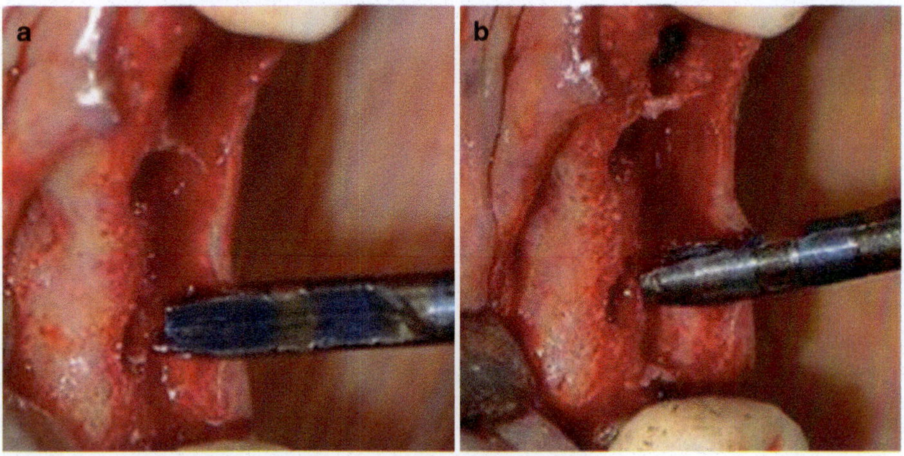

Fig. 11.11 (**a**, **b**) Microfracture of sinus floor being done with 3.5 mm reamer

material is mixed with the previously collected blood and bone harvested from the osteotomy site into a putty like consistency. A 4.0 mm bone graft syringe is used to place the graft material into the apical portion of the osteotomy. The 3.5 mm osteotome is then gently tapped pushing the material against the fractured sinus floor and Schneiderian membrane thus elevating the sinus floor (Figs. 11.12, 11.13, 11.14, and 11.15).

A 4.5 × 6 mm Bicon short implant is then inserted into the osteotomy site and then gently tapped into place until it is approximately 2 mm subcrestal (Fig. 11.16a, b).

A healing plug is then placed into the implant and the subcrestal positioned implant is covered with the remaining graft material. The mucosa is sutured and an immediate post-insertion radiograph is taken (Fig. 11.17). This radiograph shows the sinus lift with the graft material positioned at the apical portion of the implant. Compare this film with the one taken 4½ years later (Fig. 11.18).

A 5-year follow-up of a Crestal Sinus Lift shows the bone transformation and remodeling according to Wolff's Law [22]. The bone transforms from resorbable TCP augmentation material into well mineralized bone. The following radiographs shows bone transformation and crestal bone **gain** around a short Bicon implant placed following an ISL (Figs. 11.19, 11.20, 11.21, and 11.22).

The ISL has been shown to be an effective surgical technique when used in conjunction with a short or ultrashort implant. Like any sinus procedure, the ISL is not without potential complications. The most prevalent is sinus membrane perforation. Other complications include hemorrhage, infection, and chronic sinusitis. The method described has resulted in minimizing potential complications by first microfracturing the thin cortical bone of the sinus floor and then using the graft material to gently lift the floor.

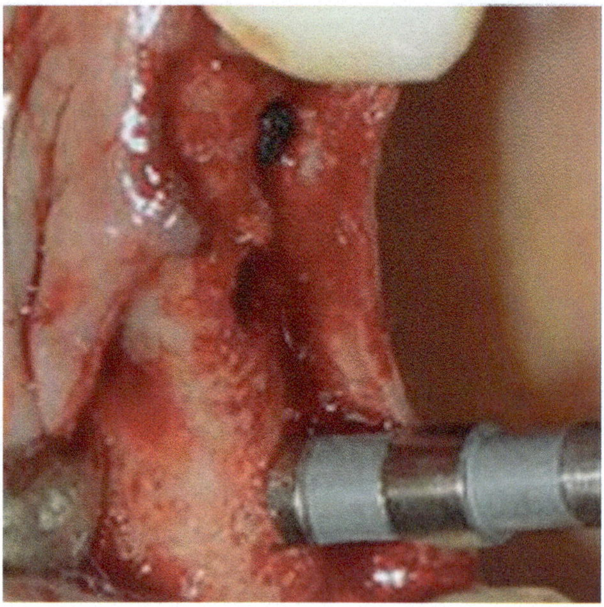

Fig. 11.12 Fracture of the sinus floor completed using a 4.0 mm osteotome

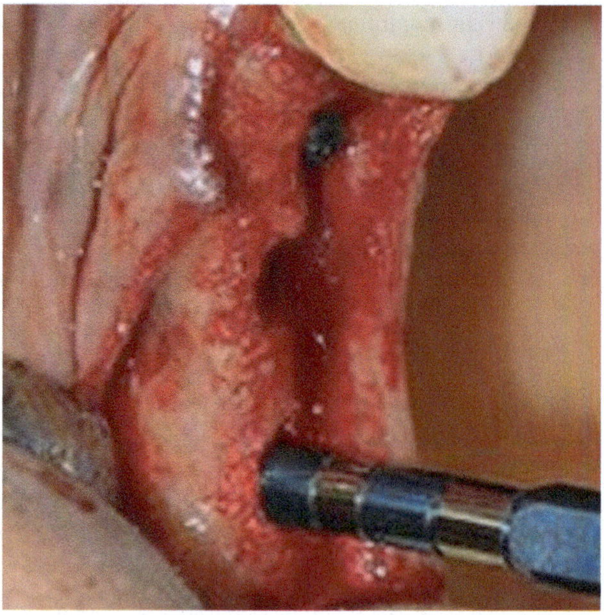

Fig. 11.13 Graft material being inserted using osteotome

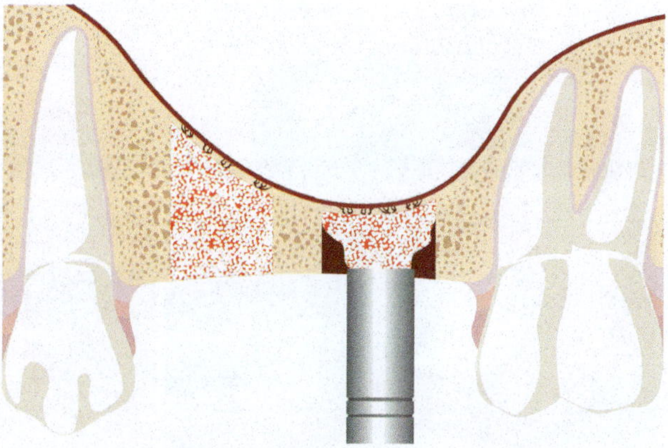

Fig. 11.14 Schematic of graft material on end of osteotome

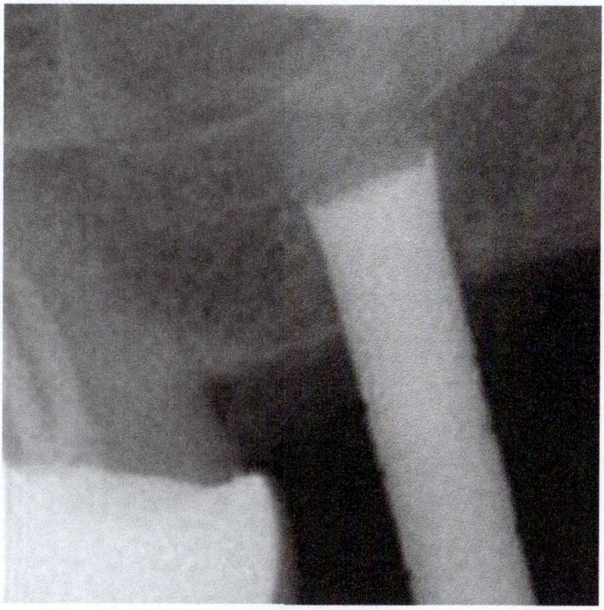

Fig. 11.15 Radiograph showing graft material at end of osteotome

The use of short and ultrashort implants in conjunction with the ISL reduces the need for an extensive osteotomy via a lateral approach. While the short and ultrashort implants can be used with the conventional lateral approach, they are more attuned to the minimally invasive ISL. The procedure is less traumatic and the patient has less swelling and less pain. In many cases, the procedure is also less costly to the patient.

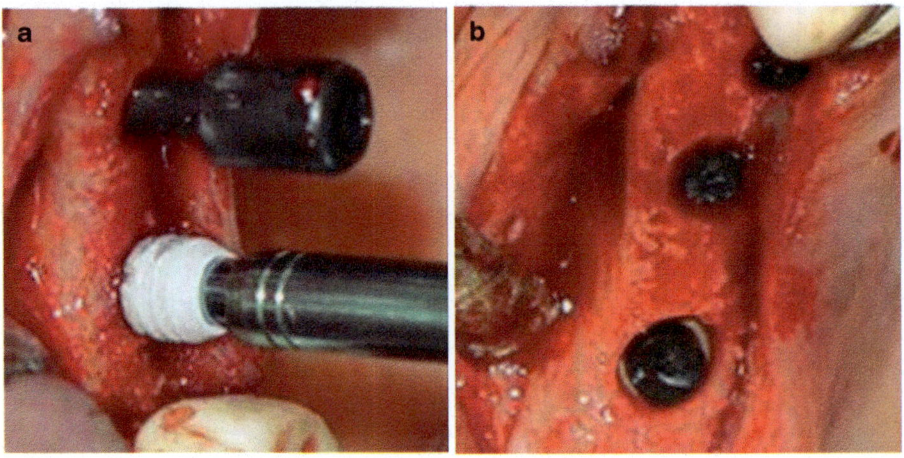

Fig. 11.16 (**a**, **b**) Short implant being placed approximately 2 mm beneath the alveolar crest

Fig. 11.17 Immediate post-surgery radiograph

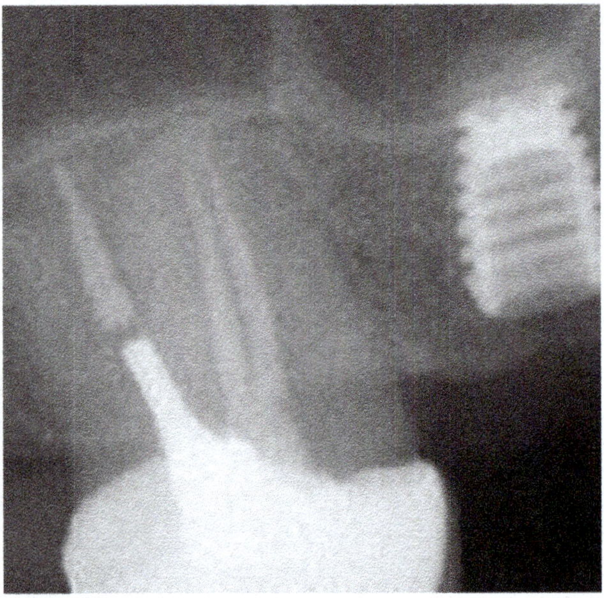

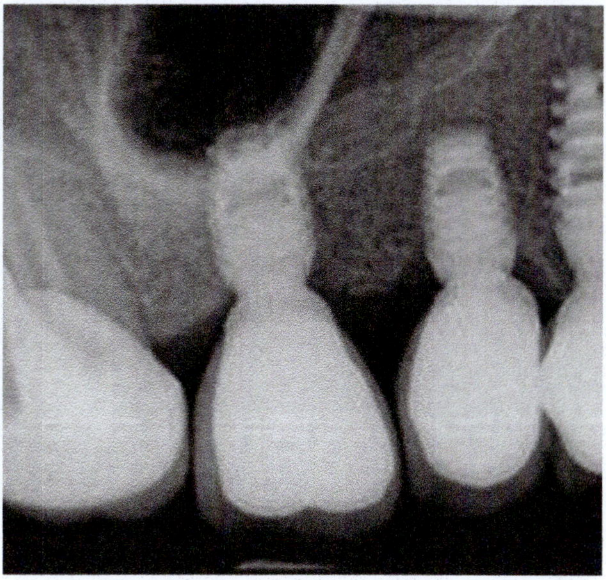

Fig. 11.18 Four and a half years later

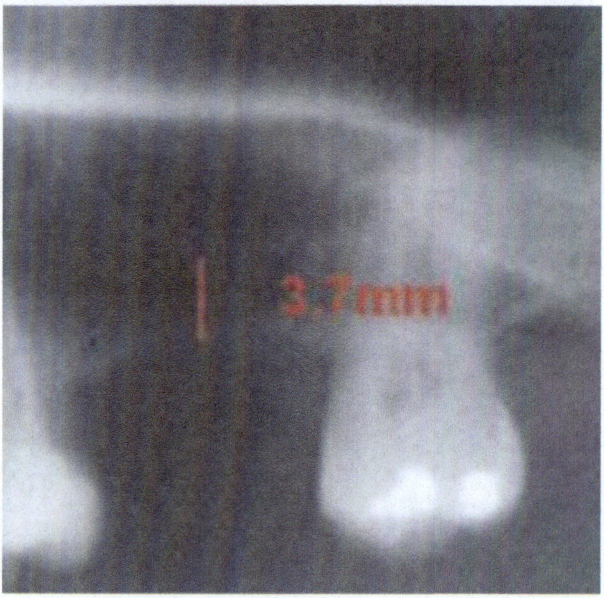

Fig. 11.19 Pre-operative radiograph showing residual bone height of 3.7 mm

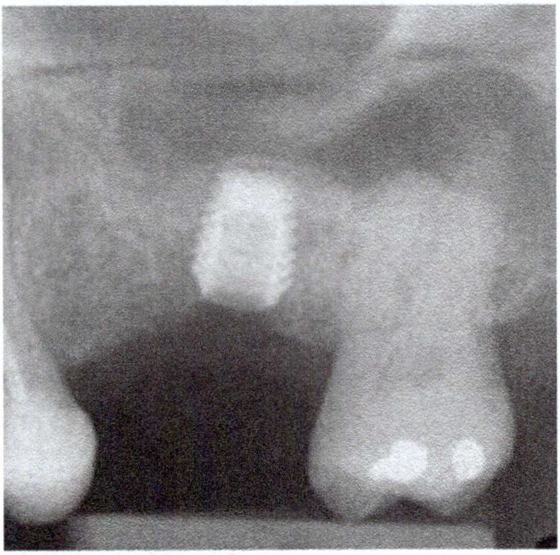

Fig. 11.20 Immediate post-insertion of a 4.0 × 5 mm Bicon implant with an ISL. Note that the implant was placed subcrestal

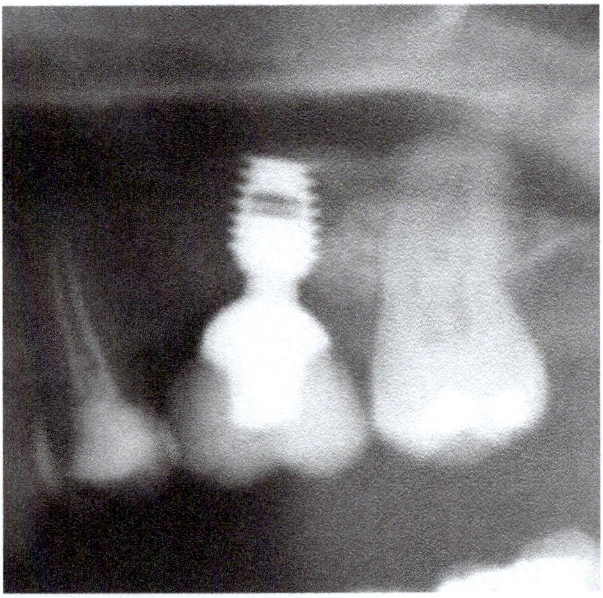

Fig. 11.21 Radiograph taken 1-year post restoration. Note the small cavity on the distal of the implant which has new mineralized bone

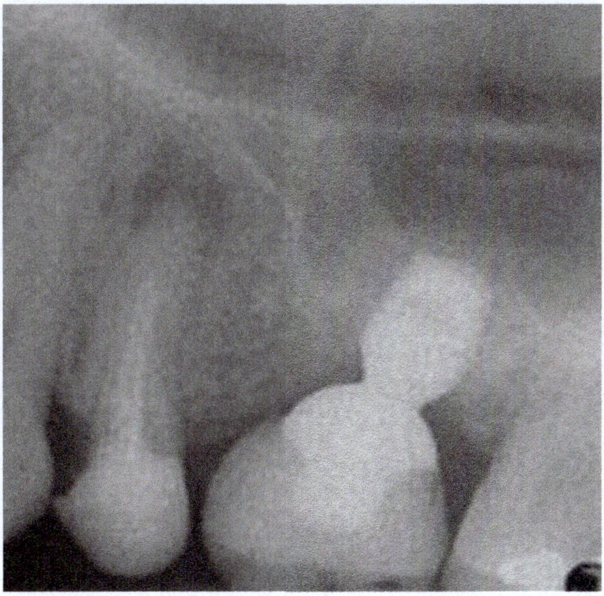

Fig. 11.22 Radiograph taken 5-years post restoration. Note the crestal bone gain around the implant plus newly formed bone at the apical portion of the implant at the sinus floor compared to the 1-year follow-up radiograph Fig. 11.21. The distal cavity also has new bone

References

1. Wagner F, Dvorak G, Nemec S, Pietschmann P, Figl M, Seemann R. A principal components analysis: how pneumatization and edentulism contribute to maxillary atrophy. Oral Dis. 2017;23:55–61.
2. Tatum OH. Lecture presented to the Alabama Implant Congress. Alabama Implant Congress. 1976. https://doi.org/10.1111/cid.12136/full.
3. Boyne PJ, James RA. Grafting of the maxillary sinus floor with autogenous marrow and bone. J Oral Surg. 1980;38(8):613–6.
4. Mellonig JT, Bowers GM, Bailey RC. Comparison of bone graft materials. Part I. New bone formation with autografts and allografts determined by Strontium-85. J Periodontol. 1981;52(6):291–6. https://doi.org/10.1902/jop.1981.52.6.291.
5. Tatum H. Maxillary and sinus implant reconstructions. Dent Clin N Am. 1986;30(2):207–29.
6. Ewers R. Maxilla sinus grafting with marine algae derived bone forming material: a clinical report of long-term results. J Oral Maxillofac Surg. 2005;63(12):1712–23. https://doi.org/10.1016/j.joms.2005.08.020.
7. AAOMS consensus conference on sinus lifts 1996.
8. Jensen O, Block M, Iacono V. Guest Editorial: 1996 sinus conference consensus conference revisited in 2016. Int J Oral Maxillofac Implants. 2016;31(3):505–8.
9. AO consensus conference on sinus lifts 2000. Int J Periodont Restorative Dent. 2001;21(15):517–23.
10. Summers RB. A new concept in maxillary implant surgery: the osteotome technique. Compendium. 1994;15(2):152, 154–6, 158 passim; quiz 162.
11. Summers RB. The osteotome technique: part 3—less invasive methods of elevating the sinus floor. Compendium. 1994;15(6):698, 700, 702–4 passim; quiz 710.
12. Ali SA, Karthigeyan S, Deivanai M, Kumar A. Implant rehabilitation for atrophic maxilla: a review. J Indian Prosthodont Soc. 2014;14(3):196–207. https://doi.org/10.1007/s13191-014-0360-4.

13. Pérez-Martínez S, Martorell-Calatayud L, Peñarrocha-Oltra D, García-Mira B, Peñarrocha-Diago M. Indirect sinus lift without bone graft material: systematic review and meta-analysis. J Clin Exp Dent. 2015;7(2):e316–9.
14. Hernández-Alfaro F, Torradeflot MM, Marti C. Prevalence and management of Schneiderian membrane perforations during sinus-lift procedures. Clin Oral Implants Res. 2008;19(1):91–8.
15. Felice P, Checchi L, Barausse C, Pistilli R, Sammartino G, Masi I, Ippolito DR, Esposito M. Posterior jaws rehabilitated with partial prostheses supported by 4.0 x 4.0 mm or by longer implants: one-year post-loading results from a multicenter randomized controlled trial. Eur J Oral Implantol. 2016;9(1):35–45.
16. Marincola M, Daher S, Ewers R, Lehrberg J. Sinus lift techniques (Chapter 12). In: The Bicon short implant. Chicago: Quintessence Publishing; 2017.
17. Cawood J, Howell R. A classification of the edentulous jaws. Int J Oral Maxillofac Surg. 1988;17:232–6.
18. Nedir R, Nurdin N, Khoury P, Bischof M. Short implants placed with or without grafting in atrophic sinuses: the 3 year results of a prospective randomized controlled study. Clin Implant Dent Relat Res. 2016;18:10–8.
19. Rammelsberg P, Mahabadi J, Eiffler C, Koob A, Galbert O. Radiographic monitoring of changes in bone height after implant placement in combination with an internal sinus lift without graft material. Clin Implant Dent Relat Res. 2015;17(Suppl 1):e267–74.
20. Ghenzi P, Tonetto G, Soldini C, Bettio E, Mortellano C, Soldini C. Dental implants with a platform switched Morse taper connection and an osteo growth induction surface. J Craniofac Surg. 2019;30(4):1049–54.
21. Lago L, da Silva L, Martinez-Silva I, Rilo B. Radiographic assessment of crestal bone loss in tissue level implants restored by platform matching compared with bone level implants restored by platform switching: a randomized, controlled, split mouth trial with 3 year follow-up. Int J Oral Maxillofac Implants. 2019;34(1):179–86.
22. Wolff J. Gesetz Der Transformation Der Knochen. Berlin: Verlag von August Hirschwald; 1892.

The Use of Short and Ultrashort Implants in Atrophic Jaws

12

Rolf Ewers, Boyd J. Tomasetti, Vincent J. Morgan, and Angelo Perpetuini

Contents

12.1 Atrophic Maxilla 179
12.2 Conclusions 191
12.3 Atrophic Mandible 192
12.4 Summary and Conclusion 202
References 202

Tooth loss results in resorption of the alveolar bone, often down to cortical bone. The amount and rapidity of resorption varies from patient to patient but eventually all alveolar and cancellous bone will resorb. Over 150 years ago, Julius Wolff, an anatomist and surgeon, observed that healthy bone adapts to loads to which it is exposed [1, 2]. He described the trabecular structures in the proximal femur based upon the load being placed on the bone [3]. Applying Wolff's law to the resorption

R. Ewers (✉)
CMF Institute Vienna, Vienna, Austria
e-mail: rolf@cmf-vienna.com

B. J. Tomasetti
Department of Oral and Maxillofacial Surgery, Denver Health and Hospitals, Denver, CO, USA

Tomasetti and McLain Oral and Maxillofacial Surgery, Littleton, CO, USA

V. J. Morgan
Bicon, Boston, MA, USA

A. Perpetuini
Dental Laboratory, Rome, Italy

Master Dental Technician, Bicon, Rome, Italy
e-mail: pperpetuini@bicon.com

B. J. Tomasetti, R. Ewers (eds.), *Short Implants*,
https://doi.org/10.1007/978-3-030-44199-9_12

of the jaws' bone is a logical consequence of tooth loss. Without the presence of a load being placed on the teeth, the mandible and maxilla will resorb.

In 1963, Atwood described a classification of atrophy in the post extraction mandible [4]. This was further developed in 1971 with inclusion of the maxilla [5]. Cawood and Howell [6], in 1988, developed a radiographic classification of the mandible and maxilla that is still in use today. Their classification describes six stages based on the amount of residual bone that is available—(I) dentate alveolar ridge, (II) early edentulous alveolus, (III) high well-rounded ridge, (IV) knife-edged ridge, (V) low well-rounded ridge, and finally (VI) low depressed alveolar ridge.

Bone atrophy has been a major concern for oral and maxillofacial surgeons and others placing implants for many decades. This was especially true when 12–15 mm and longer implants were considered the standard length for implant stability.

A variety of procedures were developed, primarily involving grafting procedures to the posterior mandible and maxilla. The most popular techniques were the sinus lift, first advocated by Tatum, and augmentation grafts that increased the vertical height of the alveolar ridge [7–9]. Other procedures that assisted the surgeon when faced with severely atrophic ridges are guided bone regeneration [10], distraction, and the horseshoe osteotomy [11]. In the vast majority of these cases, there were good long-term results [12].

Surgeons continued to look for different approaches to treating the severely atrophic edentulous maxilla and mandible. The results of this were the introductions of the zygomatic implants and the all-on-4 concept [13, 14]. The all-on-4 procedure allowed the practitioner to treat both the severely atrophic edentulous maxilla and mandible, often at the same visit. The introduction of the minimally invasive sinus augmentation allowed the surgeon to minimize both the risk and cost of these procedures [15].

The next logical step was to explore ways in which short and ultrashort implants could be used to treat those patients with severely atrophic jaws. The use of short and ultrashort implants combined with a minimally invasive sinus augmentation would further assist in minimizing the risk of augmentation and nerve lateralization procedures while at the same time lowering both the recovery time and treatment cost for the patient. While surgeons felt confident using the shorter implants, the initial concerns were with the prosthesis. The literature reflected the success of short and ultrashort implants when used to support single tooth crowns. There were initial concerns with a long crown/implant ratio when using short implants in severely atrophic areas. Multiple papers put this concern to rest [16–18].

The next step was to see if short and ultrashort implants could be used to support a full arch prosthesis in both the edentulous maxilla and mandible. And, could this be done with only four implants in each arch? Could the short implants support this fixed prosthesis? These full arch prostheses often had a long posterior cantilever that would place considerable pressure on the implants [19].

With the longer 10–15 mm implants, it was initially felt that due to the bone density, a minimum of six implants would be needed in the maxilla in order to support a full arch prosthesis [20]. The mandibular arch, with a greater bone density could do well with 4–5 implants [21]. Interestingly, zygomatic implants really have only 4–6 mm of osseointegration in the 40–50 mm long implants. To some extent, they are acting similar to short and ultrashort implants with a long crown/implant ratio.

12.1 Atrophic Maxilla

Patients between ages 53 and 84 years old with pronounced Cawood / Howell class V and VI maxillary atrophy have been treated with four short and ultrashort implants.

All patients were treated with four 4.0 × 5.0 mm ultrashort locking taper implants. In those patients with a very thin anterior maxillary ridge narrow 3.0 × 8.0 mm locking taper Bicon implants were used. In order to avoid sinus lift and ridge splitting procedures, implants were placed in the area of the maxillary tuberosities [3]. All patients were restored with metal-free prostheses made of a glass fiber-reinforced hybrid resin material under the brand name TRINIA®.

Case Studies Quattro-TRINIA®

Case I is a 73-year-old female patient with extreme Cawood/Howell class VI maxillary atrophy (Fig. 12.1a). Previously we would have treated this patient with a complex Le Fort I Horseshoe Osteotomy utilizing an iliac crest interpositional bone graft. In this case, there was sufficient bone to place four 4.0 × 5.0 mm calcium phosphate-coated Bicon Integra-CP™ implants. The implants were placed in the area of teeth numbers 4, 6, 11, and 13 without any bone augmentations during a relatively short office-based surgical procedure in local anesthesia (Fig. 12.1b).

The implants were uncovered after 6 months of healing. The osseointegration of these implants occurs by intramembranous bone healing in accordance with the callus principle [22]. Impressions were made following the uncovering of the implants, and a few days later the prosthetic wax try-in with the teeth arrangement stabilized by a single impression post (Fig. 12.2a, b).

Once the laboratory processes had been completed, the technician provided the aligned abutments on a plaster model for the cement-retained TRINIA® prosthesis

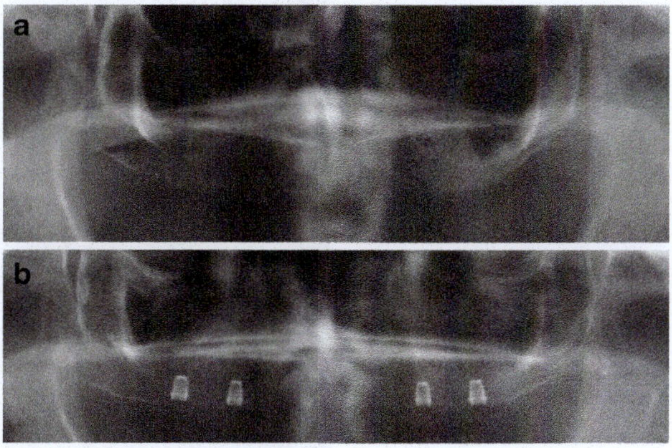

Fig. 12.1 Enlarged sections of panoramic images of the 73-year-old female patient with an atrophic maxilla (**a**) and with four inserted 4.0 × 5.0 mm Bicon Integra-CP implants (**b**)

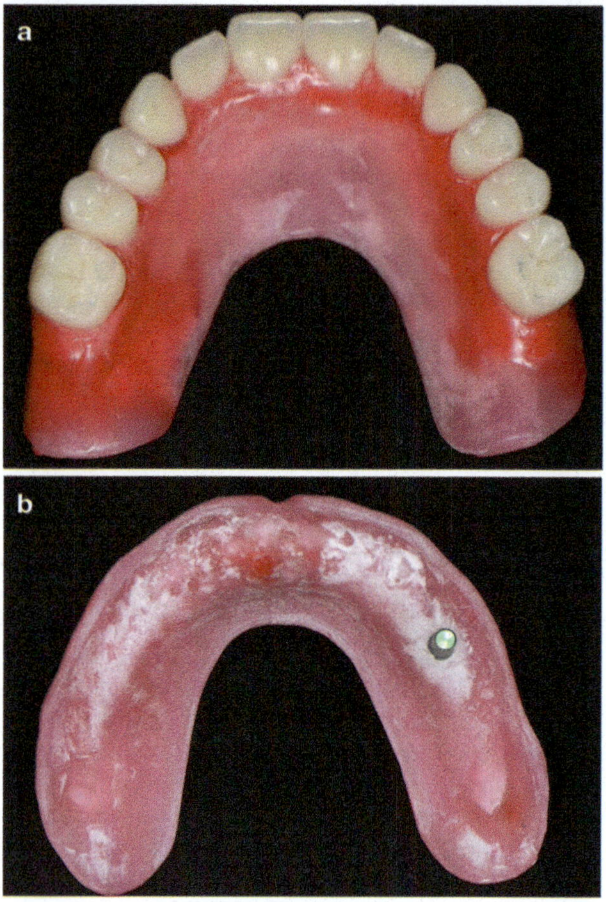

Fig. 12.2 Wax teeth arrangement with a resin base (**a**). On the ridge side, the impression post is visible, which helps to orient and stabilize the prosthesis in an implant (**b**)

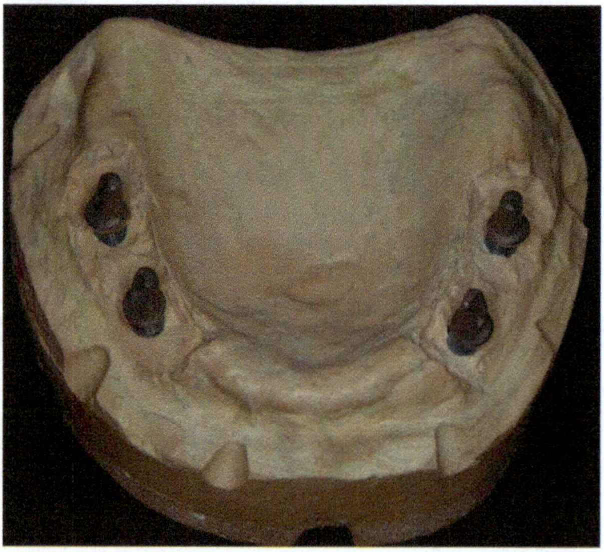

Fig. 12.3 Four parallel aligned abutments on the stone model

(Fig. 12.3) Alternatively, fixed-detachable, retentive telescopic or Locator® prostheses could have been fabricated.

The TRINIA substructure (Fig. 12.4) was fabricated by the Perpetuini dental laboratory (Cisterna di Latina/Italy) using a CAD/CAM method for the processing of a 12-unit prosthesis (Fig. 12.5).

Figure 12.6 shows the completed prosthesis with the four abutments prior to the abutments being inserted into the wells of their implants. Vaseline was applied to

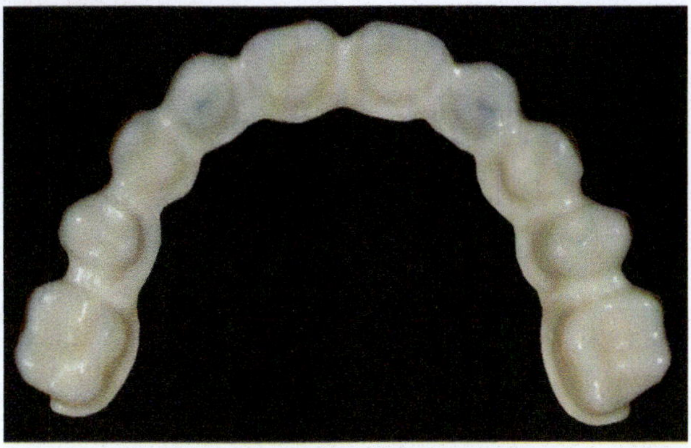

Fig. 12.4 CAD/CAM metal-free fiber-reinforced TRINIA® substructure

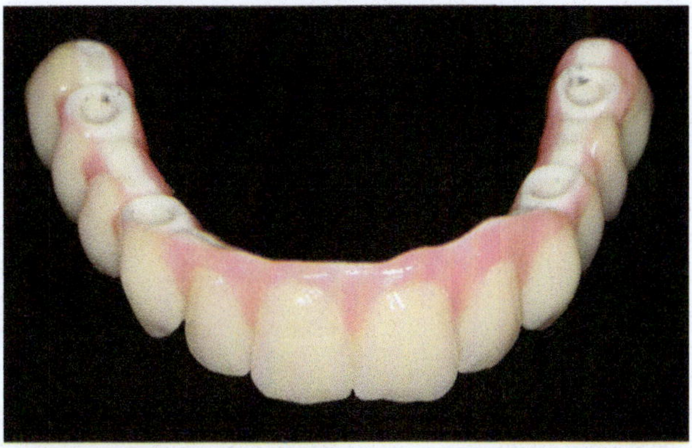

Fig. 12.5 Ridge-side view of the TRINIA prosthesis with four bores into which the abutments will be cemented

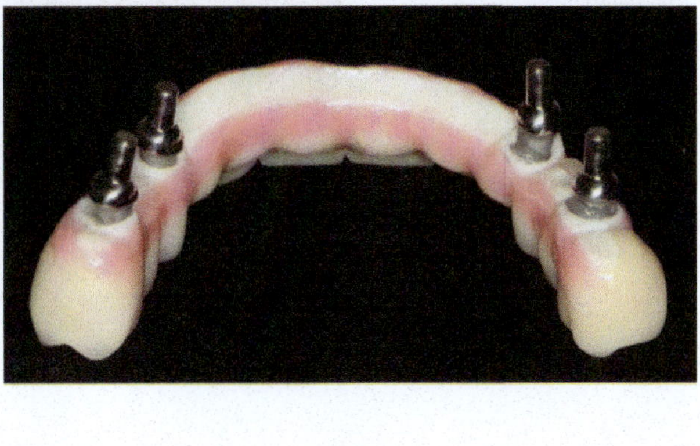

Fig. 12.6 Completed TRINIA® prosthesis with four abutments, which are to be seated and subsequently cemented into the bores of the prosthesis

the bores of the TRINIA® substructure to facilitate the removal of the prosthesis after the insertion of the abutments into their implant wells.

Figure 12.7 shows the initial try-in of the prosthesis prior to its cementation to the four definitively seated abutments.

Figure 12.8 shows the facial view of the seated 12-unit prosthesis. Figure 12.9 shows the palatal view of the palate-free prosthesis.

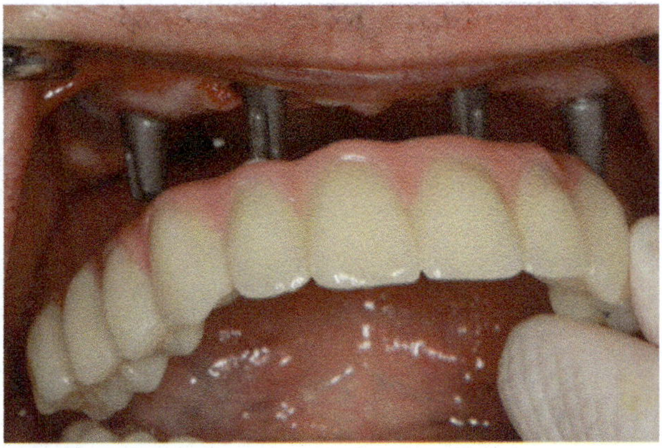

Fig. 12.7 Initial try-in of the prosthesis prior to its cementation to the four abutments with temporary cement

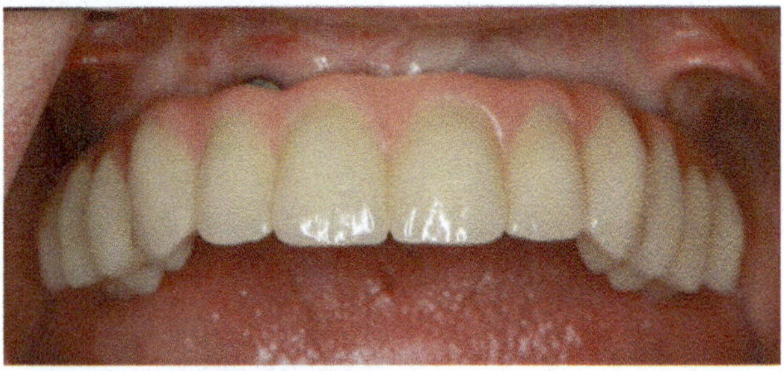

Fig. 12.8 Facial view of the seated 12-unit TRINIA prosthesis

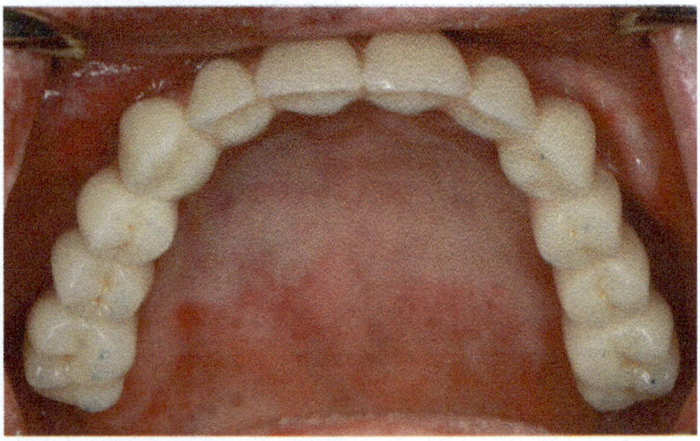

Fig. 12.9 Palatal view of the seated 12-unit prosthesis with a free palate

Figure 12.10 shows the four abutments after 5 years in function.

Despite the availability of only minimal bone in this patient's atrophic maxilla, the use of four short implants provided the benefits of a palate-free fixed prosthesis with two minor surgical procedures. The panoramic radiograph taken at the beginning of the functional loading of the prosthesis reveals good osseointegration (Fig. 12.11a), which remained unchanged after 5 years in function, as evidenced by no marginal bone loss (Fig. 12.11b).

With the TRINIA® prosthesis in the maxilla and the Locator® prosthesis, a satisfactory occlusion (Fig. 12.12) and an excellent functional result were achieved. The short and ultrashort implants have been in function for more than 5 years.

Many patients with a pronounced class V–VI maxillary atrophy in a vertical dimension, also have a very narrow posterior and anterior alveolar ridge. In this 69-year-old male patient, two narrow 3.0 × 8.0 mm Bicon Integra-CP implants were placed in the anterior region (Fig. 12.13a, b).

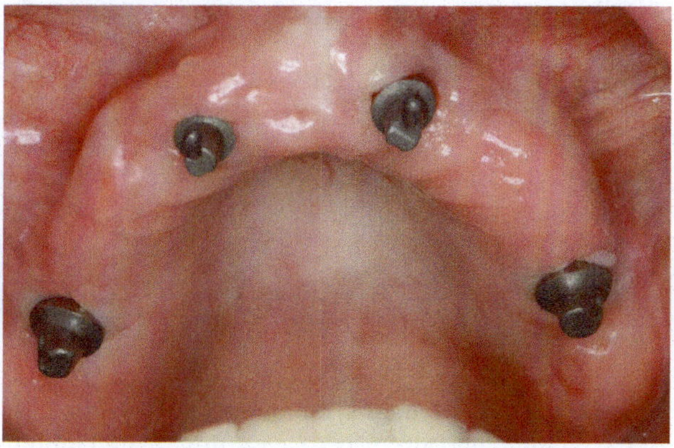

Fig. 12.10 Intraoral view of four abutments after 5 years in function

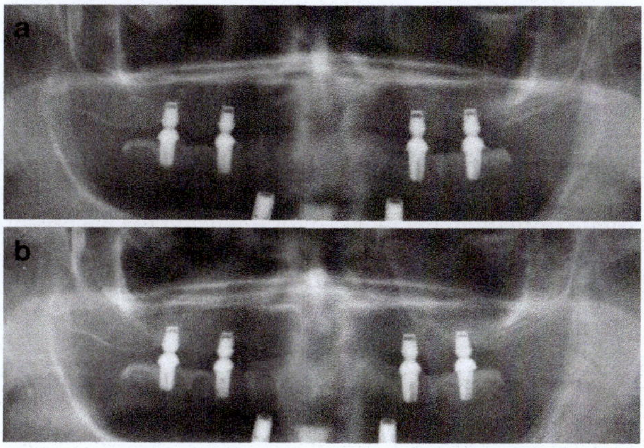

Fig. 12.11 Enlarged sections of panoramic images with the cemented prosthesis at the start of loading (**a**) and after 5 years in function (**b**)

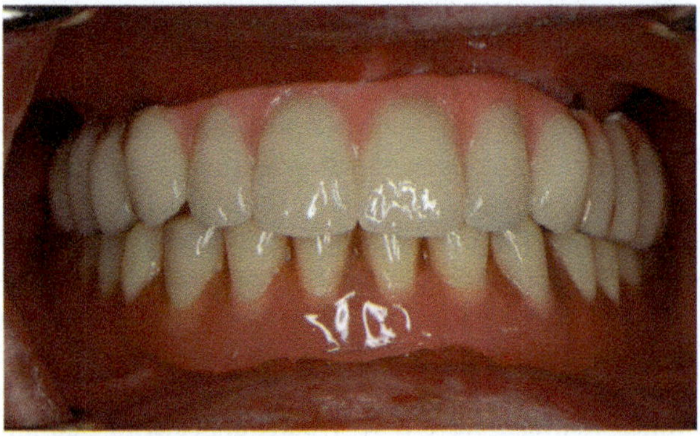

Fig. 12.12 Image of occlusion of the maxillary TRINIA® prosthesis, cemented on four implants and the mandibular Locator® prosthesis

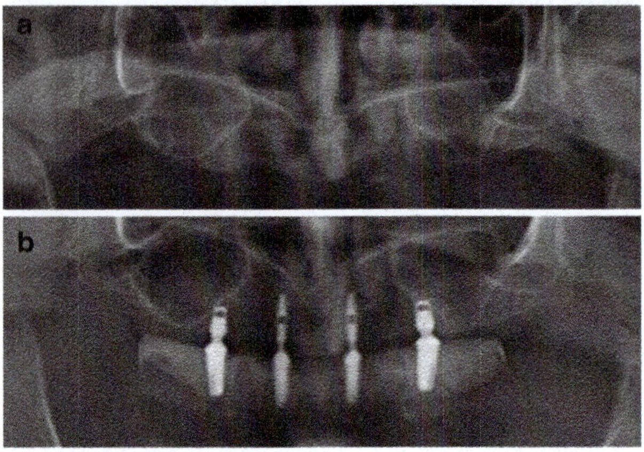

Fig. 12.13 Enlarged sections of the panoramic images of a 69-year-old male patient with extreme class V-VI maxillary atrophy (**a**) and after the insertion of two 3.0 × 8.0 mm and two 4.0 × 5.0 mm well-positioned Bicon Integra-CP implants after 6 years in function without any radiologically detectable marginal bone loss (**b**)

A lateral cephalometric radiograph reveals the challenging restorative situation of the patient, who also was successfully treated with four 4.0 × 5.0 mm mandibular Bicon implants (Fig. 12.14).

With both TRINIA® prostheses, a satisfactory occlusion and an excellent functional and esthetic result were achieved along with evidence of long-term stability over a 6-year period (Fig. 12.15).

In some cases, the alveolar crest in the premolar region is so severely resorbed (Fig. 12.16) that a split procedure is not possible. If the patient does not elect to have a major complex Le Fort I Horseshoe Osteotomy utilizing an iliac crest interpositional bone graft we prefer an Uno-TRINIA® solution. This is done by placing a single implant in the incisive foramen and the nasopalatine canal utilizing one Bicon implant and placing a single Brevis™ attached full arch TRINIA® cover denture prosthesis.

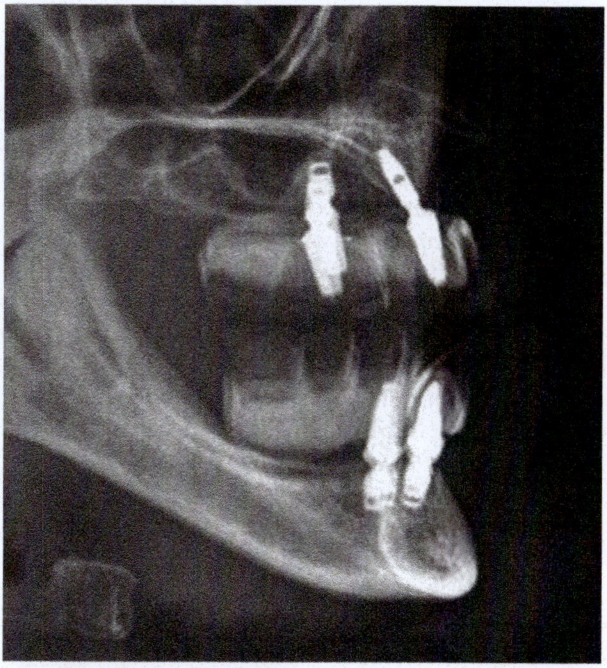

Fig. 12.14 Lateral cephalometric X-ray with implant-supported and cement-retained maxillary and mandibular TRINIA® prostheses

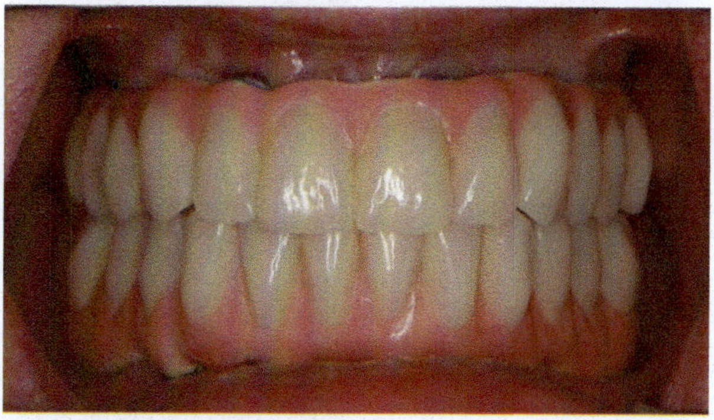

Fig. 12.15 Image of occlusion of the maxillary and mandibular TRINIA® prostheses, cemented on four implants each

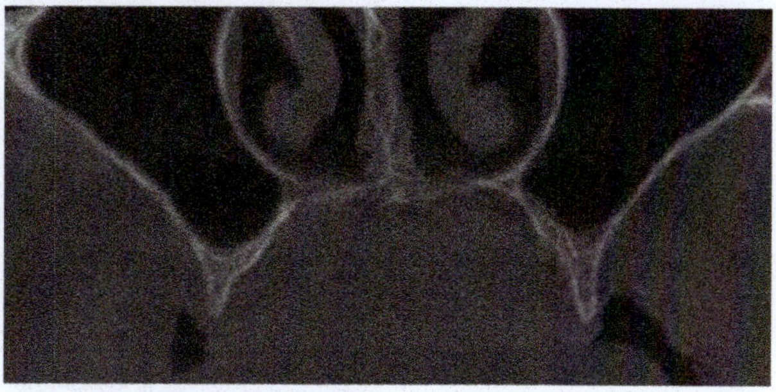

Fig. 12.16 Transverse section of a Cone Beam CT of a 75-year-old female patient with extreme alveolar crest atrophy in the premolar region

Case Study Uno-TRINIA®

The patient is a 75-year-old female with severe alveolar crest atrophy Class VI in the maxilla and Class IV–V in the mandible (Fig. 12.17). She had been edentulous since age 18! In the 57 intervening years a tremendous retro maxillary position and a mandibular anteroposition had resulted in an extreme Class III occlusion (Fig. 12.18). Due to her age and medical condition, she was not willing to have major augmentation procedures and it was decided to use a single implant for the maxilla.

Initially the maxilla was addressed and a single 4.5 × 6 mm Bicon implant was inserted through the incisive foramen into the nasopalatine canal (Figs. 12.19 and 12.20).

Three months later we inserted three 4.0 × 5.0 mm Bicon SHORT® implants into the interforaminal region of the mandible. Altogether there was a 6 month wait until the four SHORT® implants were uncovered and a 10-teeth full arch TRINIA® prosthesis for the mandible and a 14-teeth full arch cover denture TRINIA® prosthesis

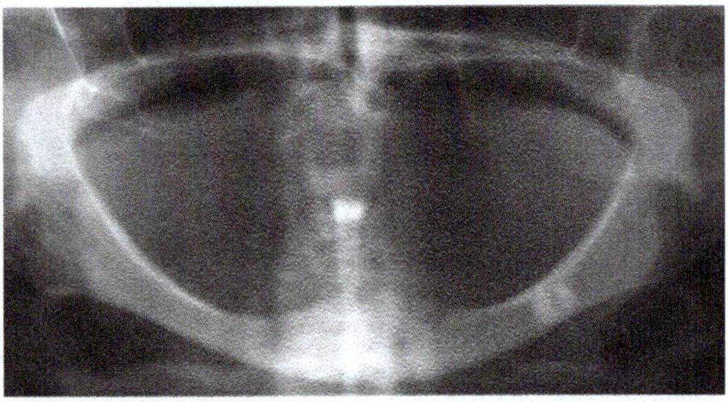

Fig. 12.17 Panoramic radiograph of this 75-year-old female patient with extreme alveolar crest atrophy in the maxilla and moderate atrophy in the mandible

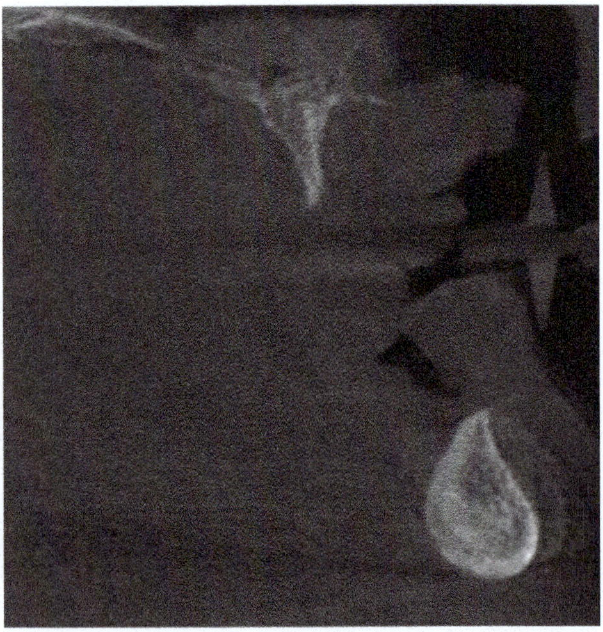

Fig. 12.18 Sagittal section of a Cone Beam CT of this 75-year-old female patient with extreme Class III occlusion due to 57 years of atrophy due to edentulism

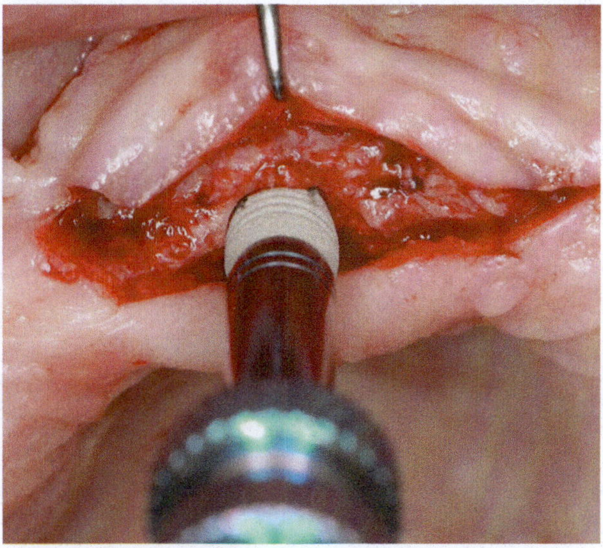

Fig. 12.19 Intraoperative view inserting the 4.5 × 6.0 mm Bicon SHORT® implant through the incisive foramen into the nasopalatinal canal

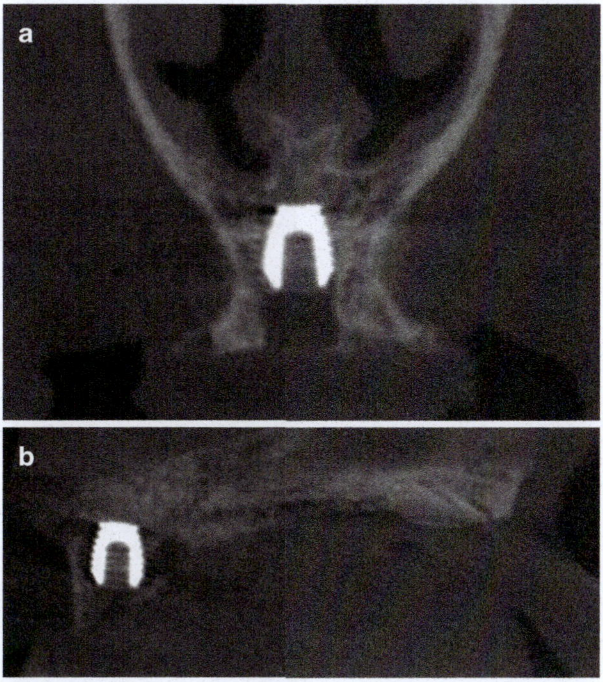

Fig. 12.20 (**a** and **b**) Cone Beam CT after inserting a 3.5 × 6.0 mm Bicon SHORT® implant into the nasopalatinal canal through the incisive canal. (**a**) Transverse view. (**b**) Sagittal view

for the maxilla were produced. Due to the extreme Class III occlusion the Perpetuini dental laboratory had to position the teeth behind the screw sleeves which resulted in a very long cantilever on both sides (Figs. 12.21, 12.22, 12.23, and 12.24).

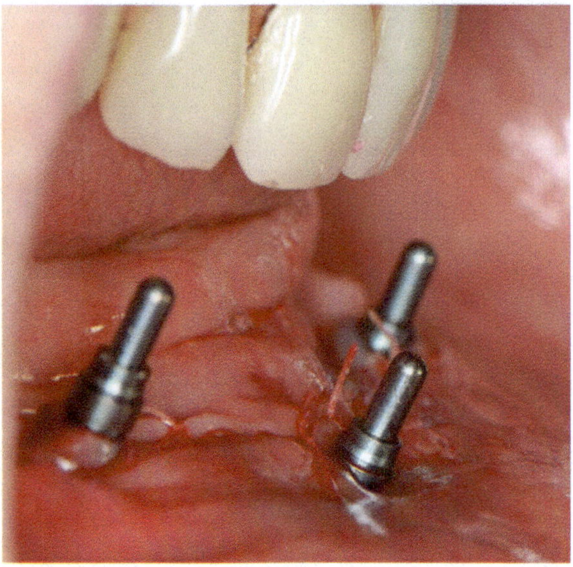

Fig. 12.21 Intraoral view after inserting three 2.5 mm titanium impression posts. Due to the Class III occlusion the titanium impression posts are located far in front of the upper central incisor teeth

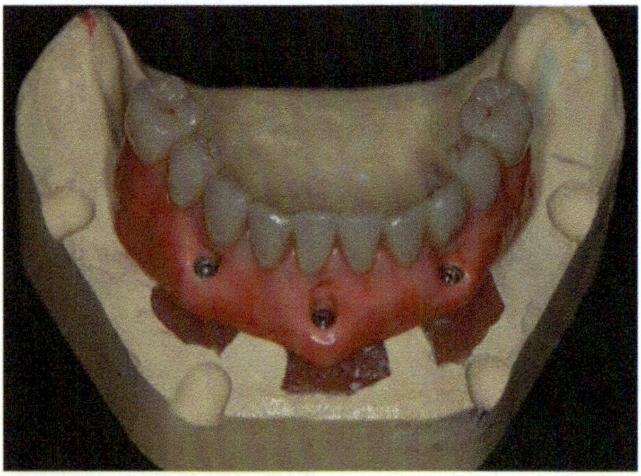

Fig. 12.22 Finalized 10-teeth full arch TRINIA® prosthesis on a plaster cast model tightened with three screws on the screw retentive abutments. The unusual position of the three screws in front of the teeth are well visible due to the Class III occlusion

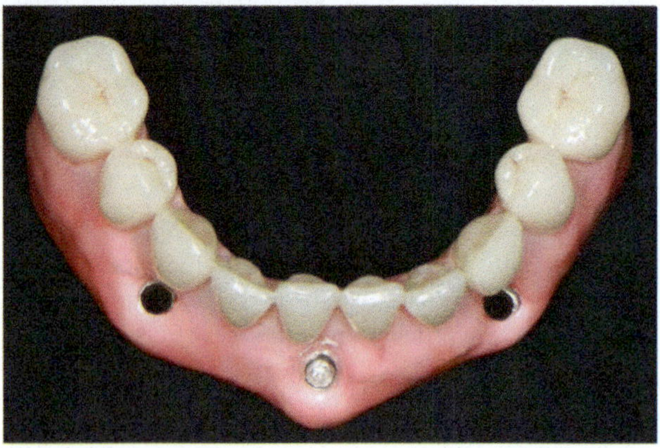

Fig. 12.23 Final 10-teeth full arch TRINIA® prosthesis with three screw sleeves in front of the teeth and a very long cantilever on both sides

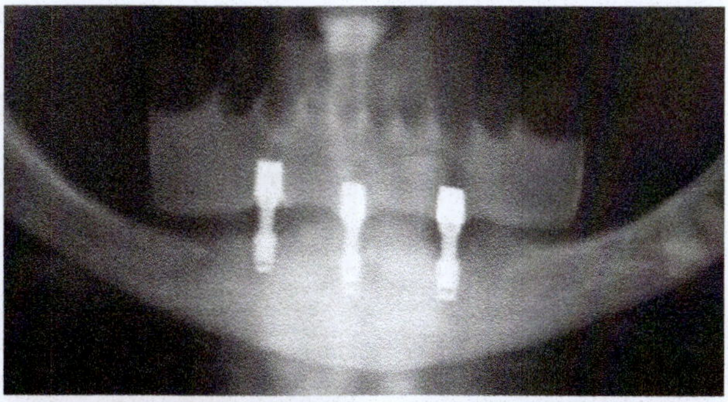

Fig. 12.24 Panoramic radiograph after fixation of the screws in the screw retentive abutments of the three 4.0 × 5.0 mm Bicon SHORT® implants with long bilateral cantilever

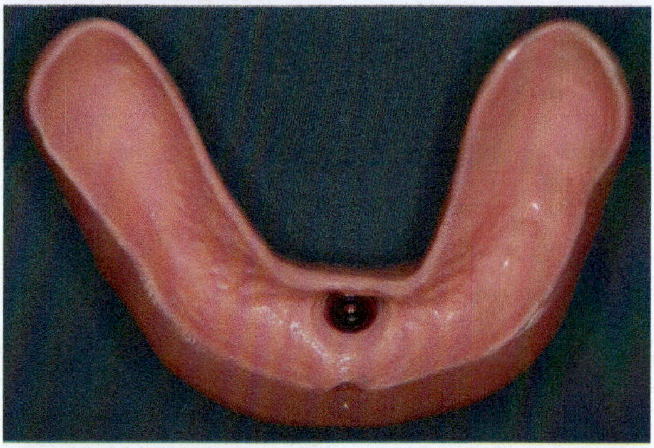

Fig. 12.25 Finalized horseshoe-like full arch TRINIA® cover denture prosthesis with one Brevis® housing in the middle

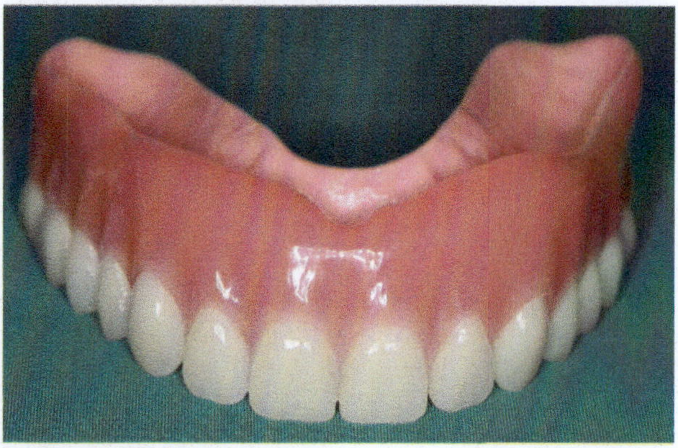

Fig. 12.26 Finalized horseshoe-like full arch TRINIA® cover denture prosthesis with 14 teeth

In the maxilla, the laboratory produced a horseshoe-like 14-teeth full arch TRINIA® denture prosthesis without coverage over the hard palate (Figs. 12.25 and 12.26).

These procedures resulted in a very satisfactory normal occlusion with an excellent esthetic outcome (Figs. 12.27, 12.28, and 12.29).

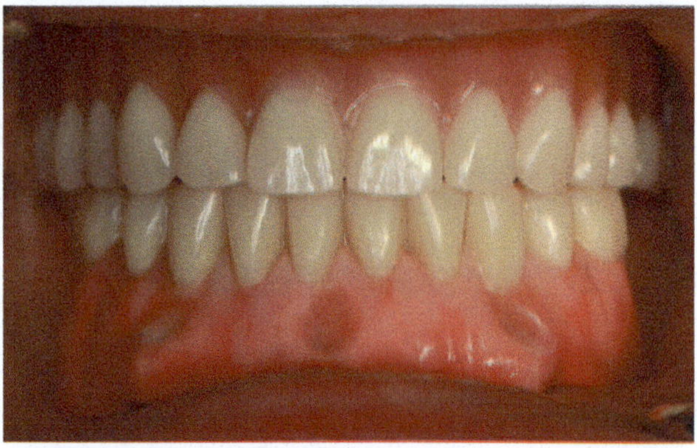

Fig. 12.27 Showing occlusion of the two full arch TRINIA® prostheses in frontal view. The three holes for the screw fixation are covered with pink resin

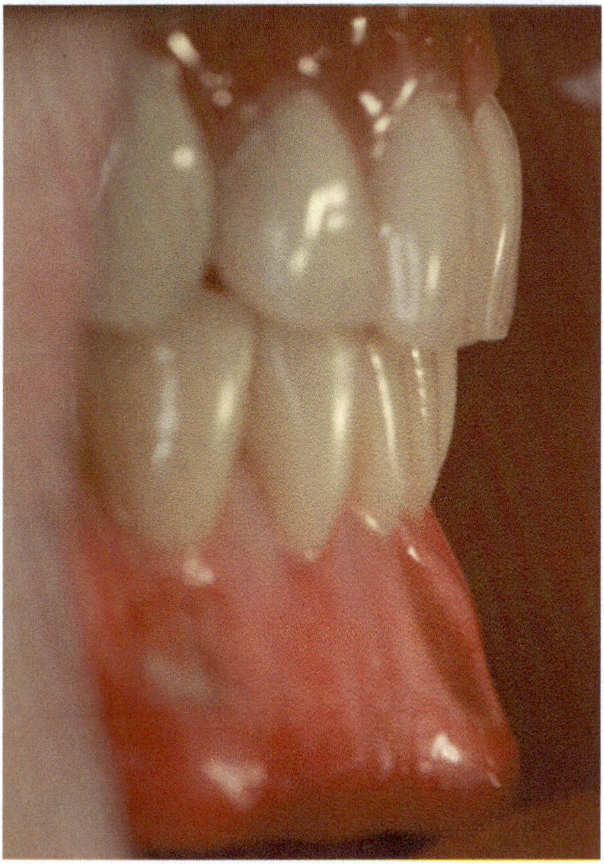

Fig. 12.28 Satisfactory occlusion of the two full arch TRINIA® prostheses in lateral view

The efficacy of treating patients with extreme maxillary atrophy without costly and time-consuming augmentation procedures by using ultrashort 4.0 × 5.0 mm and narrow 3.0 × 8.0 mm implants is well established. Restorations were completed with prostheses composed of metal-free CAD/CAM-produced fiber-reinforced hybrid resin material. In our studies, the cumulative patient-based survival

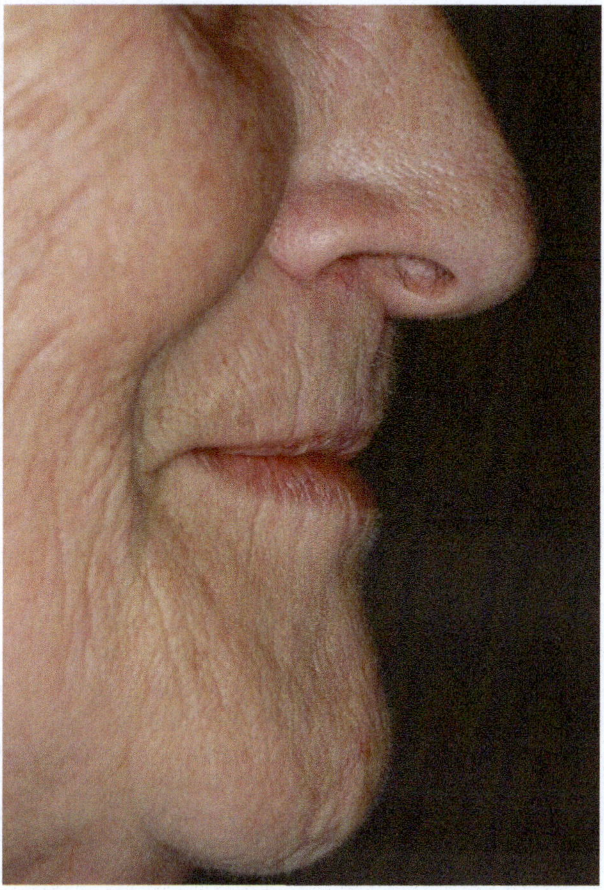

Fig. 12.29 In spite of the original extreme Class III occlusion a very satisfying esthetic result was obtained

rate (CSR) was 88.8% after 1 year. The cumulative 1-year implant-based survival rate was 97.2%. The survival rates are comparable to those of conventional long implants [23]. It is possible to treat the highly atrophic maxillae with ultrashort and narrow implants using only four implants. The results are comparable to studies by other authors. Restorations with a metal-free CAD/CAM-produced fiber-reinforced hybrid resin material does not lead to any complications. These results are very encouraging, since the extreme maxillary atrophy only required the use of narrow implants with an alveolar ridge splitting procedure or the placement of ultrashort implants with minor surgical procedures. Furthermore, the placement of implants in the tuberosities had excellent statistical results.

12.2 Conclusions

In consideration of the very difficult clinical situation of restoring highly atrophic maxilla in both the vertical and transverse dimensions, and the capability of avoiding extensive augmentation procedures, the long-term use of four ultrashort and narrow locking taper implants shows good results comparable to standard size implants with complex bone augmentations. However, long-term results with this type of atrophy are still very limited. Prospective long-term studies with a larger number of patients and implants observed over a longer period of time is necessary to make a valid recommendation.

12.3 Atrophic Mandible

The all-on-4 concept in the mandible is considered a safe treatment option for the restoration of atrophic mandibles with predictable outcomes; implant success rates and patient satisfaction is generally high. In severely atrophic mandibles Class V and Class VI however, rehabilitation with dental implants may prove to be challenging. Especially in the posterior atrophic mandible, the position of the alveolar nerve may limit the insertion of dental implants with standard lengths (8 mm and more) and limit the insertion to their classic location, the interforaminal mandibular body. In these cases, a wide range of preprosthetic treatment options exist, and bone augmentation and/or distraction procedures and lateralization of the inferior alveolar nerve have all been attempted, leaving the interforaminal implant insertion as the gold standard for most dental surgeons.

These procedures are technically demanding, time-consuming, and expensive, and may result in substantial complications. Short implants have gained in popularity during the past decade and represent a viable alternative to these procedures. Short implant survival rates are comparable with those of long implants inserted into augmented bone sites and therefore may be a preferable, less traumatic treatment option for restoration of severely atrophic mandibles. Recently, the European Association of Dental Implantologists reached a consensus that short implants in atrophic sites are a reliable treatment option whose risks are comparable with those of standard-dimension implants in combination with augmentation procedures. Still, evidence on short implants in an all-on-4 setting is limited. In a recent pilot study, we reported preliminary results of fiber-reinforced hybrid-material bridges, fixed on four ultrashort 5.0-mm implants. The aim of this study in the mandible was to evaluate the long-term outcomes of splinted ultrashort implants with full arch TRINIA® prothesis in terms of marginal bone loss and overall implant survival.

We exclusively used ultrashort calcium phosphate-coated implants with a diameter of 4.0 mm and length of 5.0 mm Bicon SHORT® implants. We have treated patients between ages 41 and 79 years old with pronounced class V and VI atrophy according to Cawood and Howell. The surgical and prosthetic protocol was the same as in the maxilla. The only difference was the uncovering, which usually took place after 3–4 months and occasionally longer [24].

A female patient, who had been edentulous for a long period underwent implant restoration at 59 years of age. The atrophic mandible, Class VI, was due to a very long period of being edentulous with a remnant bone height in the mandibular symphysis of 7 mm. (Figs. 12.30 and 12.31).

We inserted four 4.0 × 5.0 mm Bicon ultra-SHORT® implants (Fig. 12.32).

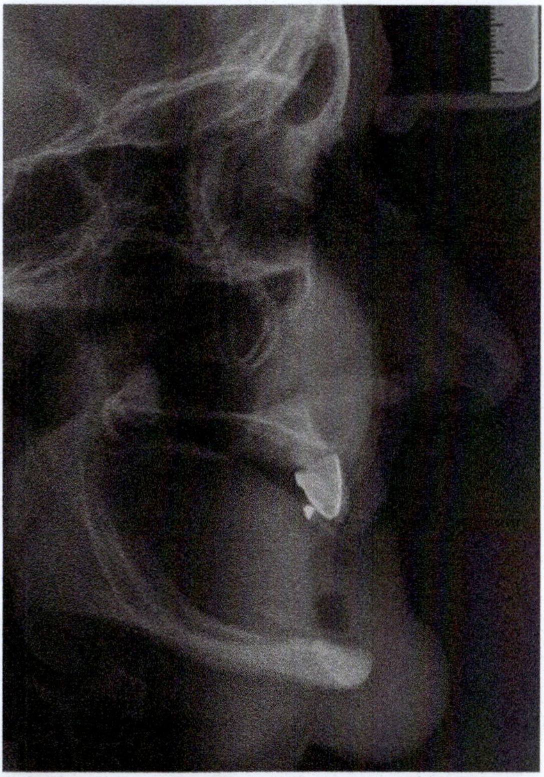

Fig. 12.30 Lateral cephalometric radiograph of a 59-year-old female patient with extreme mandibular atrophy after many decades of being edentulous

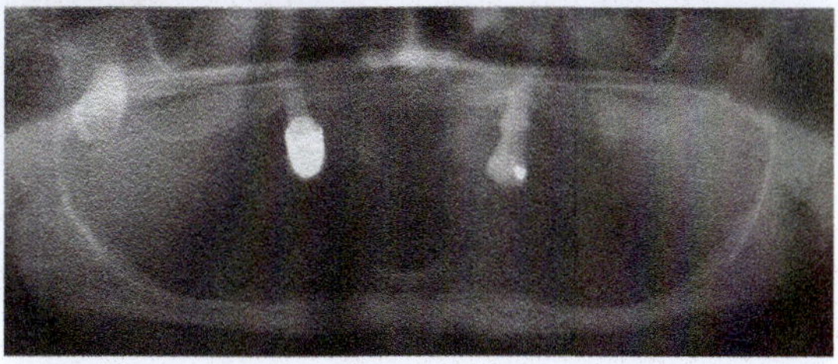

Fig. 12.31 Panoramic radiograph of a 59-year-old female patient with extreme mandibular atrophy

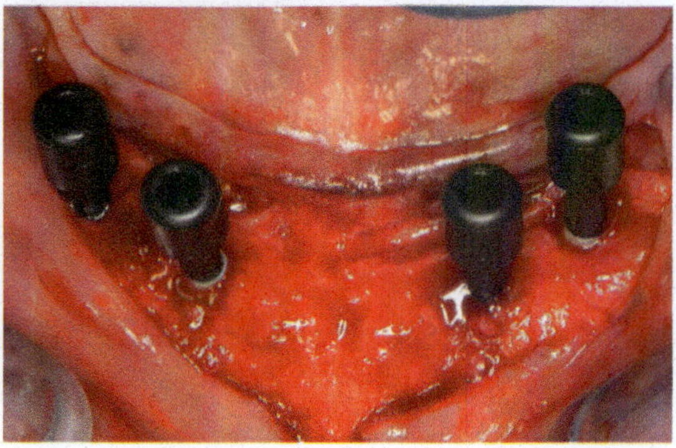

Fig. 12.32 Intraoperative view after inserting four 4.0 × 5.0 mm ultra-SHORT® Bicon implants with the four black polyethylene healing plugs still in situ

After almost 7 months, the implants were uncovered, impression and a bite registration was taken and sent to the perpetuini laboratory. About 10 days later the finalized 10-teeth full arch TRINIA® bridge prosthesis was provisionally cemented on four non-shouldered abutments (Figs. 12.33, 12.34, 12.35, and 12.36).

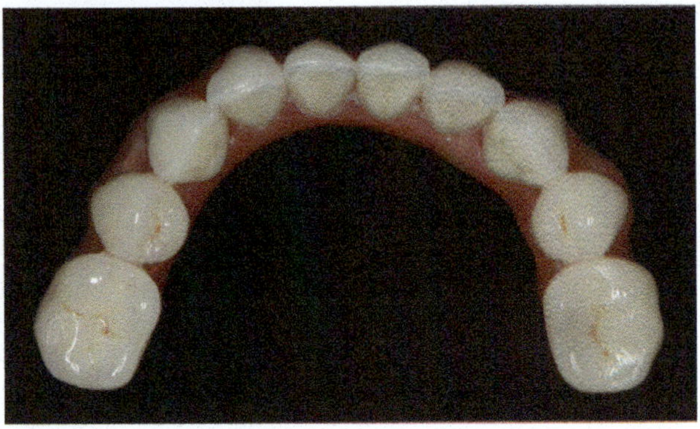

Fig. 12.33 Occlusal view of the Ceramage-facetted, 10-teeth fiber-reinforced metal-free TRINIA® full arch resin bridge prosthesis

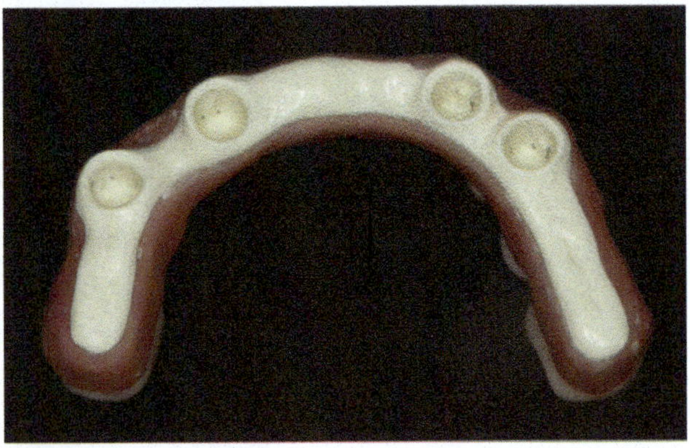

Fig. 12.34 Undersurface view of the Ceramage-facetted, 10-teeth fiber-reinforced metal-free TRINIA® full arch resin bridge prosthesis with the holes for the non-shouldered abutments

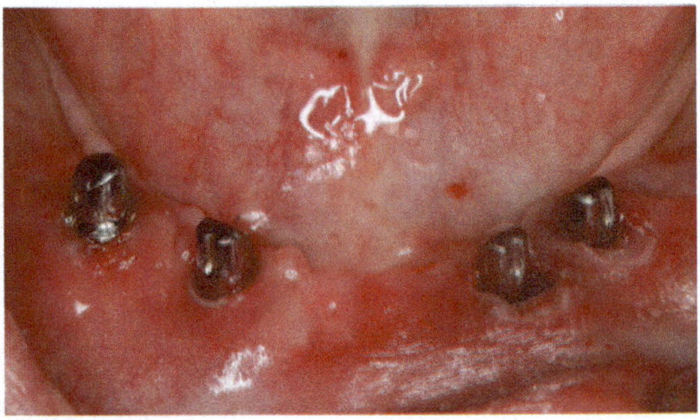

Fig. 12.35 Intraoral view of after inserting the four non-shouldered abutments ready for cementing the TRINIA® full arch bridge prosthesis

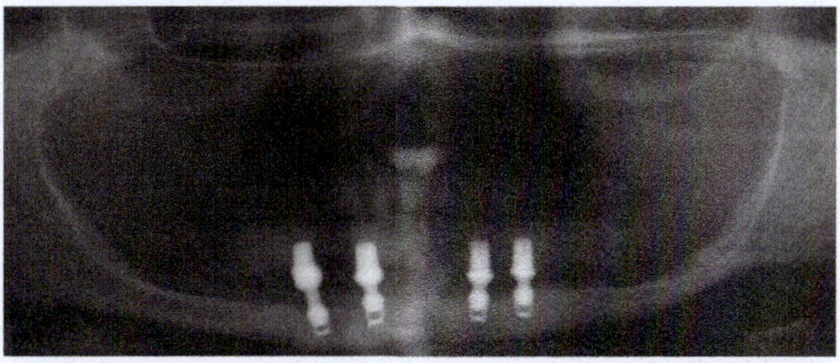

Fig. 12.36 Panoramic radiography after cementing the 10-teeth full arch TRINIA® bridge prosthesis and starting to load

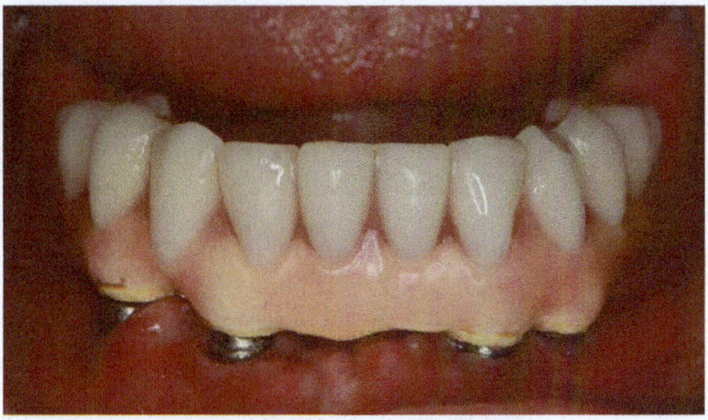

Fig. 12.37 Intraoral view at almost 7 years recall with bland mucosal appearance

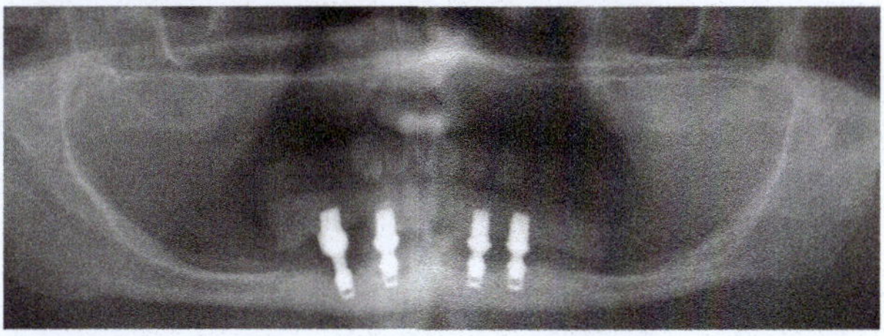

Fig. 12.38 Panoramic radiograph at almost 7 years recall. On the right posterior implant minimal marginal bone loss which is stationary since the beginning of loading this implant

At the last recall visit, after almost 7 years in function, the clinical aspect showed excellent soft tissue situation around the abutments and implants. The patient had good oral hygiene (Fig. 12.37) and the panoramic radiography showed very stable bone around the implants. The slight marginal bone loss around the right posterior implant is stationary since this implant was loaded. Due to the minimal height of the mandibular bone a subcrestal positioning of the ultra-SHORT® Bicon implant was not possible (Fig. 12.38).

A female, 55-year-old, edentulous patient was treated by placing ultrashort implants after a mandibular body fracture. More than 1 year earlier, an osteosynthesis plate had been removed. After 3 months, the implants were uncovered, and osseointegration was assessed. The left anterior implant, although thought to be osseointegrated when uncovered, progressively loosened and was removed just before prosthetic restoration. The lost implant had been placed directly into the former position of the outermost left osteosynthesis screw (Fig. 12.39). The bridge was permanently cemented on three implants. The patient did not want the removed implant to be replaced.

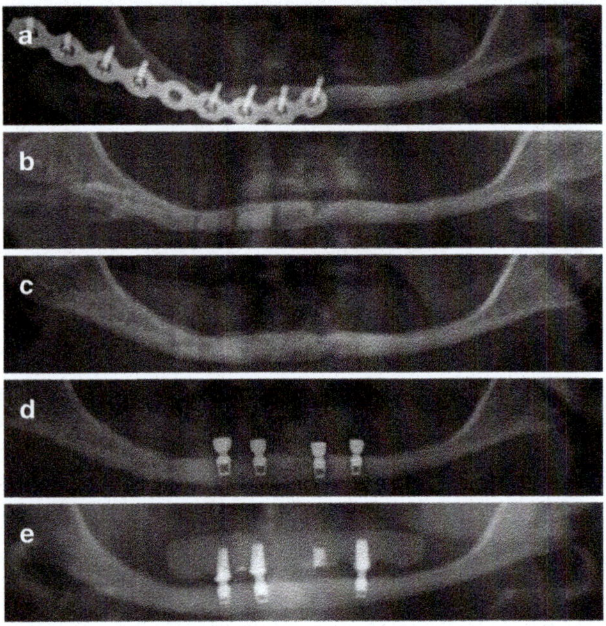

Fig. 12.39 (**a–e**) Sections of panoramic radiographs showing a stable osteosynthesis treatment after fracture of the right horizontal ramus of the mandible (**a**) Situation after metal removal (**b**). Healed situation several months later (**c**). Situation after insertion of four 4.0 × 5.0 mm Bicon SHORT® implants and after uncovering and inserting four titanium healing abutments (**d**). After final temporary cement fixation of the full arch TRINIA® bridge prosthesis after removal the non osseointegrated left medial implant (**e**). Note that this implant was inserted in the region of a former osteosynthesis screw hole

Clinical photographs and panoramic radiograph was taken 8 years after permanent restauration on three implants had been inserted (Figs. 12.40 and 12.41).

Fig. 12.40 Intraoral view at 8-year recall with bland, infection-free periimplant mucosa around the three abutments and implants

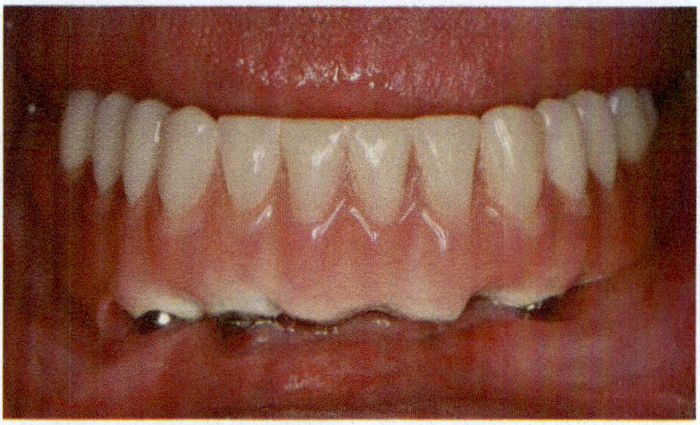

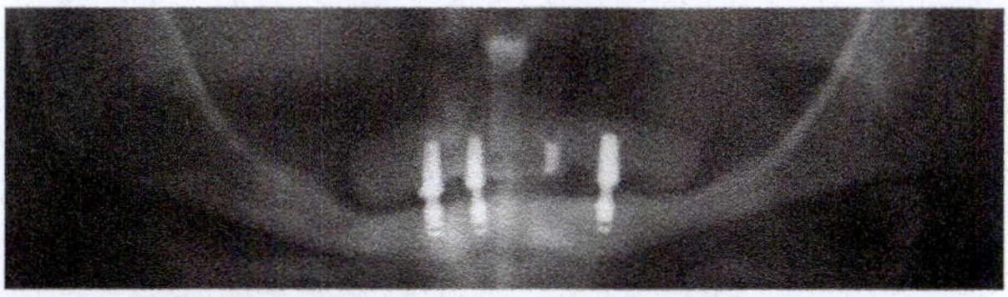

Fig. 12.41 Panoramic radiograph at 8-year recall with no peri implant crestal bone loss and stable functional situation loaded only on three ultrashort 4.0 × 5.0 mm Bicon SHORT® implants

12.3.1 Trio-TRINIA®

After experiencing a good result with three implants as noted with the previous patient, we decided to change our study design to only three ultrashort 4.0 × 5.0 mm SHORT® Bicon implants also in the mandible.

Case Studies Trio-TRINIA®

A 60-year-old patient had three ultrashort 4.0 × 5.0 mm SHORT® Bicon implants placed in the atrophic mandible. Three months later we uncovered the three implants and subsequently three 2.5-mm-thick titanium impression posts with their corresponding blue plastic impression sleeves were inserted (Fig. 12.42).

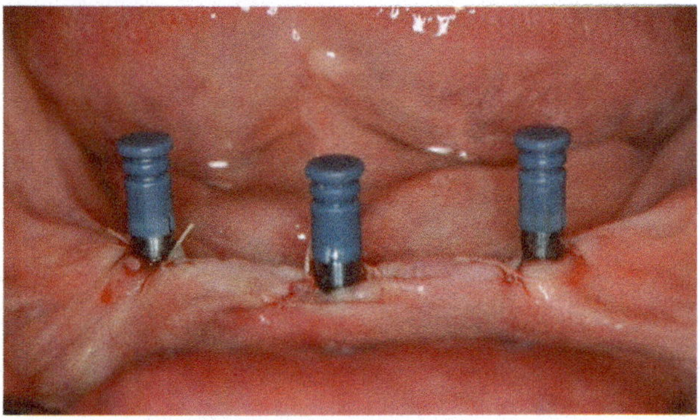

Fig. 12.42 Intraoral view after uncovering the implants and inserting three 2.5-mm-thick titanium impression posts with their corresponding blue Plastic Impression Sleeves

A full arch implant-level transfer impression and a bite registration were taken and sent to the Perpetuini Laboratory. After consultation with the lab and restoring dentist, we decided to produce a TRINIA® full arch bridge prosthesis with retentive copings. After receiving the plaster model and the finalized TRINIA® prosthesis (Figs. 12.43 and 12.44) a special abutment insertion jig (Fig. 12.45) was used to assist in seating the abutments in the desired position.

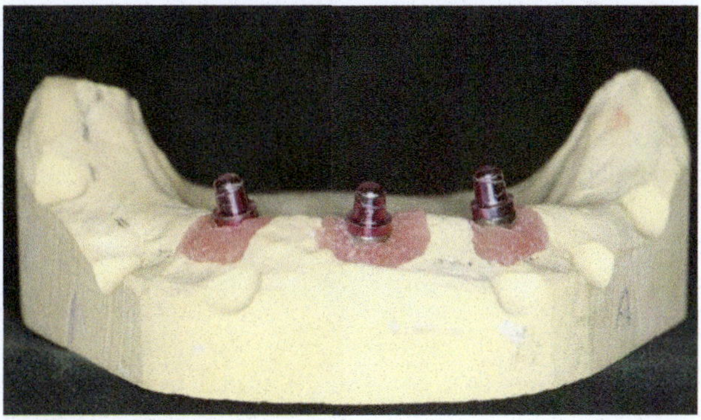

Fig. 12.43 Stone model with three abutments and three Prefabricated Retentive Telescoping Copings

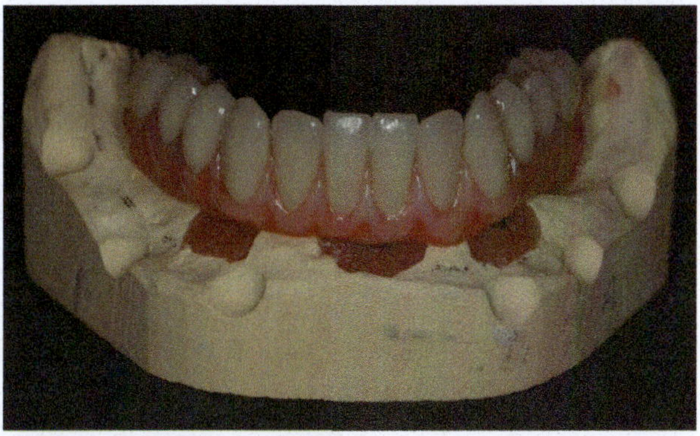

Fig. 12.44 Finalized 12-teeth full arch TRINIA® bridge prosthesis on stone model

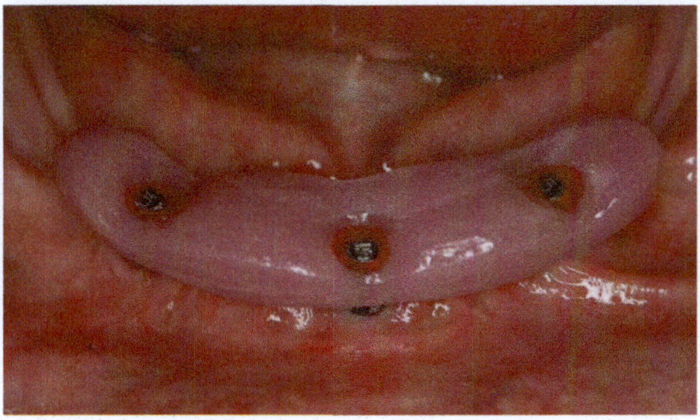

Fig. 12.45 Resin positioning jig after positioning and seating the prefabricated telescoping abutments into the desired position

After tapping the abutments into the right position, the three Prefabricated Retentive Telescoping Copings are positioned over the well-positioned abutments (Fig. 12.46).

Now the Telescoping Copings are fixed with light cured resin into the full arch TRINIA® bridge prosthesis (Fig. 12.47).

The radiologic control with the panoramic radiograph reveals a very satisfactory result (Fig. 12.48).

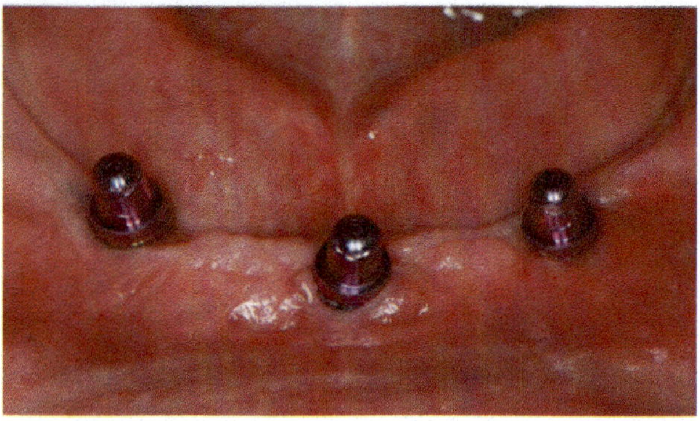

Fig. 12.46 Three seated Prefabricated Retentive Telescoping Copings of the seated and tapped abutments

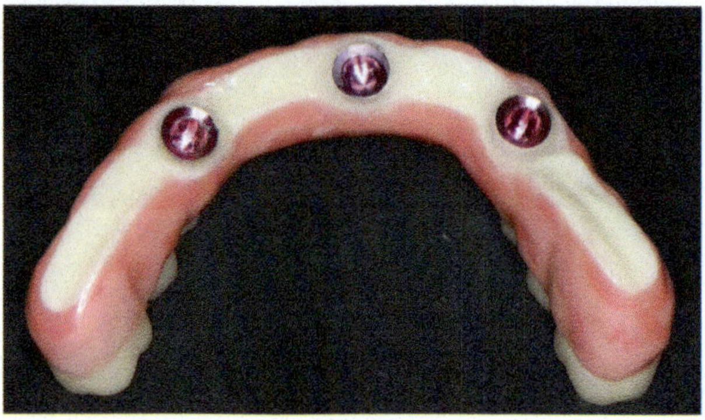

Fig. 12.47 Undersurface view with three light cured resin fixed Prefabricated Retentive Telescoping Copings in the desired position

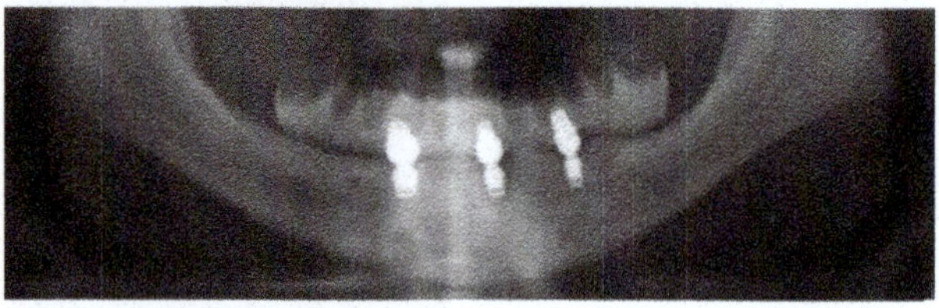

Fig. 12.48 Panoramic radiograph after inserting the abutments and fixing the telescoping full arch TRINIA® bridge prosthesis. Starting to load

The 2-year recall revealed both the clinical and radiological aspects to be a good result with no functional difficulties (Figs. 12.49 and 12.50).

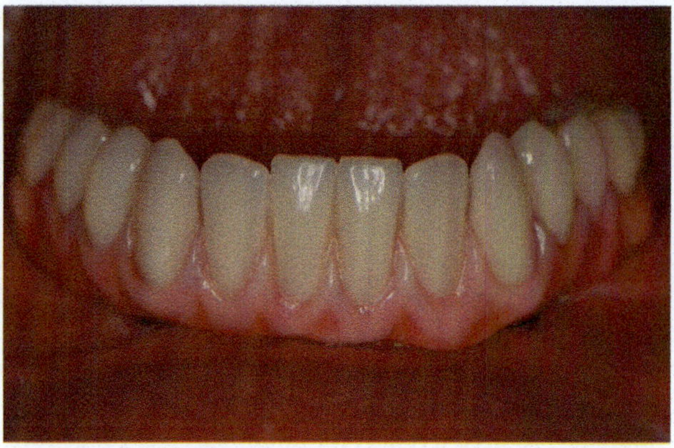

Fig. 12.49 Intraoral view of the full arch TRINIA® prosthesis at 2-year recall

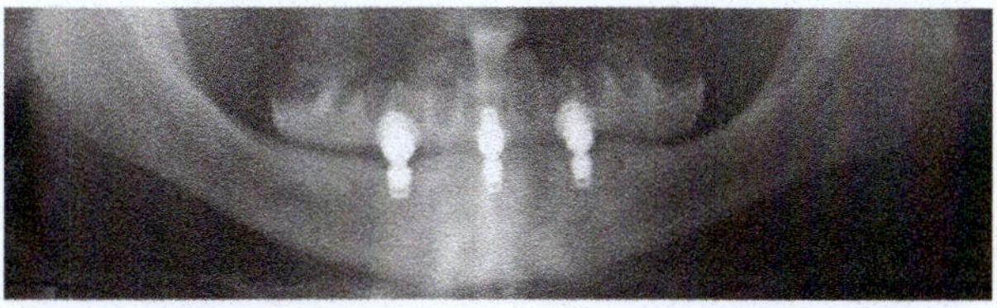

Fig. 12.50 Panoramic radiograph at 2-year recall

12.4 Summary and Conclusion

These studies in the maxilla and mandible showed the efficacy of treating patients with extreme maxillary atrophy without costly and time-consuming augmentation procedures by using ultrashort 4.0 × 5.0 mm, 4.5 × 6.0 mm, and narrow 3.0 × 8.0 mm implants. Implants were restored with prostheses of metal-free CAD/CAM-produced fiber-reinforced hybrid resin material TRINIA®. The survival rates of these Bicon SHORT® implants are comparable to those of conventional long implants. This demonstrates that it is possible to treat highly atrophic jaw with ultrashort and narrow implants using only four, three, or even only one implant.
The results are comparable to studies by other authors. Furthermore, this study shows that restorations with a metal-free CAD/CAM-produced fiber-reinforced hybrid resin material does not lead to any complications. These results for the maxilla and mandible are very encouraging, since also the extreme maxillary atrophy only required the use of SHORT® implants and in the thin alveolar crest narrow implants with an alveolar ridge splitting procedure. The placement of ultra-SHORT® implants required a relatively minor surgical procedure when compared to extensive bone grafting procedures prior to implant placement. Additionally, the postsurgical recovery was usually easier and the cost savings to the patient were considerable.

References

1. Wolff J. The law of bone remodeling. Berlin: Springer; 1986 (translation of the German 1892 edition).
2. Frost HM. Wolff's law and bone's structural adaptations to mechanical usage: an overview for clinicians. Angle Orthod. 1994;64(3):175–88.
3. Wolff J. The classic: on the inner architecture of bones and its importance for bone growth. Clin Orthop Relat Res. 2010;468(4):1056–65.
4. Atwood DA. Postextraction changes in the adult mandible as illustrated by microradiographs of midsagittal sections and serial cephalometric roentgenograms. J Prosthet Dent. 1963;13:810–24.
5. Atwood DA. Reduction of residual ridges: a major oral disease entity. J Prosthet Dent. 1973;17:747–54.
6. Cawood JL, Howell RA. A classification of the edentulous jaws. Int J Oral Maxillofac Surg. 1988;17:232–6.
7. Tatum H. Lecture presented to the Alabama Implant Congress 1976.
8. Tatum H. Maxillary and sinus implant reconstruction. Dent Clin N Am. 1986;30(2):207–29.
9. Boyne PJ, James RA. Grafting of the maxillary sinus floor with autogenous marrow and bone. J Oral Surg. 1980;38(8):613–6.
10. Buser D, Brägger U, Lang NP, Nyman S. Regeneration and enlargement of jaw bone using guided tissue regeneration. Clin Oral Implants Res. 1990;1(1):22–32.
11. Watzinger F, Ewers R, Millesi W, Kirsch A, Glaser C, Ackerman KL. Horseshoe LeFort I osteotomy in conjunction with endosteal implants—a medium term follow up study. Int Oral Maxillofac Surg. 1966;25(6):424–9.
12. Ewers R. Maxilla sinus grafting with marine algae derived bone forming material: a clinical report of long term results. J Oral Maxillofac Surg. 2005;63(12):1712–23.
13. Malevez C, Daeleman P, Adriaenssens P, Durdu F. Use of zygomatic implants to deal with resorbed posterior maxillae. Periodontology. 2000;33(1):82–9.

14. Maló P, Rangert B, Nobre M. 'All-on-Four' immediate-function concept with Brånemark system implants for completely edentulous mandibles: a retrospective clinical study. Clin Implant Dent Relat Res. 2003;5:2–9.
15. Summers R. A new concept in maxillary implant surgery: the osteotome technique. Compendium. 1994;15(2):152–4.
16. Bairdi H, Schulte J, Kovacs A, Weed M, Chuang SK. Crown-to-implant ratio of short length implants. J Oral Implantol. 2010;36:425–33.
17. Atieh MA, Zadeh H, Atanford C, Cooper L. Survival of short dental implants for treatment of posterior partial edentulism: a systematic review. Int J Oral Maxillofac Implants. 2012;27:1323–31.
18. Hadzik J, Krawiec M, Slawecki K, Kunert-Keil C, Dominak M, Gedrange T. The influence of the crown-implant ratio on the crestal bone level and implant secondary stability—36 month clinical study. BioMed Res Int. 2018; Article ID 4246874.
19. Bevilacqua M, Tealdo T, Pera F, Menini M, Mossolov A, Drago C, Pera P. Three-dimensional finite element analysis of load transmission using different implant inclinations and cantilever lengths. Int J Prosthodont. 2008;21(6):539–42.
20. Fischer K, Stenberg T. Three year data from a randomized, controlled study of early loading of single stage dental implants supporting maxillary full arch prostheses. Int J Oral Maxillofac Implants. 2006;21(2):245–52.
21. Heydecke G, Zwahlen M, Nicol H, Nisand D, et al. What is the optimal number of implants for fixed reconstructions: a systematic review. Clin Oral Implants Res. 2012;23(Suppl 6):217–28.
22. Lehrberg J, Coehlo P. Biologic response to dental implants. In: Morgan V, editor. The Bicon short implant. Chicago: Quintessence Publishing; 2017. p. 37–47.
23. Wagner F, Seemann R, Marincola M, Ewers R. Fixed, fiber-reinforced resin fixed prostheses on four short implants in severely atrophic maxillas: 1-year results of a prospective cohort study. J Oral Maxillofac Surg. 2018;76(6):1194–9. https://doi.org/10.1016/j.joms.2018.02.001. Epub 2018 Feb 19.
24. Seemann R, Wagner F, Marincola M, Ewers R. Fixed, fiber-reinforced resin bridges on 5.0-mm implants in severely atrophic mandibles: Up to 5 years' follow-up of a prospective cohort study. J Oral Maxillofac Surg. 2017. pii: S0278–2391(17)31465–9. https://doi.org/10.1016/j.joms.2017.11.043.

Restorative Techniques for Bicon Short® Implants

13

Kristina Pisarik, Angelo Perpetuini, Laura Murcko, Katherine Morgan, Drauseo Speratti, Muneki Hirayama, and Jordyn Hollingsworth

K. Pisarik
Bicon, Boston, MA, USA

Implant Dentistry Centre, Boston, MA, USA

A. Perpetuini (✉)
Master Dental Technician, Bicon, Rome, Italy

Dental Laboratory, Rome, Italy
e-mail: pperpetuini@bicon.com

L. Murcko · K. Morgan
Implant Dentistry Centre, Boston, MA, USA
e-mail: lmurcko@bicon.com; kmorgan@idcboston.com

D. Speratti
Bicon, Boston, MA, USA

Midwestern University College of Dental Medicine, Glendale, AZ, USA

Midwestern University College of Dental Medicine, Downers Grove, IL, USA
e-mail: dsperatti@bicon.com

M. Hirayama
Implant Dentistry Centre, Boston, MA, USA

Bicon, Tokyo, Japan
e-mail: mhirayama@bicon.com

J. Hollingsworth
Midwestern University College of Dental Medicine, Downers Grove, IL, USA
e-mail: jhollingsworth42@midwestern.edu

B. J. Tomasetti, R. Ewers (eds.), *Short Implants*,
https://doi.org/10.1007/978-3-030-44199-9_13

Contents

13.1 Crown-to-Implant Ratio 206
13.2 Factors of Bone Gain Versus Bone Loss 208
13.3 Bicon Restorations: Design and Technique 211
13.4 Single-Unit Restorations 214
13.5 Prosthetic Restorations and TRINIA® 274
13.6 Conclusion 311
References 313

Although the restorative stage may be considered by some clinicians to be the easiest stage of an implant treatment, care and precision must not be overlooked. To hasten through the final restorative phase would be to negate previous efforts, such as the tissue-preserving incisions for anterior crowns at the uncovering stage. The crown is the only visible part of an implant for patients, thus the aesthetics are critical in terms of patients' concerns; however, in addition to the importance of a restoration's appearance is its functionality. The appropriate seating of a crown into its implant is integral to its prosthetic mechanics, which in turn influences the success of the implant, since it is the implant that depends on the restoration to transfer occlusal forces to the surrounding bone.

In terms of Bicon SHORT® Implants, the restorative stage is simplified through the cementless and screwless properties of the implant-abutment connection, and the 360 degrees of abutment positioning. Additionally, the design feature of the locking taper implant-abutment-interface (IAI) creates a bacterial seal, which prevents contamination of the implant well and micro-movement of the abutment. Although Bicon has offered a range of abutments varying in shape and size, the most versatile and most commonly used is the Universal Abutment. The height of the Universal Abutment prosthetic post is 4.0 mm, which offers adequate stability to support any restoration, yet maintains as much space as possible for the optional addition of material for aesthetics. Possibly the most effective aspect of the Universal Abutment is its hemispheric base: With its geometry modeled after that of a natural tooth, it has the capability to create a similar emergence profile, allowing for soft tissues to grow in their usual manner.

Before delving too deeply into the advantages of Bicon-specific restorations, it is important to understand the techniques involved with short implant restorations, and how and why those restorations work.

13.1 Crown-to-Implant Ratio

The most jarring imagery that some new users of short implants struggle to come to terms with is that of a little implant holding a restoration potentially five times its length or more. It may seem like a counterintuitive idea, but the crown-to-implant ratio (CIR) is not a direct conversion of the crown-to-root ratio (CRR)

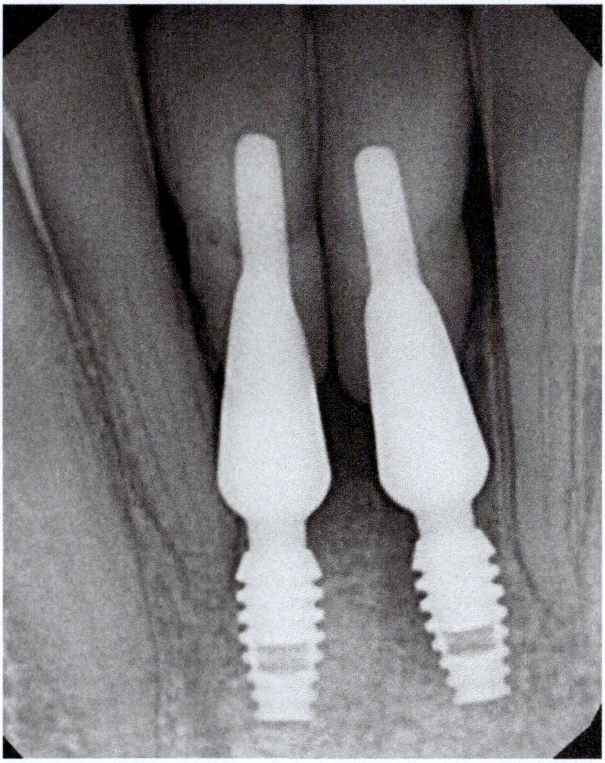

Fig. 13.1 Post-insertion radiograph of two implants with a crown-to-implant ratio (CIR) of 3.0 mm

[1]. The CRR is a standard 1:2 ratio with the root at twice the length of the crown; however, there are variables such as the bone and periodontal ligament, which can sustain an increase in occlusal forces without fracturing the tooth. Up to a certain point, bone will adapt to the increased stresses distributed by the periodontal ligament by growing thicker and denser—that is, in the absence of periodontal disease. In the case of periodontal disease, increased occlusal stresses will result in bone loss, which is why increased occlusal stresses are often regarded in a negative way.

Likewise, the large CIR of short implants receives skepticism despite radiographic evidence proving otherwise (Figs. 13.1 and 13.2). Furthermore, it is harder to extract an ankylosed tooth with a 3.0 mm root than it is to extract a tooth with a 28 mm root, and a deciduous molar with only a 3.0 mm root can function for decades. The same process of bone adaptation that occurs when a natural tooth free of periodontal disease experiences an increase in occlusal forces also occurs for bone surrounding an implant. If the forces were to exceed the implant's limitation, it would not result in bone loss; rather, the material of the crown may fracture, as would the crown of a natural tooth. Furthermore, bone needs to be continuously stimulated in order to remain strong, so it is a specious notion that an increased load on an implant would be detrimental to the bone [2]. In fact, studies have shown a correlation between implants with increased loading and crestal

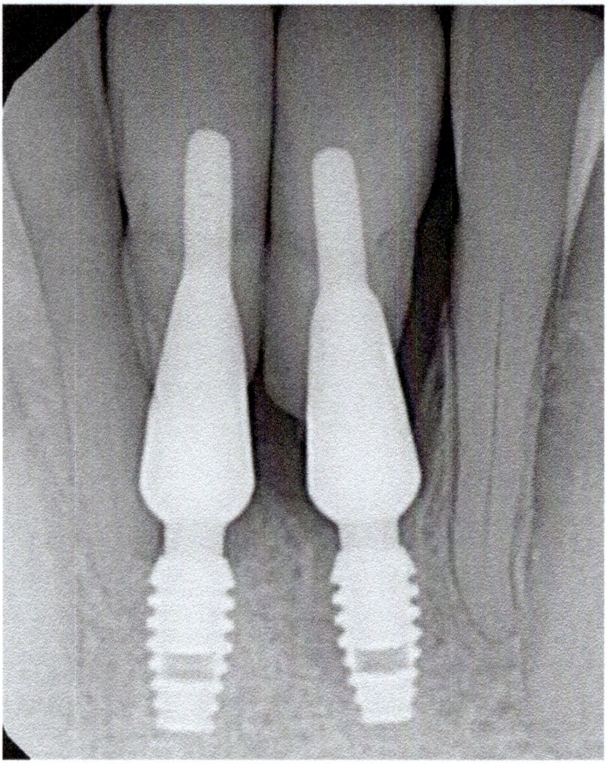

Fig. 13.2 1.5-year post-insertion radiograph of bone gain around two implants with a CIR of 3.0 mm

bone growth [3, 4]. Figures 13.3 and 13.4 present the resultant bone gain around short implants after years with a CIR of 2 or more. Despite several positive findings among short implants, it is important to note that not all implants will have the same effect on bone [5]. Variables such as implant design, size, and material can all factor into the gain or loss of bone, as found in a multivariate analysis by Urdaneta et al. [6].

13.2 Factors of Bone Gain Versus Bone Loss

Material is perhaps the most obvious factor in affecting bone levels, but it is fortunately not an irreversible one in cases of bone loss. Where titanium has been associated with reports of bone growth, composite has conversely been associated with bone loss. Thus, it is critical that the titanium base of an abutment not be covered with composite material for aesthetic purposes; an exposed metal margin is not as dire as bone loss. However, should composite on an implant's abutment base have a deleterious effect on the bone, the abutment can be easily replaced and bone potentially regained.

Another variable that the aforementioned study found to be associated with bone gain is an implant coating of hydroxyapatite (HA), the calcium phosphate (CP), and

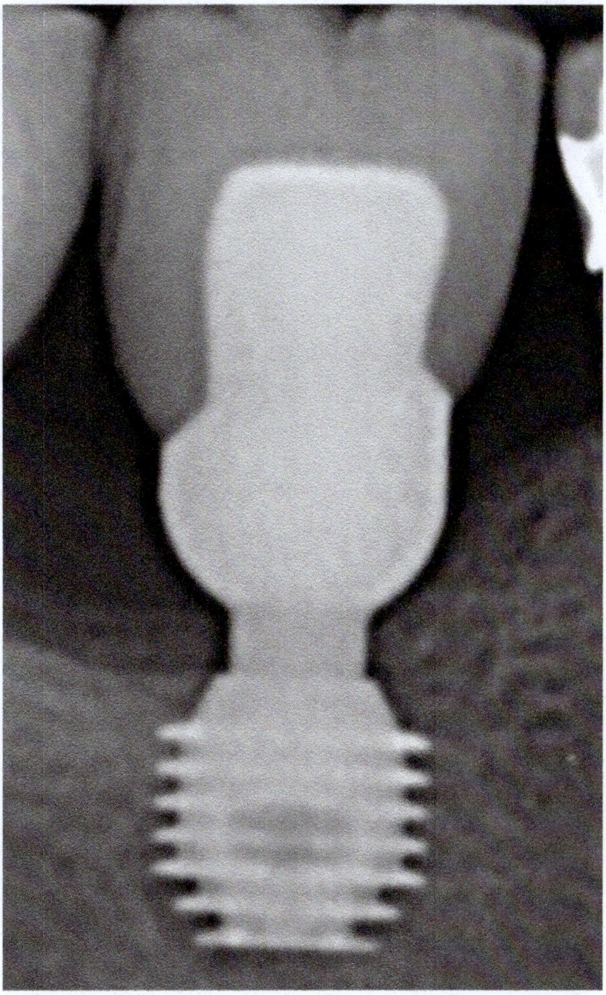

Fig. 13.3 Post-insertion radiograph of an implant with a CIR of 2.0 mm

primary mineral found in natural teeth. Considering that HA is naturally occurring in teeth and bone, it is reasonable to believe that HA- or CP-coated implants would have a positive influence on the surrounding bone. This idea is supported by long-term clinical evidence of the multivariate investigation, which found bone gain to take place specifically after the implant's crown insertion, as well as by several studies [7–10]; however, another factor to be considered in conjunction with the HA coating is the implant design [11, 12]. For example, the plateau root form design of the Bicon implant preserves the HA coating because only the tips of its fins come into contact with the osteotomy or extraction socket during implant placement (Figs. 13.5 and 13.6) [4]. Not only does the design of the finned implant disrupt less bone during placement, but its conservation of the HA coating maximizes the bone's mineralization.

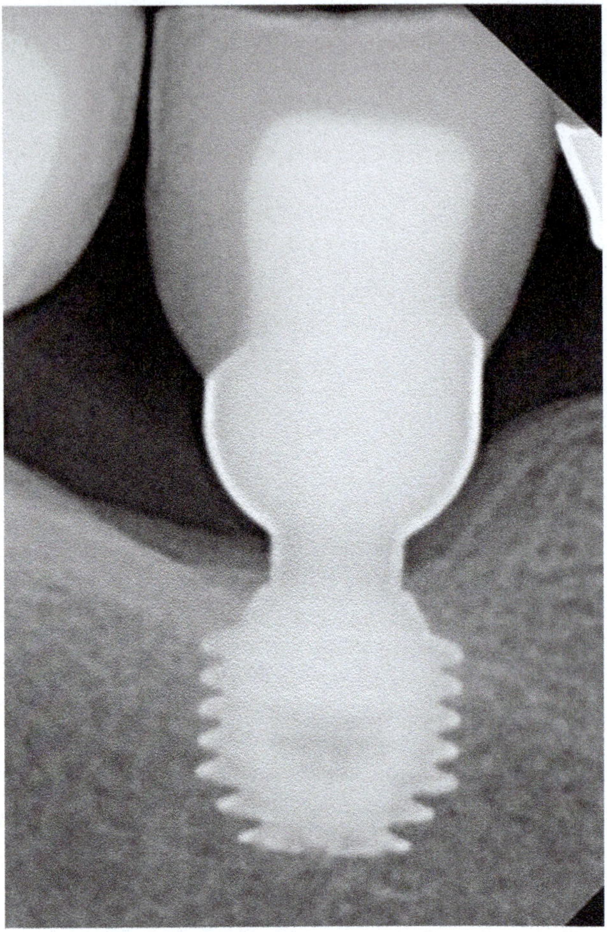

Fig. 13.4 Seven-year post-insertion radiograph of bone gain around an implant with a CIR of 2.0 mm

In addition to the design of the implant, the design of the abutment is an important factor to be considered for affecting bone levels. The hemispheric base of the Bicon abutment has been consistently present in reports of bone gain. The geometry of this design causes compressive forces to be transmitted to the bone around the implant-abutment interface in a phenomenon known as platform switching [13]. As stated previously, increased loading of a short implant in a healthy mouth is not harmful to the bone and can even provide the stimulation necessary to maintain its strength. The hemispheric base works in such a way that it distributes the occlusal forces around the implant rather than absorbing excessive impact at one point.

Size (of the implant and the abutment) is another source to be considered with bone gain and loss. Clinical evidence of the multivariate analysis suggests that bone responds better to shorter implants than it does to longer implants (Figs. 13.7, 13.8, and 13.9); however, it also indicates that the optimal size of an implant depends on the area that it is placed in the mouth [4]. No matter the implant's location, the

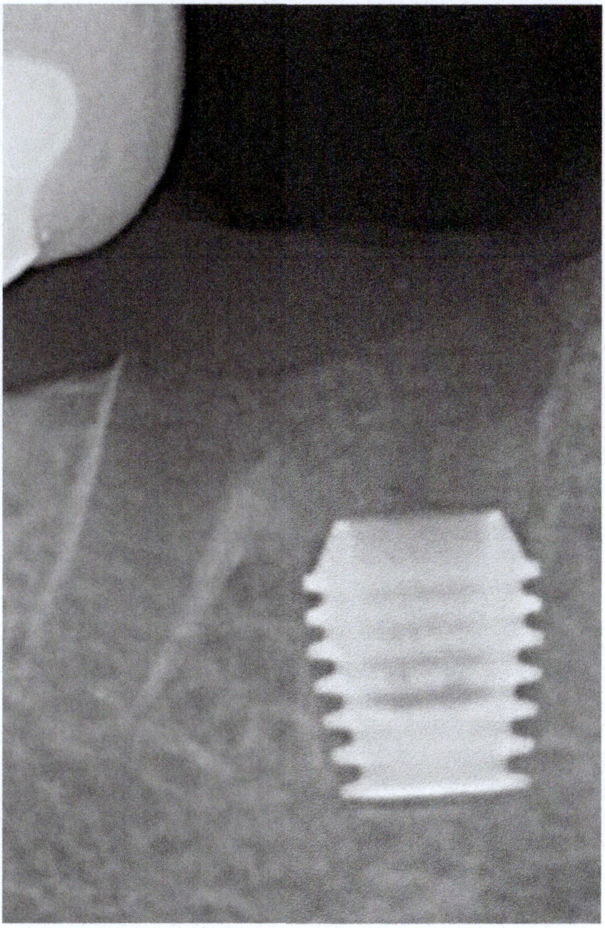

Fig. 13.5 Postoperative radiograph of a plateau-root form implant seated in an extraction socket. Note that only the tips of the fins touch the socket walls, since the implant was tapped in without torque, preserving the HA coating of the implant

minimal size capable of withstanding the masticatory forces is preferable, as it means less disruption of the bone. Bone preservation must be prioritized; therefore, steps should be taken from the beginning of the procedure to ensure a result of bone gain rather than bone loss.

13.3 Bicon Restorations: Design and Technique

For more than 30 years, Bicon implants have been known for their short and "ultra-short" sizes, and their screwless and cementless restorative system. The 1.5° locking taper implant-abutment connection can eliminate the risk of extraneous cement leaking into the area surrounding the implant by the extraoral cementation of the crowns. The single-unit integrated abutment crown (IAC) is another restoration that provides for the avoidance of intraoral cementation and extraneous cement. The

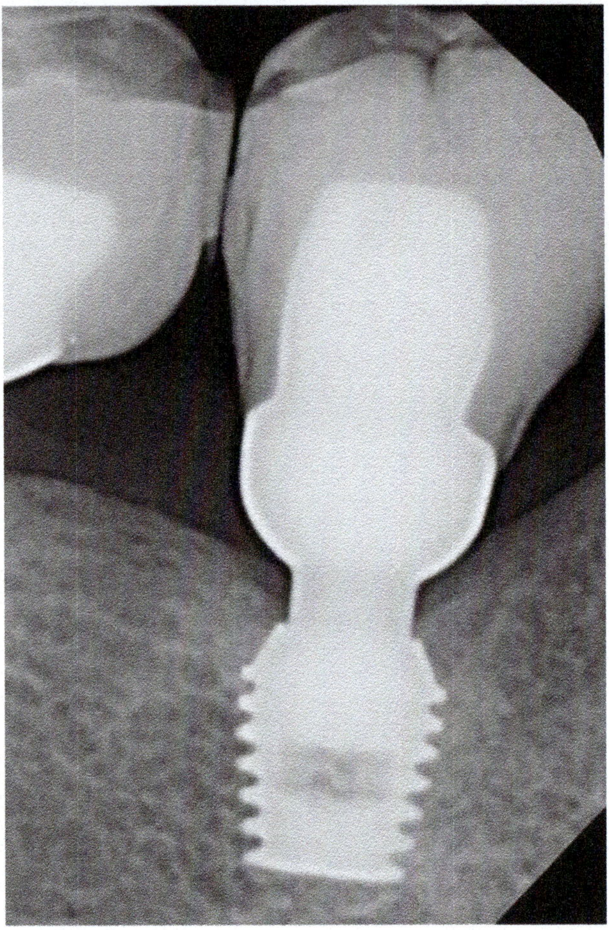

Fig. 13.6 Four-year postoperative radiograph of a plateau-root form implant with bone gain between the fins of the implant

IAC is comprised of an abutment and layers of polyceramic material bonded together by chemical agents. The single-unit IAC offers 360° of universal positioning, as well as the capability for its polyceramic material to be readily modified chairside. The Bicon implant-abutment is comprised of a two-part, locking taper and bacterially sealed connection between the implant and abutment-crown. Although the connection is simple, it is essential that the restorative steps be followed with knowledge and care. For this reason, in the remainder of this chapter we will discuss the basic restorative techniques for the Bicon system, from single-unit restorations to full arch prostheses.

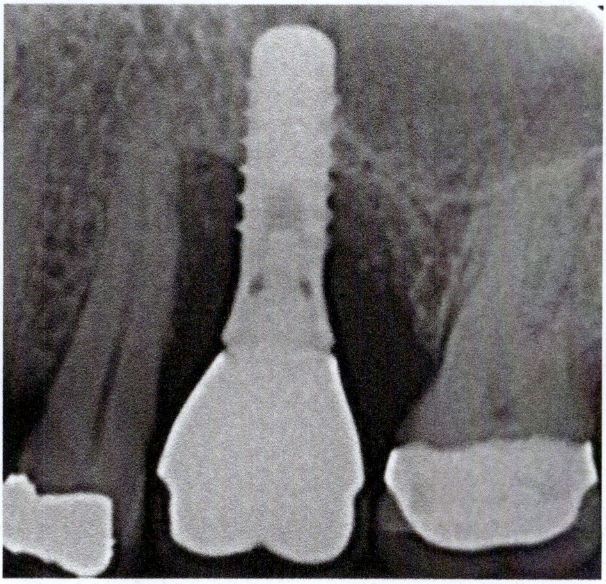

Fig. 13.7 Radiograph of bone loss around a ~4.1 × 12 mm screw-retained implant prior to its explant and replacement by a 6.0 × 5.7 mm HA-coated implant 5 months later

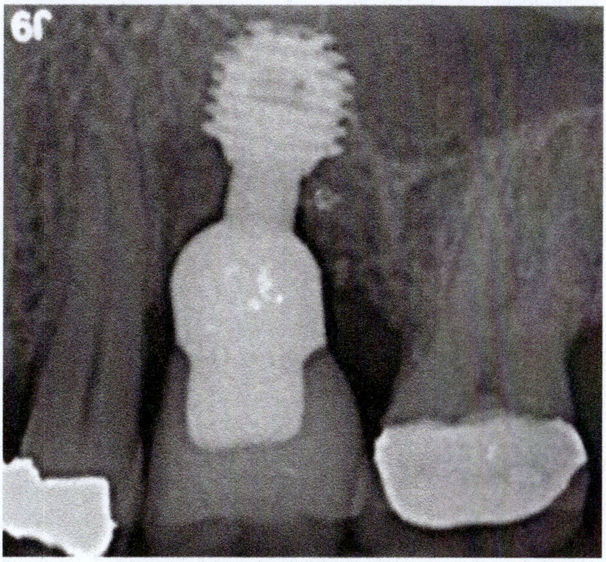

Fig. 13.8 Post-insertion radiograph of a 6.0 × 5.7 mm HA-coated implant with its crown

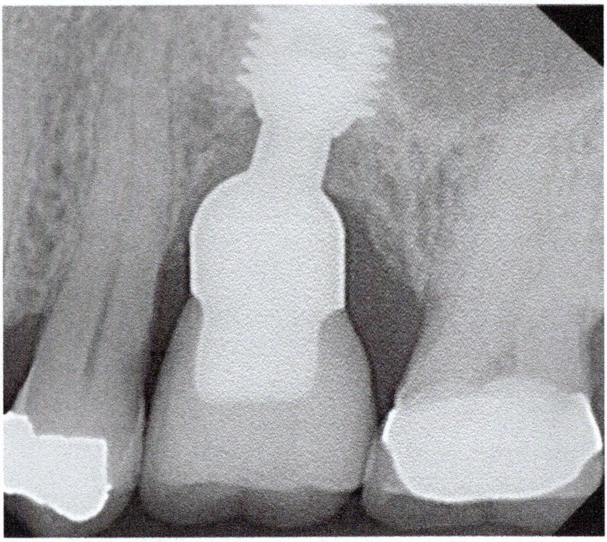

Fig. 13.9 2.8-year post-insertion radiograph of bone gain around a 6.0 × 5.7 mm HA-coated implant and its crown

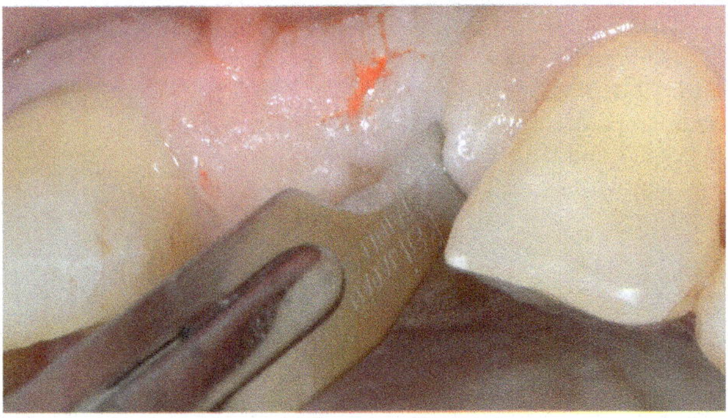

Fig. 13.10 A slight incision is being made to facilitate the uncovering of the implant

13.4 Single-Unit Restorations

The first restorative step for the two-stage technique begins at the second-stage surgical visit, usually 3–4 months after the implant placement, when the implant is uncovered. Once a Bicon implant is uncovered, the black polyethylene plug, which was inserted into the implant well at the time of placement, is removed (Figs. 13.10 and 13.11). After the removal of the healing plug, a guide pin is inserted into the implant well to confirm osseointegration of the implant by being grasped and moved apically and laterally (Fig. 13.12). Lateral movement of the guide pin indicates that additional time may be needed for osseointegration, whereas apical or vertical movement indicates that the implant is not integrated and should be removed.

After the implant's stability has been confirmed, a sulcus former of the same diameter as the intended abutment should be rotated around the guide pin to remove any interfering soft and hard tissues (Figs. 13.13 and 13.14). Sulcus formers can be

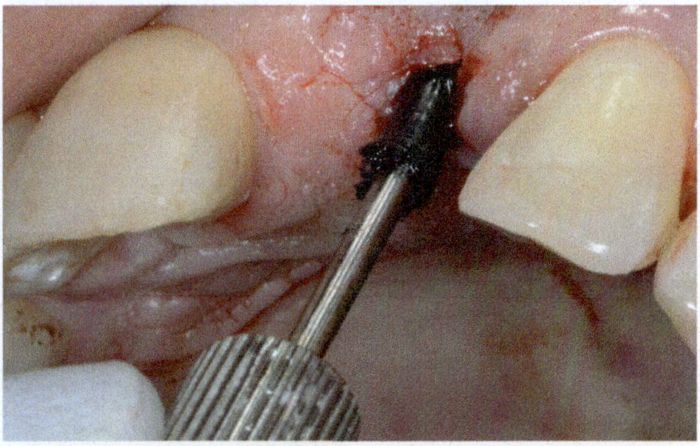

Fig. 13.11 A healing plug removal instrument is being used to retrieve the polyethylene healing plug from the well of the implant

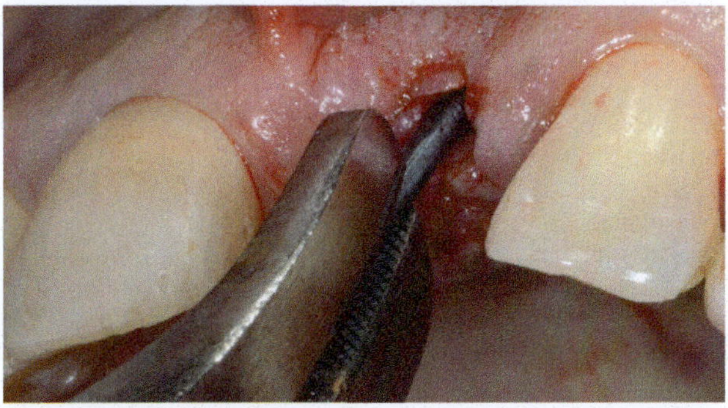

Fig. 13.12 Carbide tips are being used to pull on the guide pin to confirm the implant's osseointegration

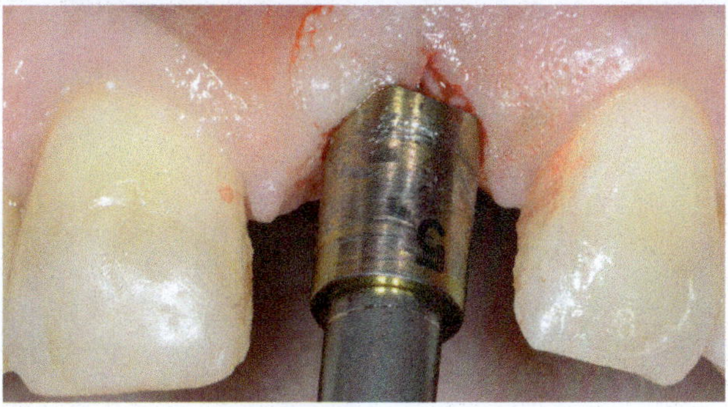

Fig. 13.13 A gold 5.0 mm sulcus former is being rotated on a guide pin to shape the sulcus to the diameter of the intended abutment

attached to a threaded handle, a threaded instrument adapter, or a threaded knob, which is often more appropriate for posterior areas (Fig. 13.15). An occlusal registration and full arch impression is then ready to be made using one of five techniques: conventional or digital implant-level, and direct (without a sleeve), indirect (with a sleeve), or digital abutment-level. A conventional implant-level impression is the most commonly used technique, involving a titanium impression post seated in the well of the implant, capped with an acrylic impression sleeve (Figs. 13.16 and 13.17).

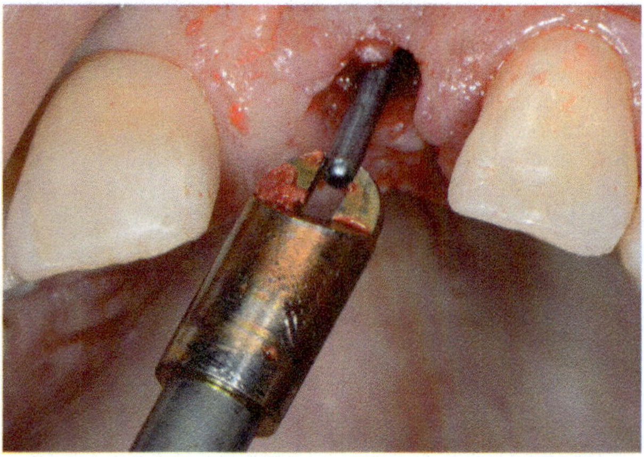

Fig. 13.14 A gold 5.0 mm sulcus former removes soft and hard tissues from the implant well

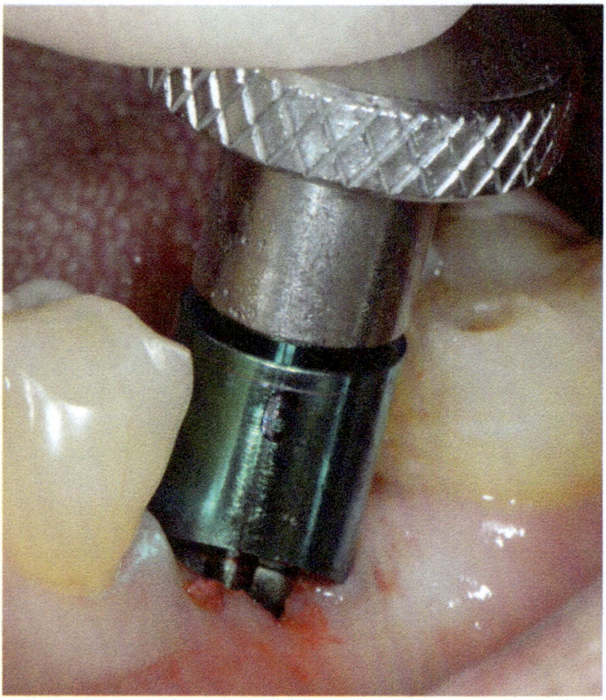

Fig. 13.15 A green 6.0 mm sulcus former attached to a threaded knob is being used for a mandibular posterior implant

Impression material is injected around the sleeve and post before a full tray of impression material is inserted for 4 min (Fig. 13.18). Once the impression material hardens, the tray is removed and the acrylic sleeve—captured within the impression—is lifted off of the impression post (Fig. 13.19). If the impression post were to be removed with the acrylic sleeve, another impression must be taken to ensure an accurate recording of the implant's position. This same technique is used for the occlusal registration,

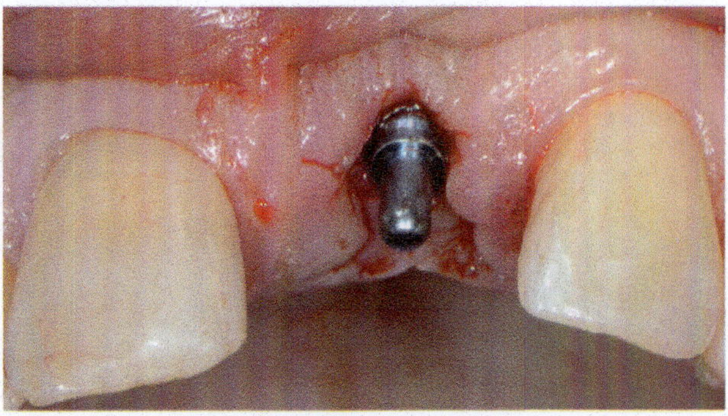

Fig. 13.16 A blue 2.0 mm titanium impression post is seated in the well of an implant for the fabrication of a conventional implant-level impression

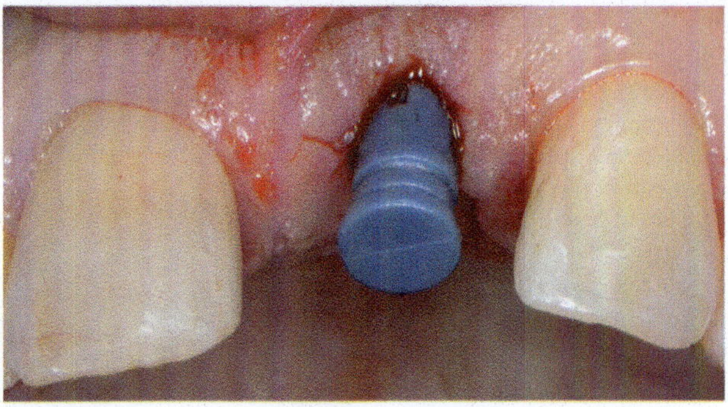

Fig. 13.17 A blue acrylic impression sleeve is seated on its impression post

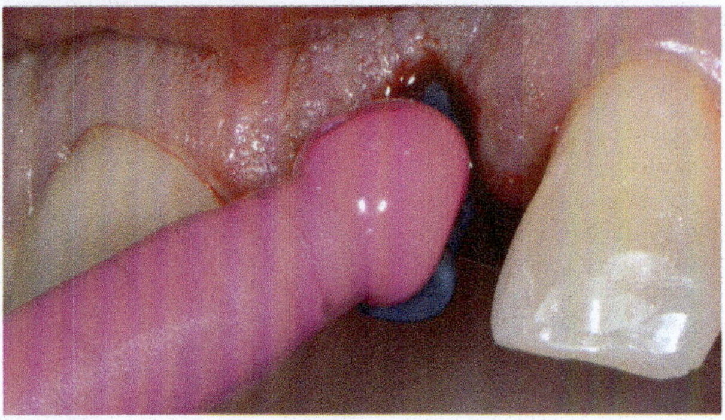

Fig. 13.18 Impression material is being applied around the impression sleeve

although the occlusal registration material is applied all along the occlusal surface of the arch before the patient is asked to close on it for approximately 30 s. An abutment-level impression works in a similar manner, but instead of an impression post, a Universal Abutment (of the same size and profile to be used for the IAC) is seated in the well of the implant alone (to be impressed directly), or capped by an abutment-level impression sleeve (to be impressed indirectly) (Figs. 13.20, 13.21, 13.22, and 13.23). Digital impressions require a bit more equipment and diligence. Similarly to the impression post, a scan flag or an abutment is inserted into the implant. The flag is

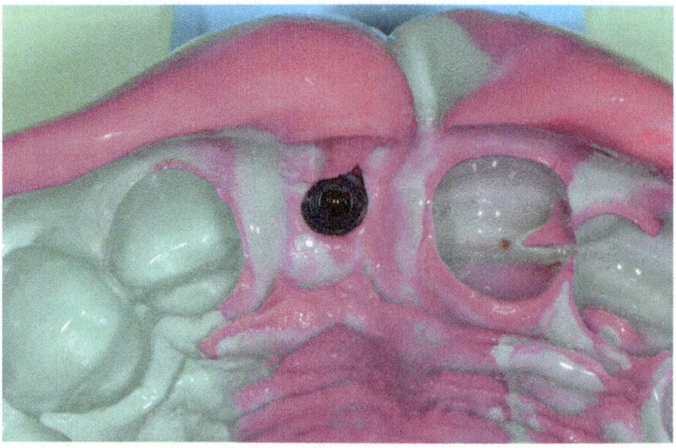

Fig. 13.19 A blue impression sleeve is captured within a full arch implant-level transfer impression

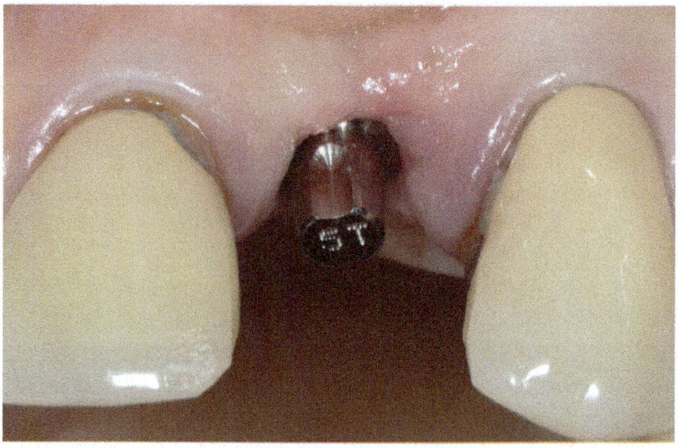

Fig. 13.20 A 5 Tall Profile (5T) Universal Abutment is seated in the well of an implant for the fabrication of an indirect abutment-level impression

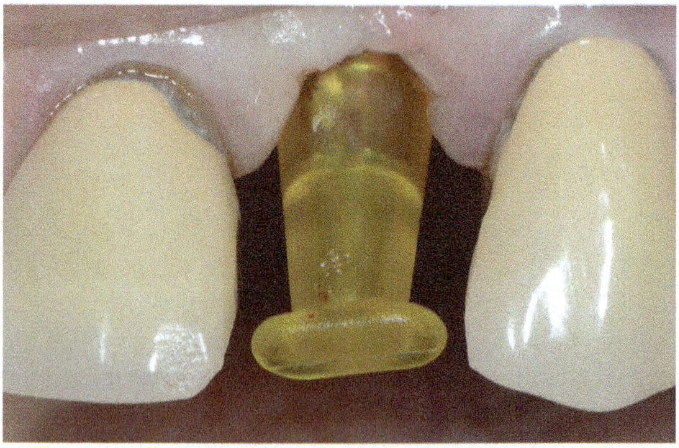

Fig. 13.21 A yellow 5-5T Universal Abutment impression sleeve is seated on its Universal Abutment

scanned by means of a scanning instrument, which is connected to a computer with corresponding scanning software. Once the scanning is initiated, the instrument must be moved all around the area of the flag and its adjacent teeth as the instrument

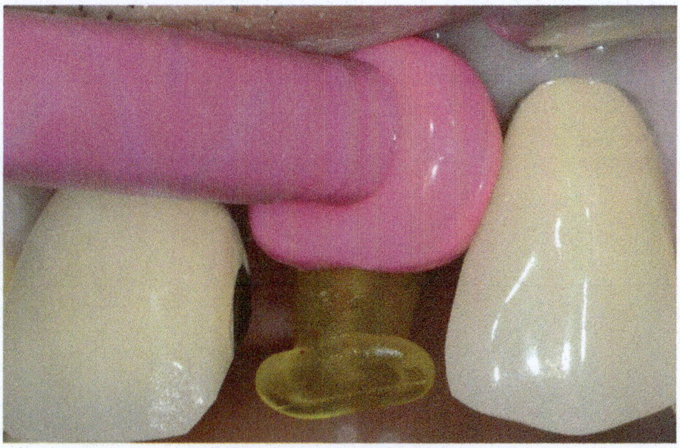

Fig. 13.22 Impression material is being applied around the impression sleeve

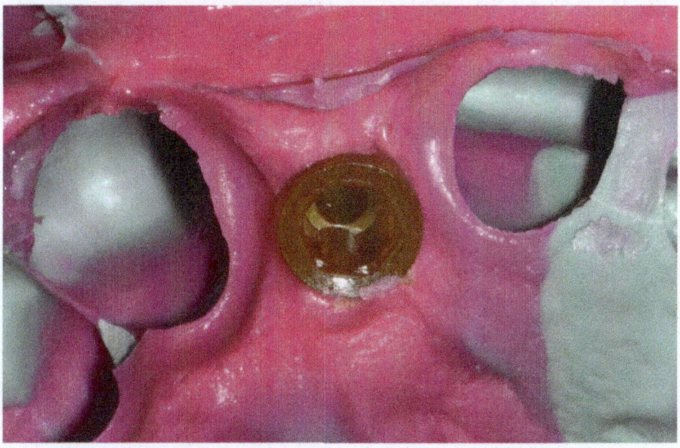

Fig. 13.23 A yellow Universal Abutment impression sleeve is captured within a full arch indirect abutment-level transfer impression

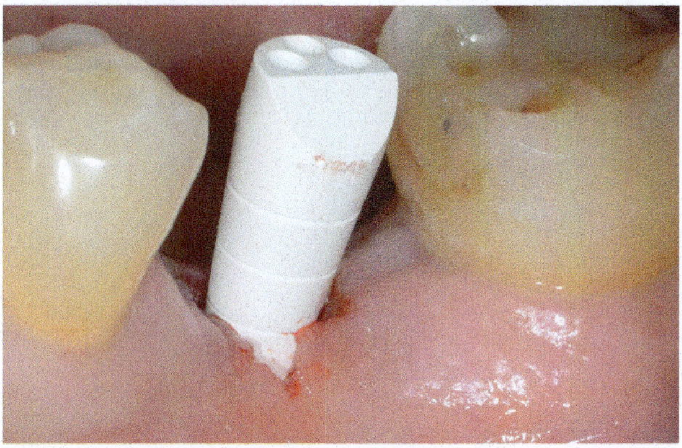

Fig. 13.24 A digital scan flag is seated in the well of an implant for the fabrication of a digital implant-level impression

automatically records images (Figs. 13.24 and 13.25). It is best to capture the three-dimensional image of the flag in as few images as possible to send unambiguous data for the software to process. An advantage of digital scanning is that the image can be

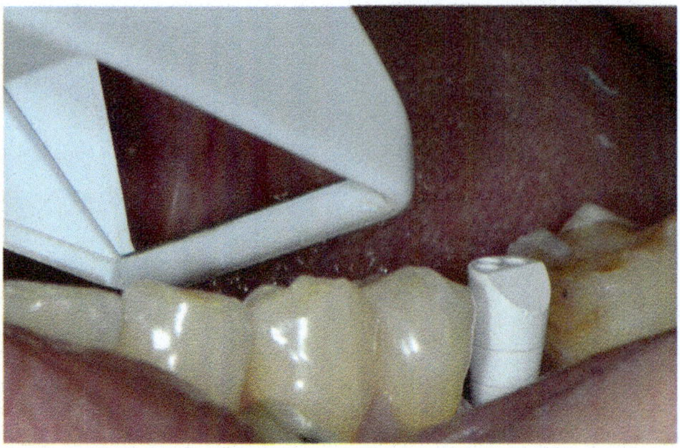

Fig. 13.25 A scanning instrument is being moved around as it automatically records images of the scan flag

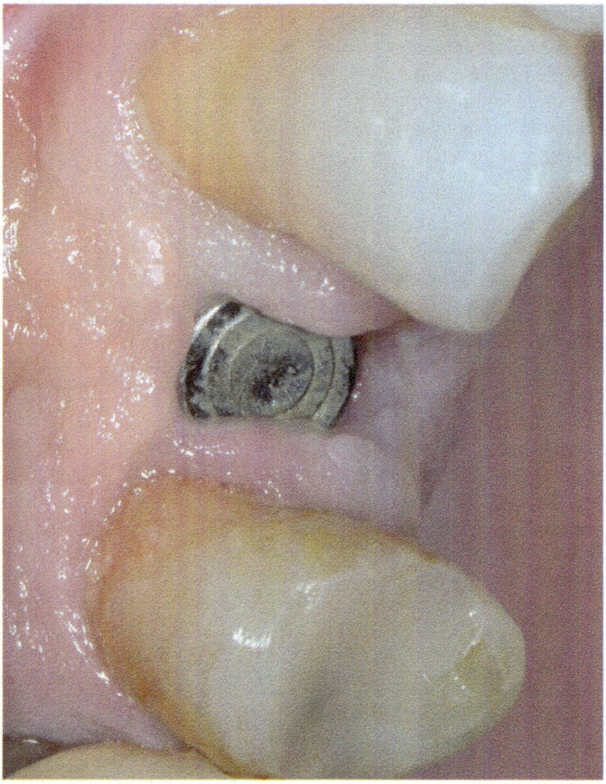

Fig. 13.26 A titanium temporary abutment is seated in an implant prior to its removal

sent directly from the scanning software to CAD/CAM milling software; however, the time saved in delivery is only efficient if the scanning itself takes 4 min or less and results in as accurate a scan image as a physical transfer impression.

Once the laboratory has fabricated an IAC based on the impression, the restorative visit can be scheduled. The IAC may be inserted immediately upon removal of the temporary abutment, which can be either twisted or tapped out with forceps (Figs. 13.26, 13.27, and 13.28). If tissue interference is suspected, a sulcus former

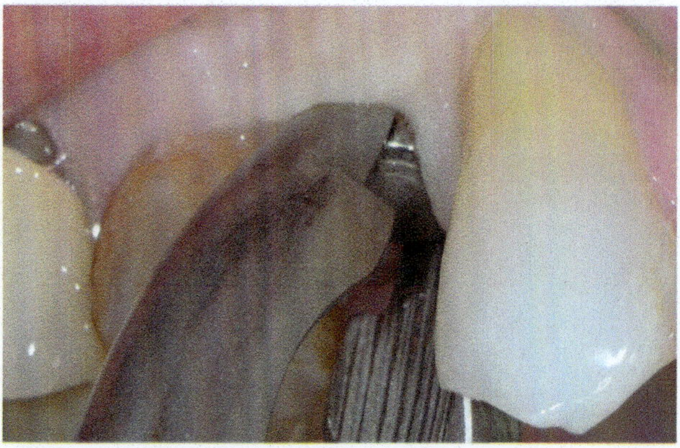

Fig. 13.27 Forceps grip the hemispheric edge of the temporary abutment to remove it from its implant

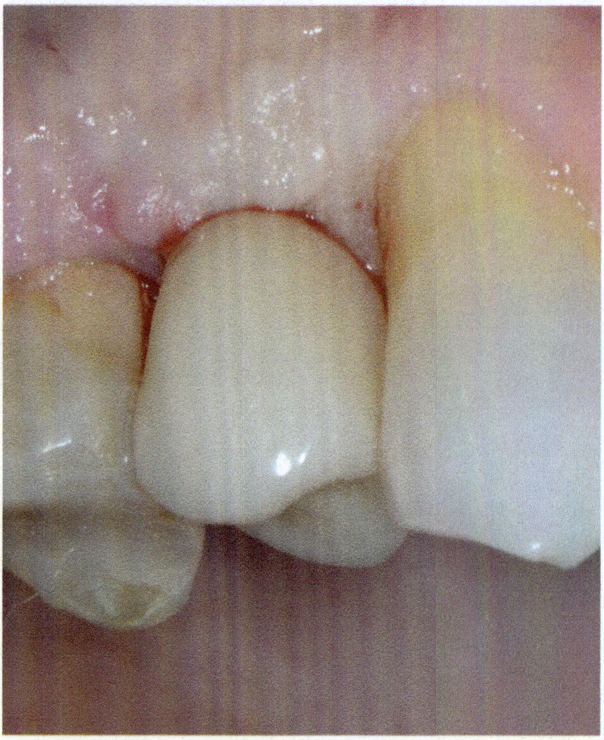

Fig. 13.28 Blanching is evident upon insertion of the crown, indicating a need to remove impinging tissues from the sulcus

may be rotated on a guide pin in the well of the implant, as was done at the uncovering stage. After all of the impinging tissue has been removed, the IAC may be inserted (Figs. 13.29 and 13.30). Initially, finger pressure can be used to insert the IAC, but it must also be tapped or occlusal pressure applied to affirm definitive seating. For anterior implants, a thermoplastic resin orientation jig must be used to direct seating forces in the same trajectory of the implant prior to definitive seating. Definitive seating is performed through the use of a mallet tapped against a threaded handle, which is attached to a thermoplastic seating jig customized to fit into the

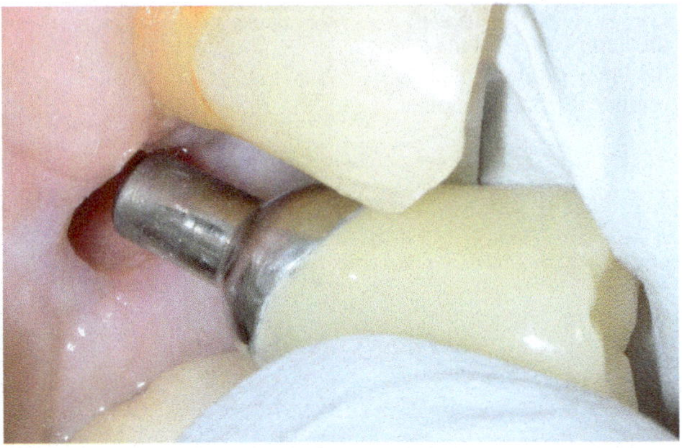

Fig. 13.29 An IAC is being inserted into a clean implant well

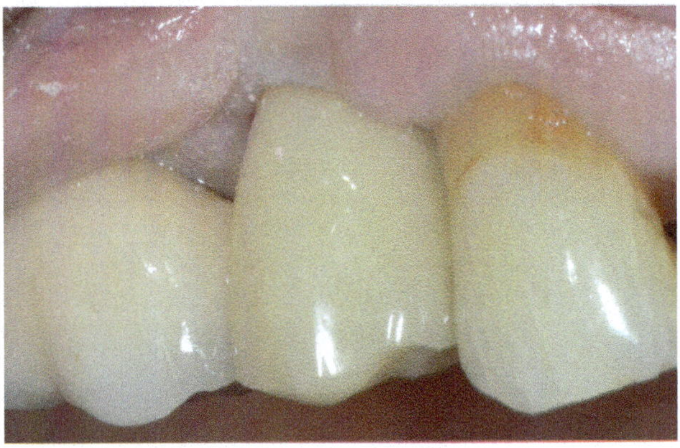

Fig. 13.30 View of an IAC immediately after its insertion

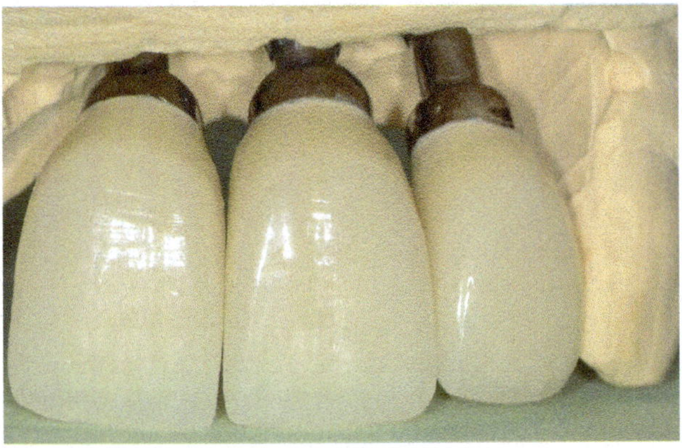

Fig. 13.31 Three anterior IACs seated in a stone model

incisal edge of the crown (Figs. 13.31, 13.32, 13.33, 13.34, 13.35, 13.36, and 13.37). The customized seating jig, fabricated from resin and using a crown alignment device, is an integral asset of the Bicon restorative process because it ensures that

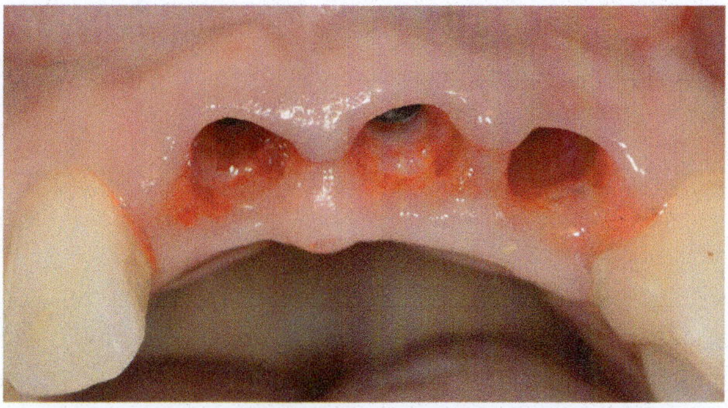

Fig. 13.32 View of three sulci

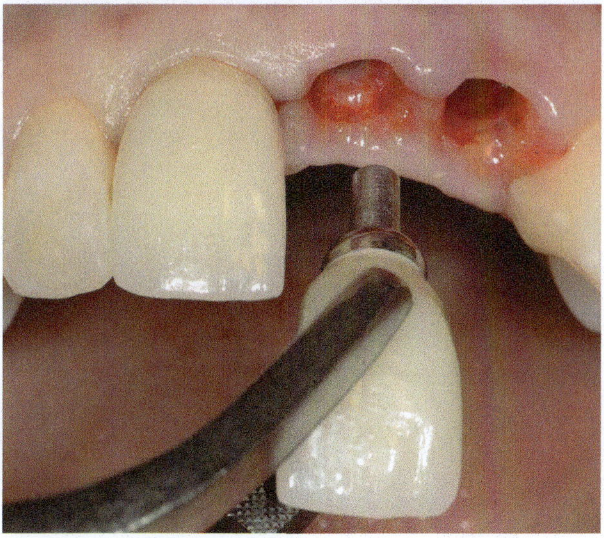

Fig. 13.33 An IAC is being inserted with carbide tips

the locking taper connection is engaged and that the seating forces are being distributed in the direction of the long axis of the implant and abutment. The laboratory procedure for fabricating a customized thermoplastic seating jig is addressed in detail in *The Bicon Short Implant*. For posterior cases, customized thermoplastic seating jigs are unnecessary for seating an IAC; instead, the patient can apply occlusal pressure on a cotton roll or a cotton tip applicator, and as an additional measure, a mallet can be used to tap a plastic abutment on a threaded handle in the direction of the long axis of the implant (Figs. 13.38 and 13.39).

As with any crown insertion, the interproximal and occlusal contacts should be verified after the definitive seating of the IAC. The interproximal contacts are usually addressed first, since they are significant indicators of whether the locking taper connection is fully engaged. The feel and sound of dental floss can indicate the status of the interproximal contacts. Due to the ease of polyceramic as a crown material, adjusting the contacts of an IAC is not a time-consuming issue: If the contacts are too passive, polyceramic material can be easily added to the IAC chairside,

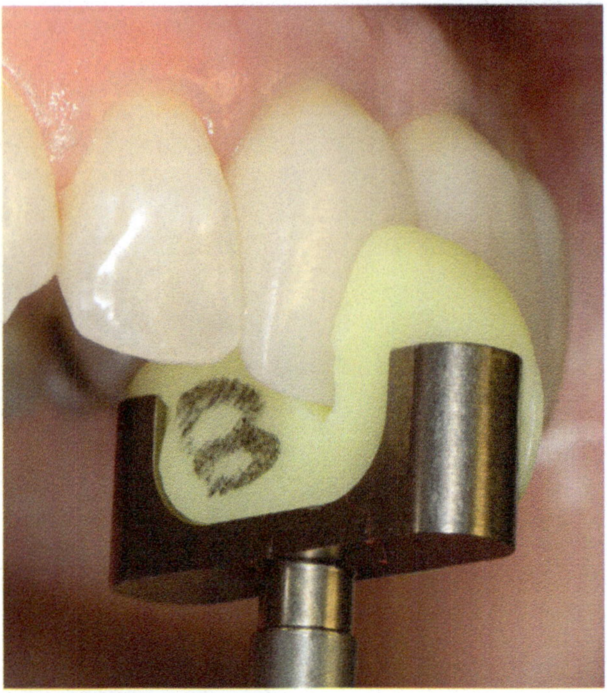

Fig. 13.34 A customized seating jig is being used to definitively seat the IAC for Tooth #8

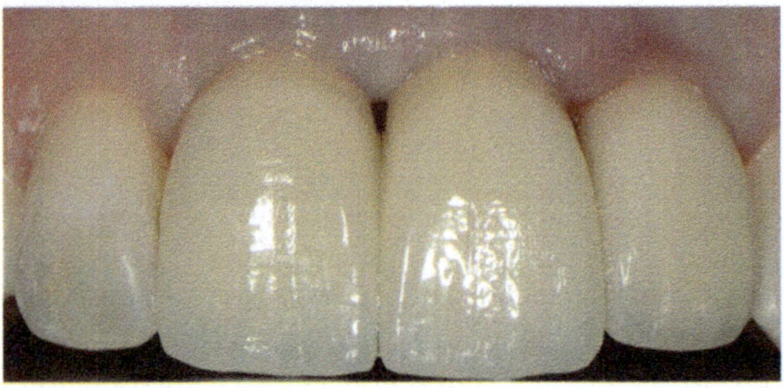

Fig. 13.35 Three definitively seated maxillary incisor IACs

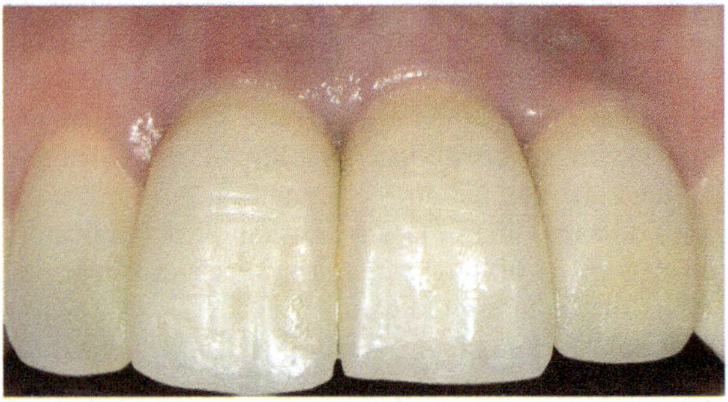

Fig. 13.36 One-year post-insertion view of three maxillary incisor IACs

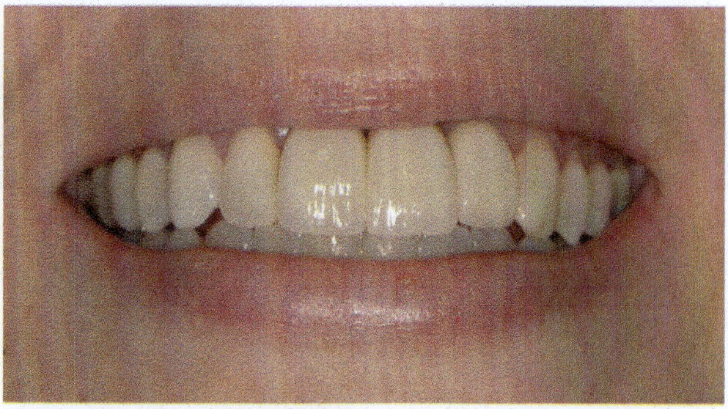

Fig. 13.37 Patient's smile with three maxillary incisor IACs

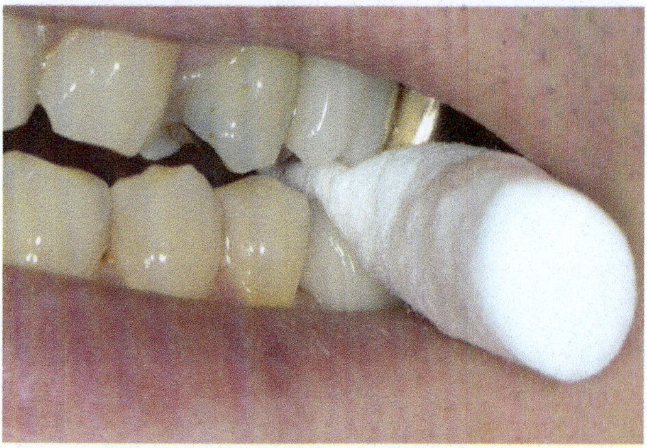

Fig. 13.38 A mandibular molar IAC is being seated with occlusal pressure from a cotton roll

and if the contacts are too tight, excessive material can be removed from the IAC with either a metal finishing strip or polishing bur (Figs. 13.40, 13.41, and 13.42). The occlusal contacts can be checked with articulating paper, which leaves ink on the higher areas of contact. A series of polishing burs (in a progression from hard to soft) can be used to adjust the occlusal contacts in the same manner as the interproximal contacts (Figs. 13.43, 13.44, 13.45, 13.46, 13.47, and 13.48). If the contacts have been accounted for but there still seems to be interference, the hard and soft tissues of the implant's sulcus should be evaluated; it is possible that additional sulcus reaming may be necessary. If soft tissue interference is suspected, a relieving incision can be made, preferably on the palatal-oblique side to preserve the papillae.

The final step of an IAC insertion is to take a radiograph to ensure complete seating within the implant. It should be noted that on a radiograph, complete seating appears differently for each implant well size. For example, a 2.0-mm-wide well will have approximately two plateau spaces between its bottom and the abutment post; a 2.5-mm-wide well will have approximately one plateau space between its bottom and the abutment post; and a 3.0-mm-wide well will have approximately two plateau spaces between its bottom and the abutment post (Figs. 13.49, 13.50, and 13.51). Figures 13.52, 13.53, 13.54, 13.55, 13.56, 13.57, 13.58, 13.59, 13.60,

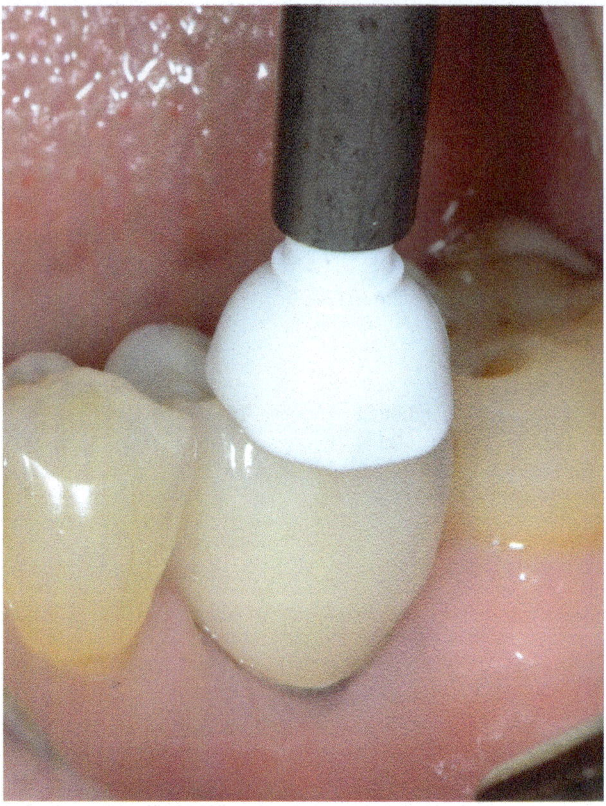

Fig. 13.39 A mandibular molar IAC is being tapped with a plastic abutment on a threaded handle

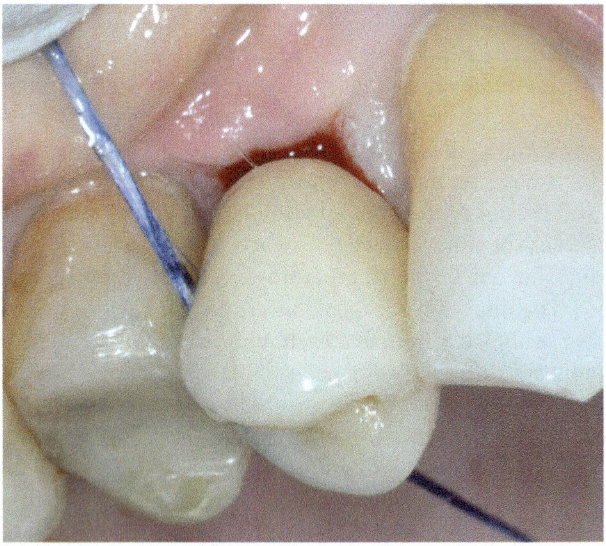

Fig. 13.40 Floss marked with blue ink is being used to check the interproximal contacts

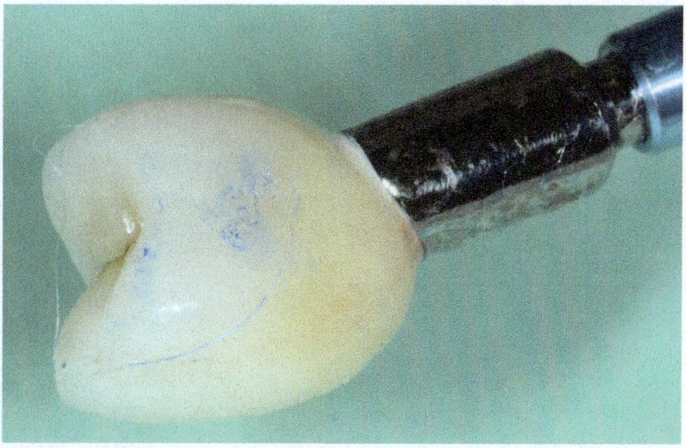

Fig. 13.41 Blue ink marks a point of high interproximal contact on the IAC

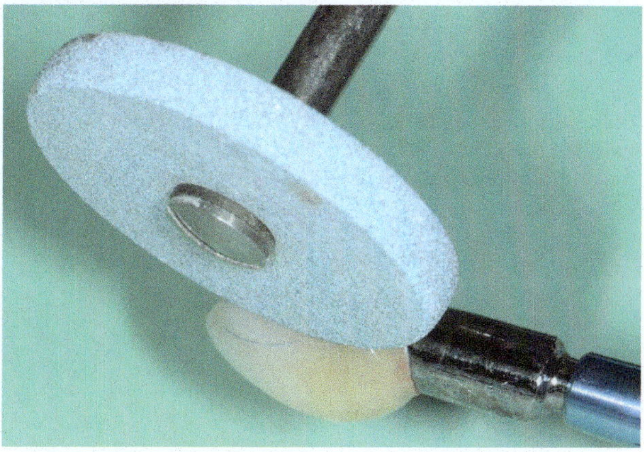

Fig. 13.42 A coarse wheel is being used to adjust the point of high contact on the IAC

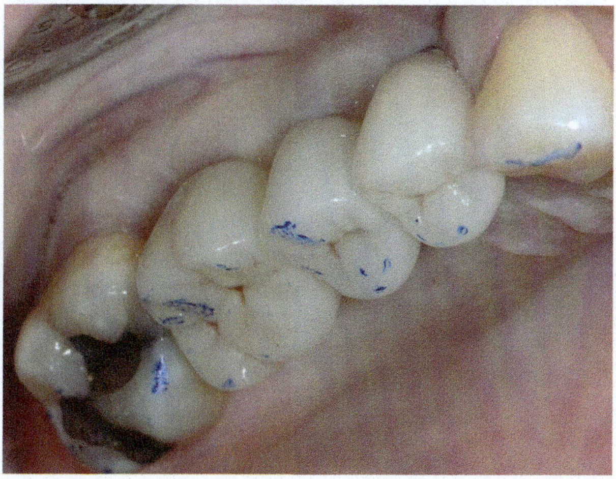

Fig. 13.43 Blue ink marks the occlusal contacts for three maxillary IACs

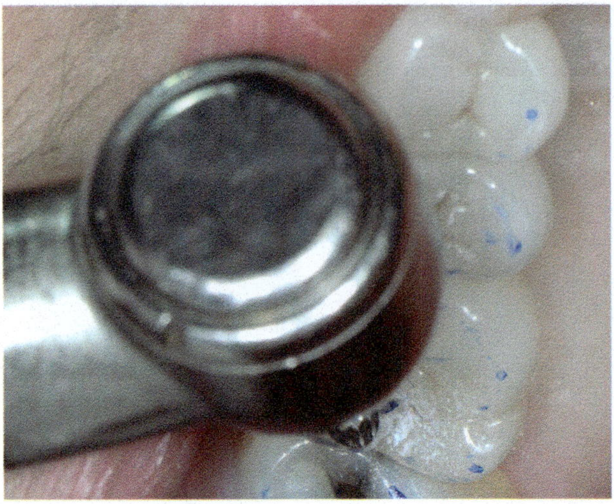

Fig. 13.44 Points of high occlusal contact are being polished intraorally with a slow-speed bur

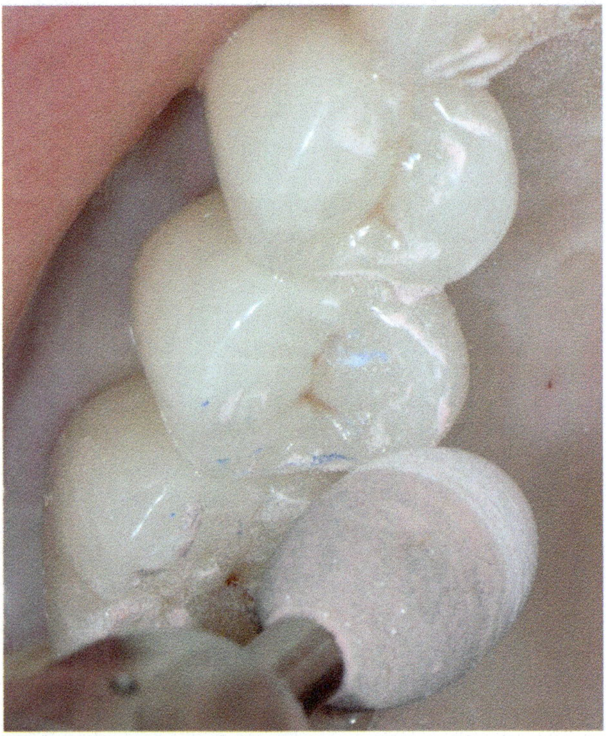

Fig. 13.45 Points of high occlusal contact are being polished intraorally with a pink rubber bur

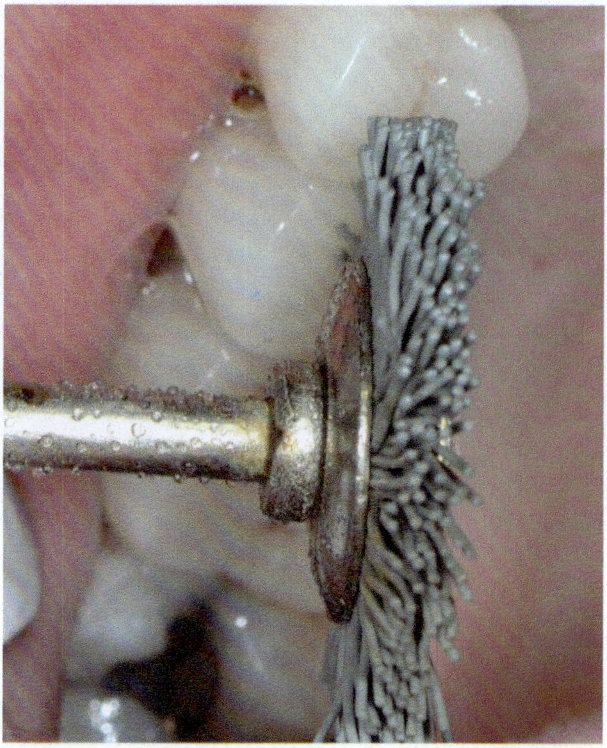

Fig. 13.46 Points of high occlusal contact are being polished intraorally with a silicone brush

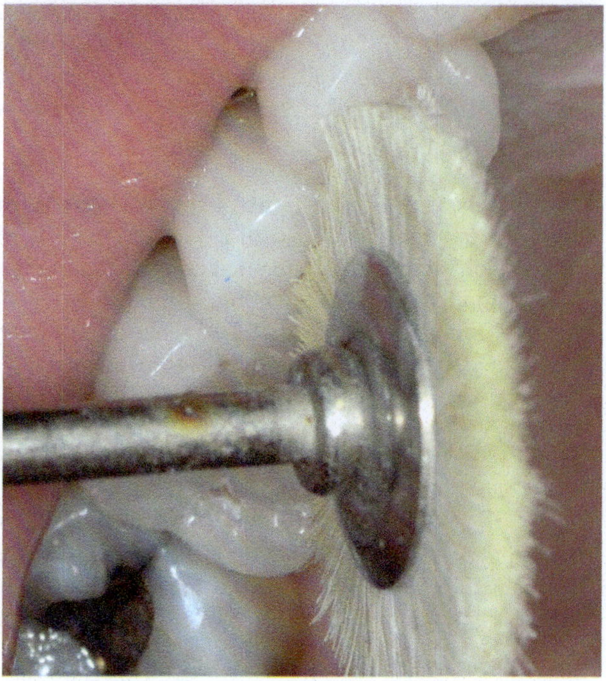

Fig. 13.47 Points of high occlusal contact are being polished intraorally with a bristle brush

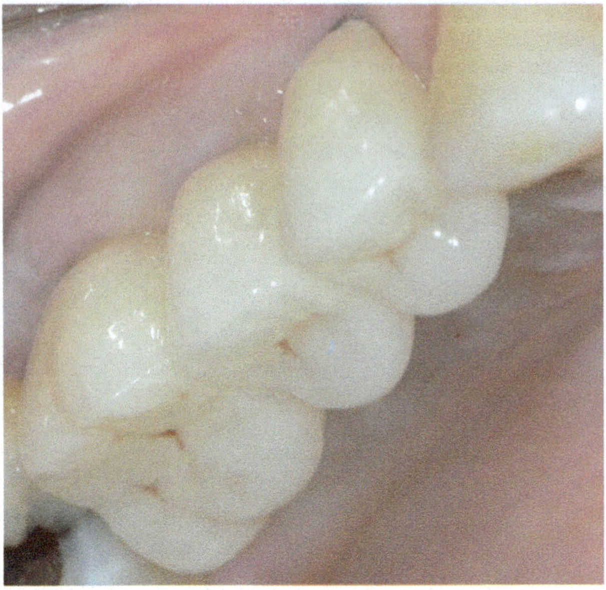

Fig. 13.48 View of three polished maxillary IACs

13.61, 13.62, 13.63, 13.64, 13.65, 13.66, 13.67, 13.68, 13.69, 13.70, 13.71, 13.72, 13.73, 13.74, 13.75, 13.76, 13.77, 13.78, 13.79, 13.80, 13.81, 13.82, 13.83, 13.84, 13.85, 13.86, 13.87, 13.88, 13.89, 13.90, 13.91, 13.92, 13.93, 13.94, 13.95, 13.96, 13.97, 13.98, 13.99, 13.100, 13.101, 13.102, 13.103, 13.104, 13.105, 13.106, 13.107, 13.108, 13.109, 13.110, 13.111, 13.112, 13.113, 13.114, 13.115, 13.116, 13.117, 13.118, 13.119, 13.120, 13.121, 13.122, 13.123, 13.124, 13.125, 13.126, 13.127, 13.128, 13.129, 13.130, 13.131, 13.132, 13.133, 13.134, 13.135, 13.136, 13.137, 13.138, 13.139, 13.140, 13.141, 13.142, 13.143, and 13.144 demonstrate the restorative techniques for maxillary and mandibular treatments in different regions of the mouth.

IAC Case 1: Mandibular Central Incisor IACs Within a Limited Space

Two 3.0 × 6.0 mm implants with 2.0 mm wells were placed in the limited space of a 59-year-old woman's missing mandibular central incisors (Figs. 13.52 and 13.53). After 4 months of osseointegration, a semi-lunar incision was made to uncover the implants (Figs. 13.54 and 13.55). A healing plug removal instrument was used to extract the polyethylene healing plugs from the wells of the implants, and guide pins were inserted in their place (Figs. 13.56 and 13.57). Once the integration of the implants was confirmed, a full arch implant-level transfer impression was taken (Figs. 13.58, 13.59, 13.60, and 13.61). The site was sutured and white healing abutments were inserted into the implants for the duration of the healing period (Fig. 13.62). Note that the healing abutments were modified with a bur in order to attain complete seating within their implants due to the tight interproximal space. Customized thermoplastic resin seating jigs were used to definitively seat the IACs upon their insertion (Fig. 13.63). Due to an open contact, the right IAC was removed

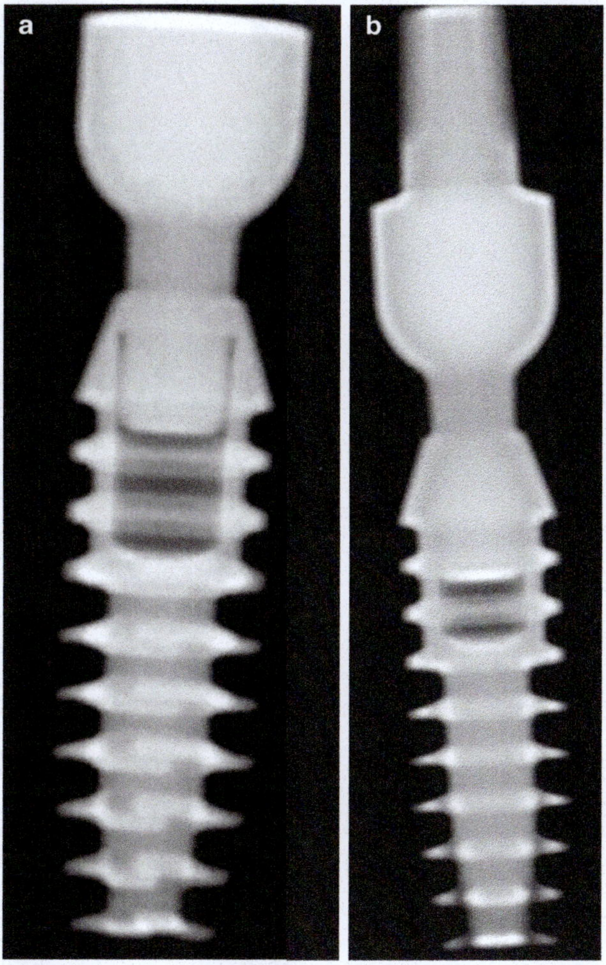

Fig. 13.49 Comparison radiographs of a 2.0 mm Temporary Abutment (**a**) and a Universal Abutment (**b**). Note the discrepancy of the space between the bottom of the implant wells and the different posts

for modification. The surface of the crown was polished with a coarse wheel prior to the application of modeling liquid and polyceramic material (Figs. 13.64, 13.65, 13.66, and 13.67). The crown was then polished again to smooth the surface where material was added, and a diamond strip was used to make final adjustments to verify appropriate interproximal contacts (Figs. 13.68, 13.69, 13.70, 13.71, 13.72, 13.73, and 13.74). A post-insertion radiograph verified complete seating of the two IACs (Fig. 13.75).

IAC Case 2: Maxillary Molar IAC and Alternative Crown Options

A maxillary left first molar in a 23-year-old man was extracted and replaced with a 6.0 × 6.0 mm implant with a 3.0 mm well (Figs. 13.76, 13.77, 13.78, and 13.79). After 4 months of healing, a radiograph was taken (Fig. 13.80). The implant was also uncovered for the making of a full arch indirect abutment-level impression, which

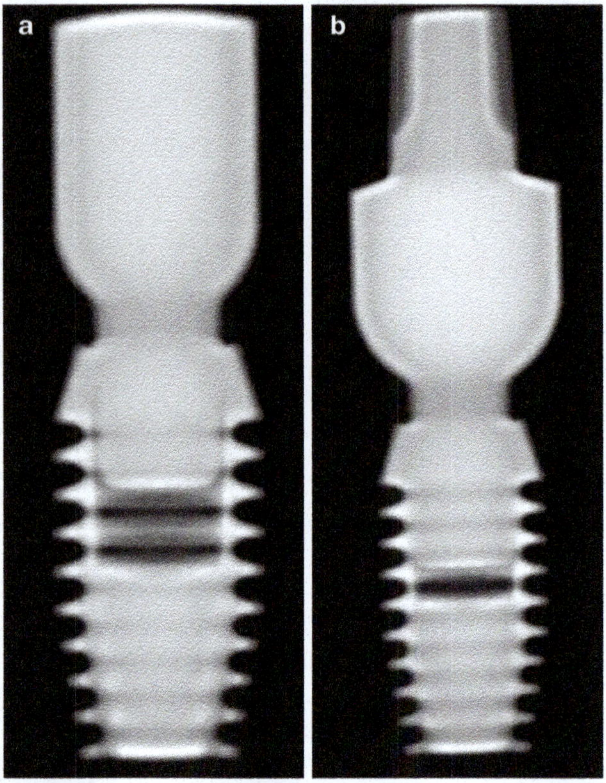

Fig. 13.50 Comparison radiographs of a 2.5 mm Temporary Abutment (**a**) and a Universal Abutment (**b**). Note the discrepancy of the space between the bottom of the implant wells and the different posts

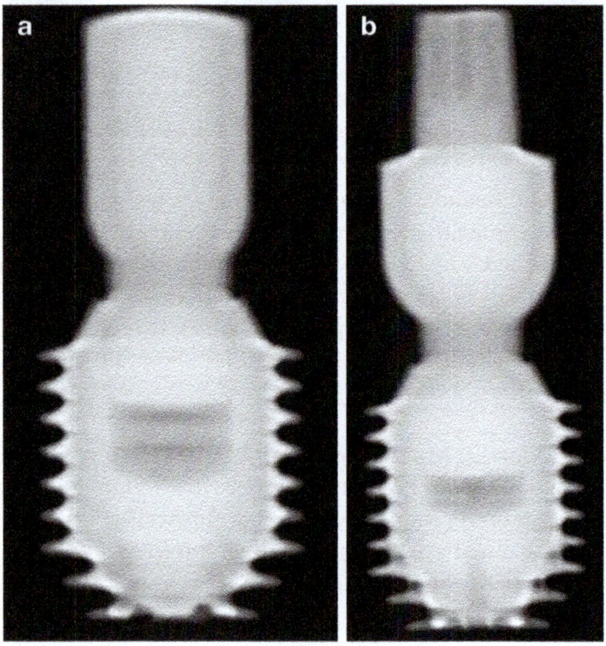

Fig. 13.51 Comparison radiographs of a 3.0 mm Temporary Abutment (**a**) and a Universal Abutment (**b**). Note the discrepancy of the space between the bottom of the implant wells and the different posts

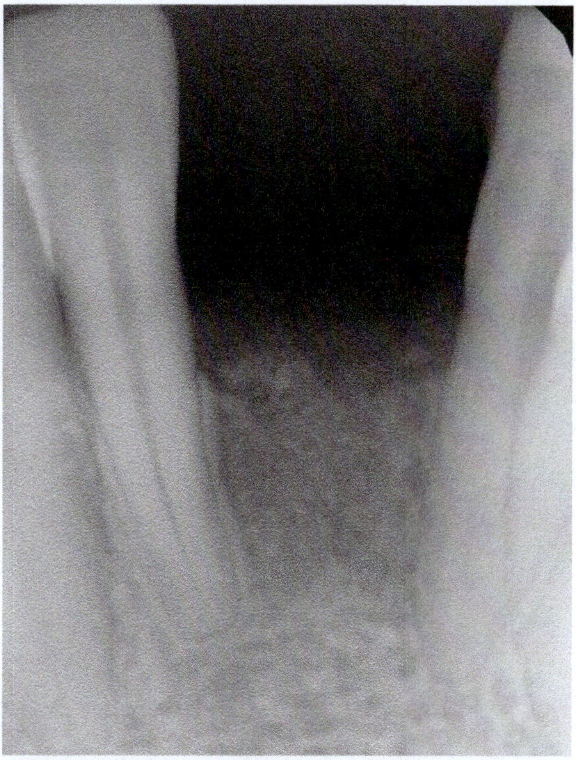

Fig. 13.52 Preoperative radiograph of limited space for mandibular central incisor implants

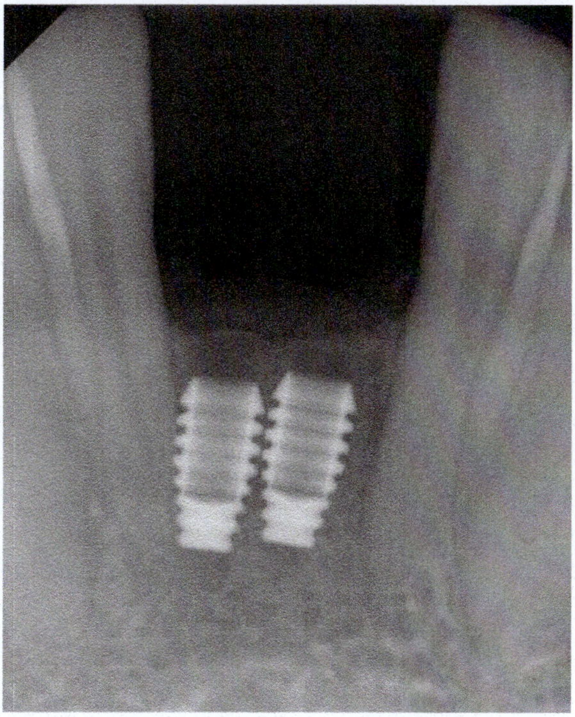

Fig. 13.53 Postoperative radiograph of two 3.0 × 6.0 mm implants with 2.0 mm wells

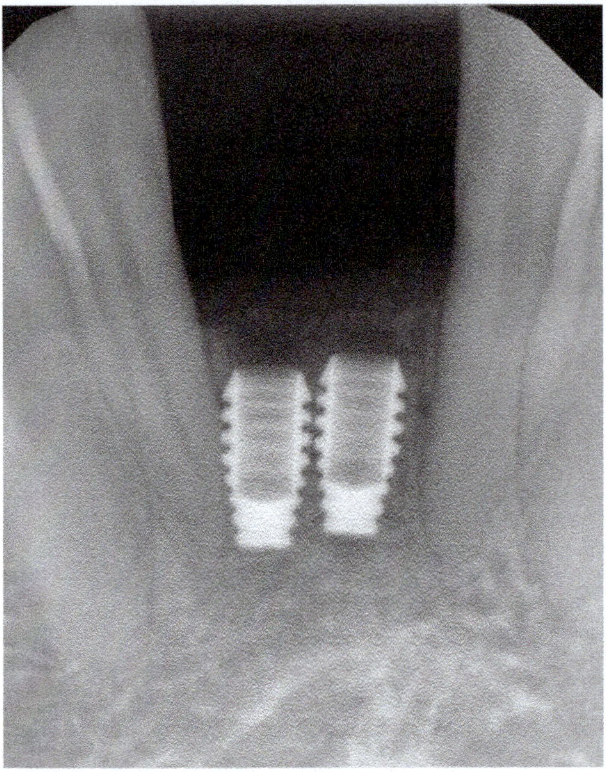

Fig. 13.54 Four-month postoperative radiograph prior to the uncovering of the implants

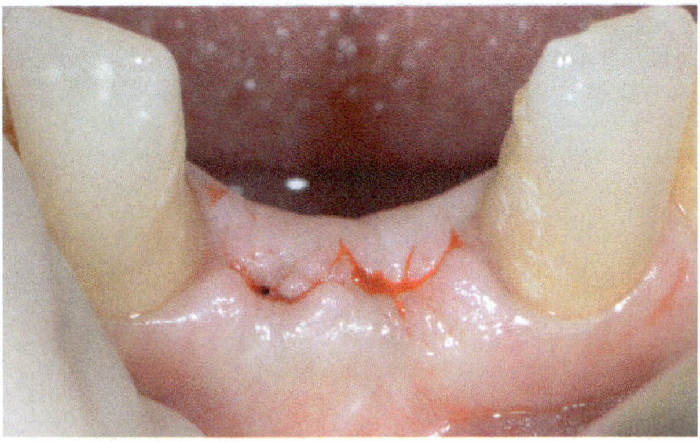

Fig. 13.55 View of semilunar incision to uncover the implants after 4 months of osseointegration

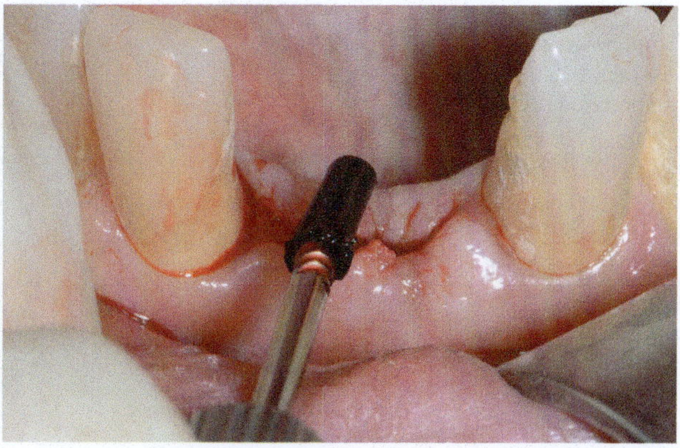

Fig. 13.56 A healing plug removal instrument is being used to retrieve the polyethylene healing plug from its implant well

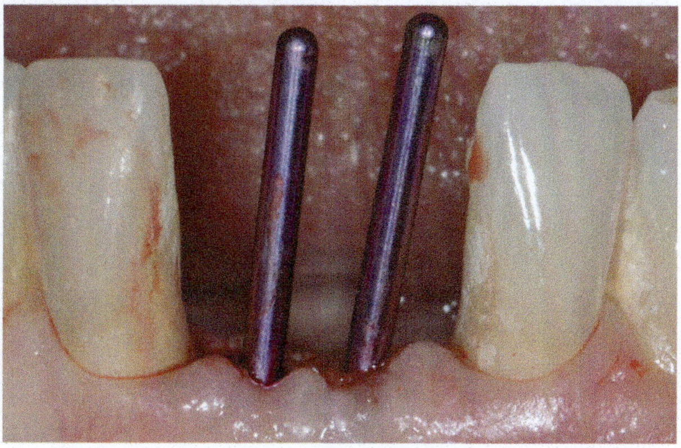

Fig. 13.57 Two violet 2.0 mm guide pins seated in their implant wells to confirm osseointegration

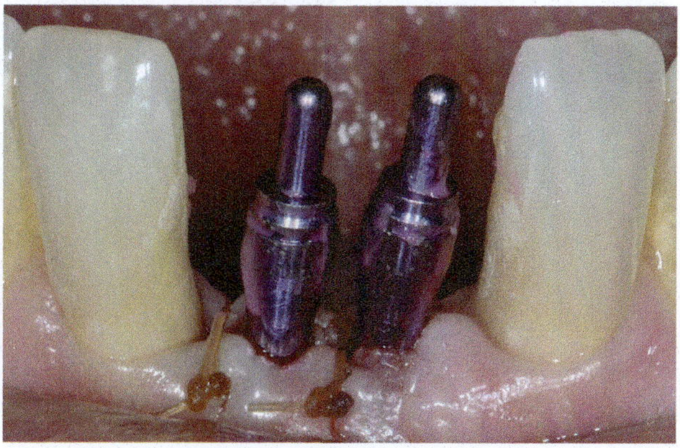

Fig. 13.58 Two violet 2.0 mm titanium impression posts seated in their implant wells

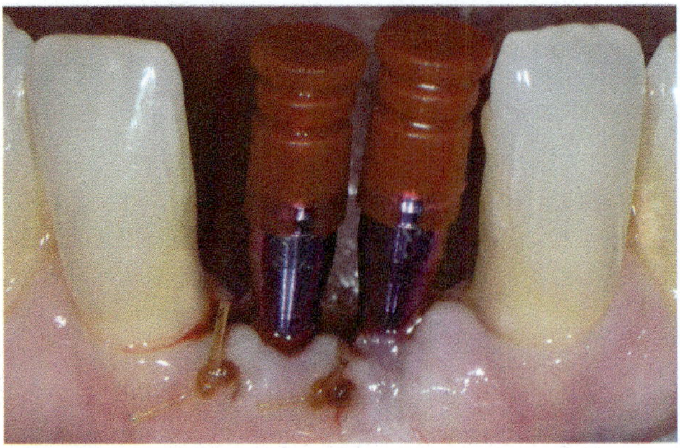

Fig. 13.59 Red acrylic impression sleeves seated on their respective impression posts

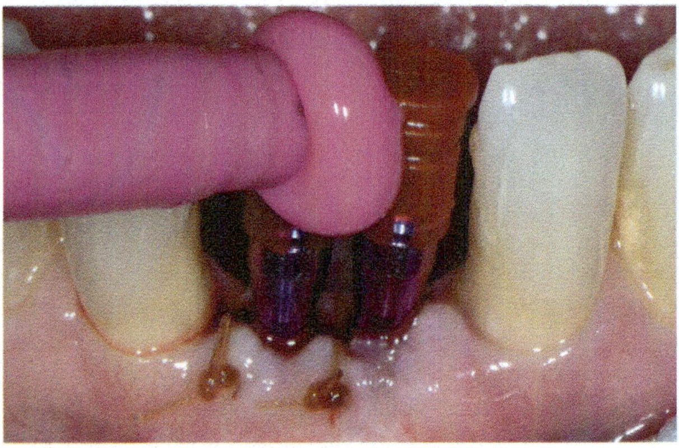

Fig. 13.60 Impression material is being applied around impression sleeves

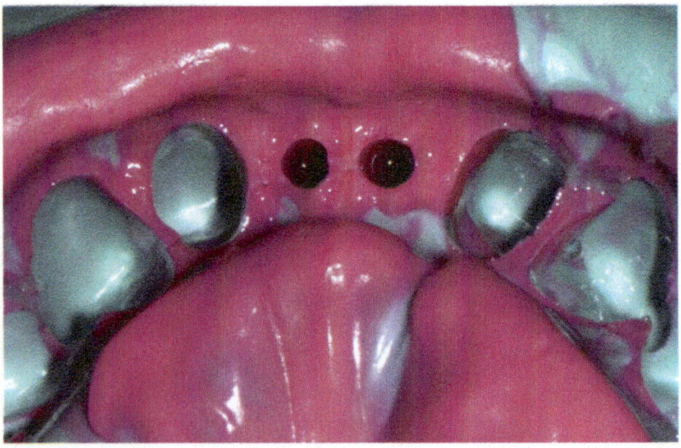

Fig. 13.61 Two red impression sleeves captured within a full arch implant-level transfer impression

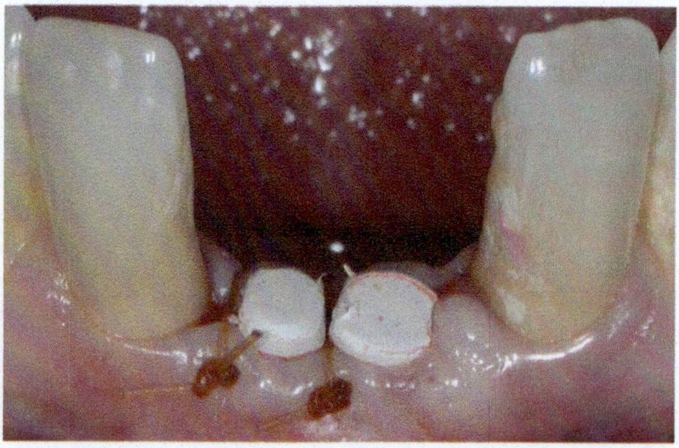

Fig. 13.62 Two modified healing abutments seated in their implants to maintain the sulci for the period prior to the restorative visit

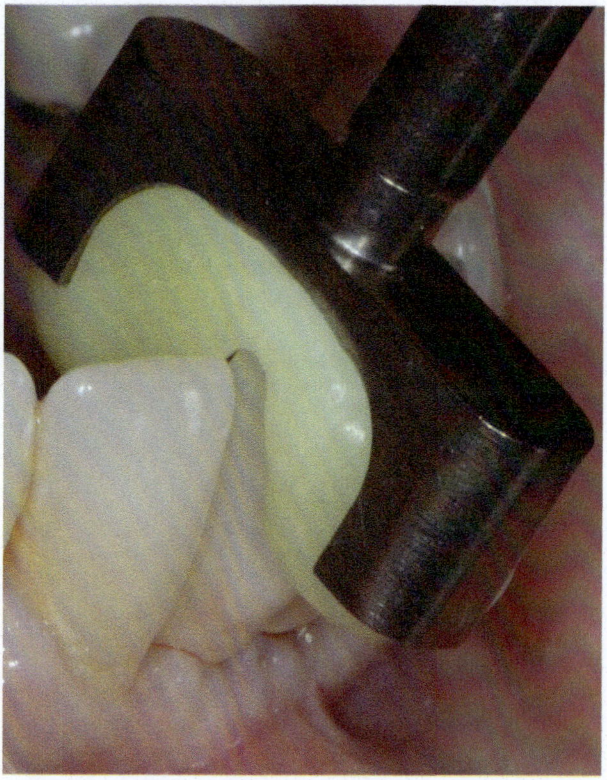

Fig. 13.63 A customized seating jig is being used to seat the mandibular left central incisor IAC

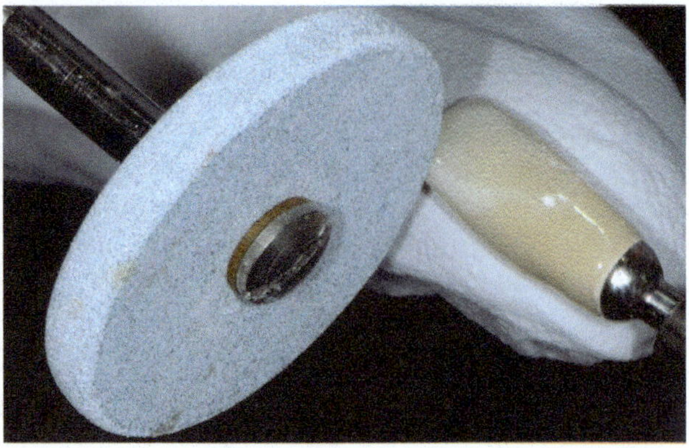

Fig. 13.64 A coarse wheel is being used to polish the surface of the IAC for the bonding of additional polyceramic material

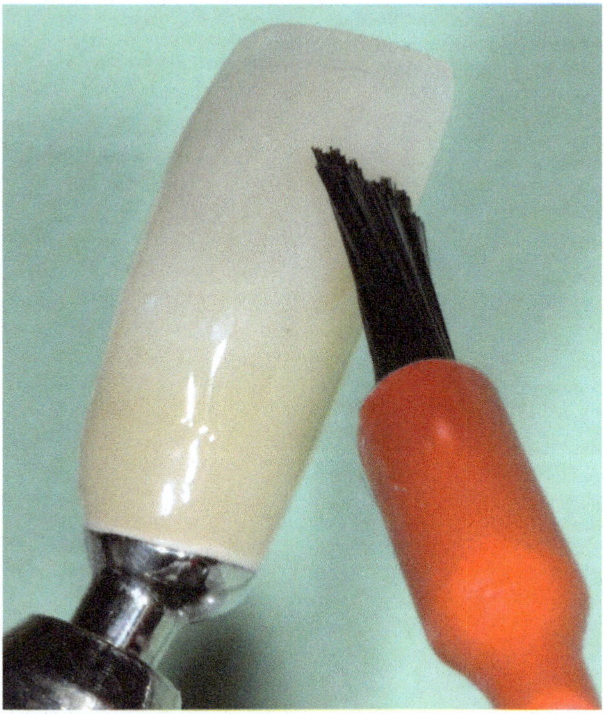

Fig. 13.65 Modeling liquid is being applied to the IAC

would be used in the laboratory with a Universal Abutment transfer die to fabricate the crown (Figs. 13.81, 13.82, and 13.83). The patient was discharged with a 6 Standard Profile Universal Abutment, which was covered by a white healing cap, to provide a temporary placeholder sufficient for its posterior location (Figs. 13.84 and 13.85). Subsequently, the IAC was inserted and definitively seated with both a cotton roll and a cotton tip applicator (Figs. 13.86, 13.87, 13.88, and 13.89). Blue ink markings indicated satisfactory occlusal contacts, and a post-insertion radiograph

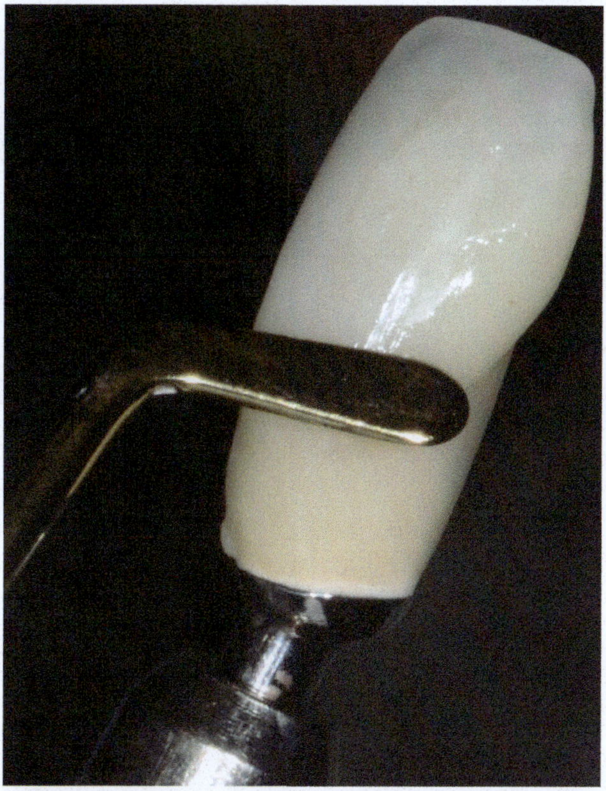

Fig. 13.66 Polyceramic material is being added to the IAC

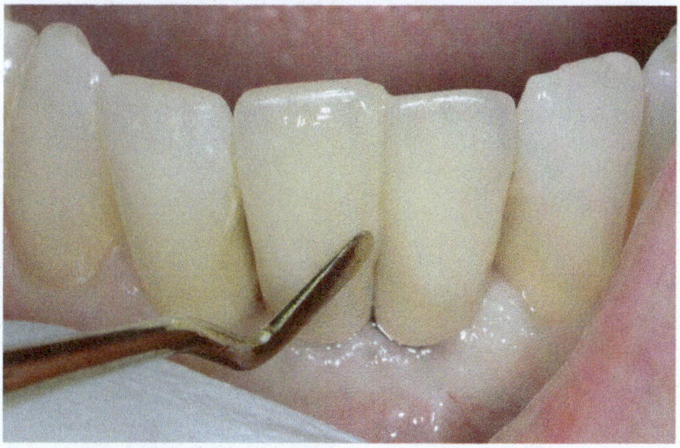

Fig. 13.67 Additional polyceramic material is being shaped intraorally to accomplish appropriate interproximal contact with the adjacent IAC

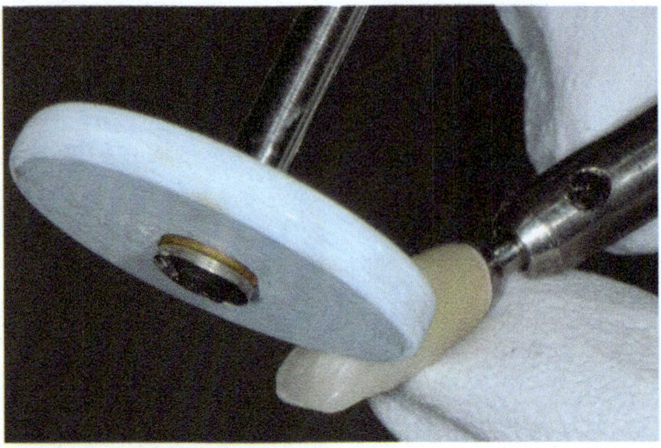

Fig. 13.68 A coarse wheel is being used as the first in a series of polishing brushes and wheels to smooth the surface of the modified IAC

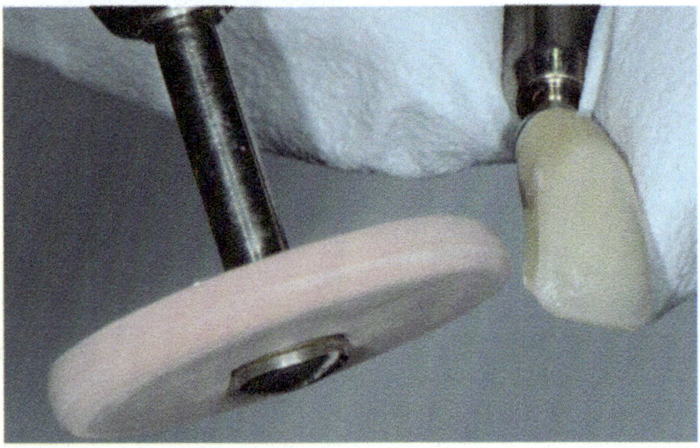

Fig. 13.69 A pink rubber wheel is being used to polish the surface of the modified IAC

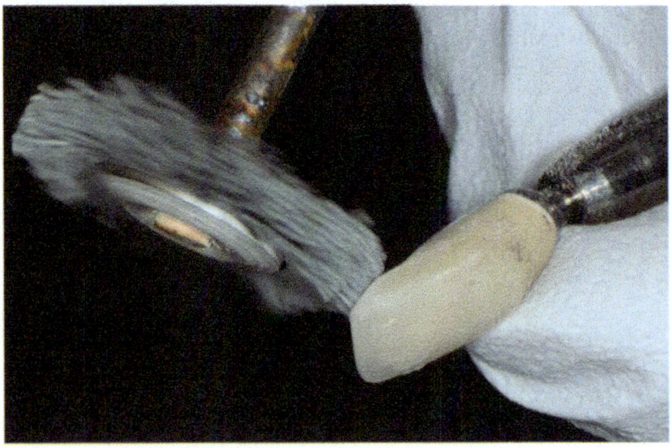

Fig. 13.70 A silicone brush is being used to polish the surface of the modified IAC

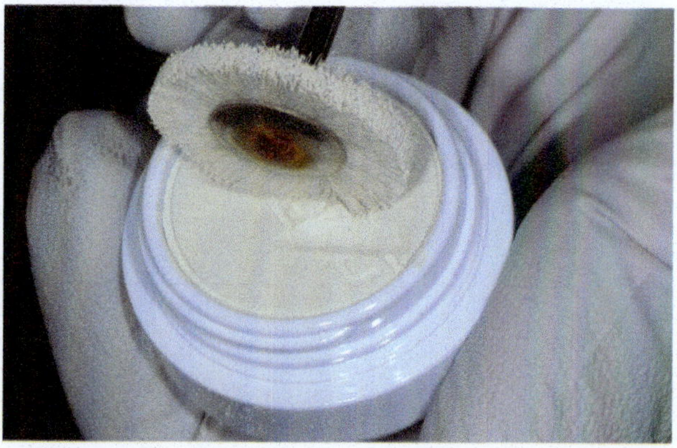

Fig. 13.71 A bristle brush with diamond paste is being used to polish the surface of the modified IAC

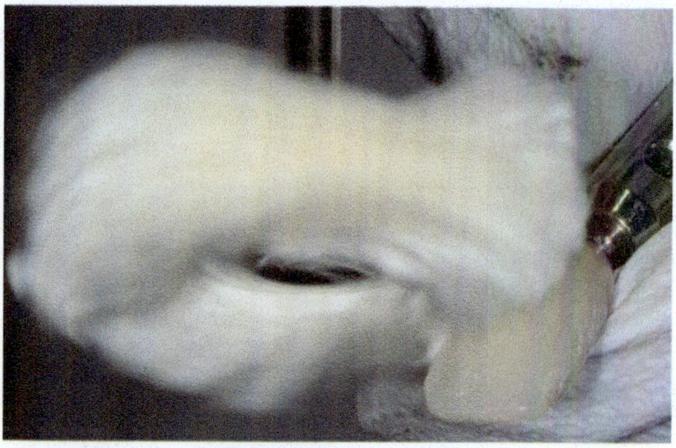

Fig. 13.72 A cotton wheel is being used to polish the modified IAC

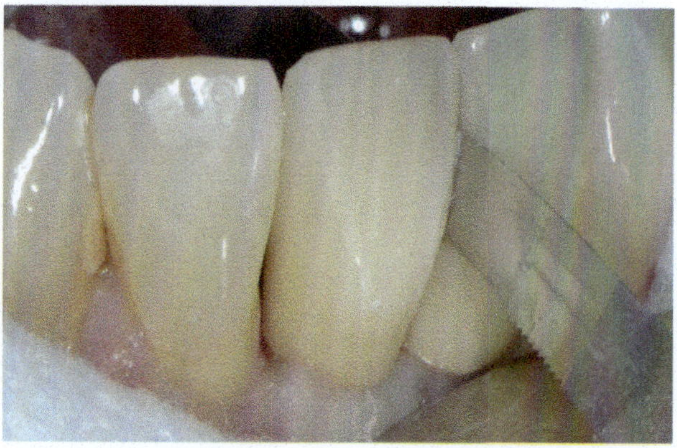

Fig. 13.73 A diamond strip is being used to make final adjustments to the interproximal contacts

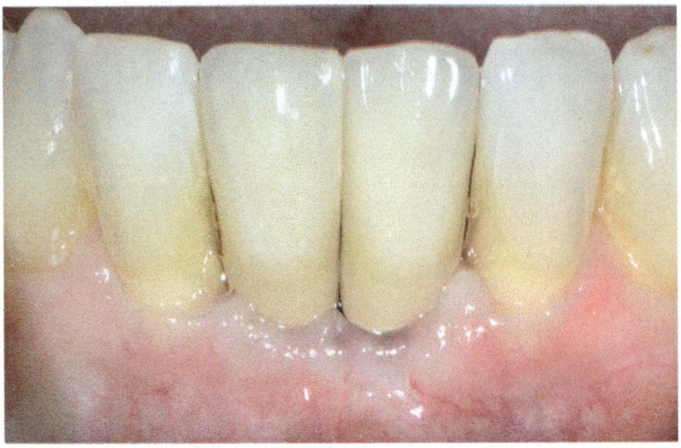

Fig. 13.74 Post-insertion view of two mandibular central incisor IACs

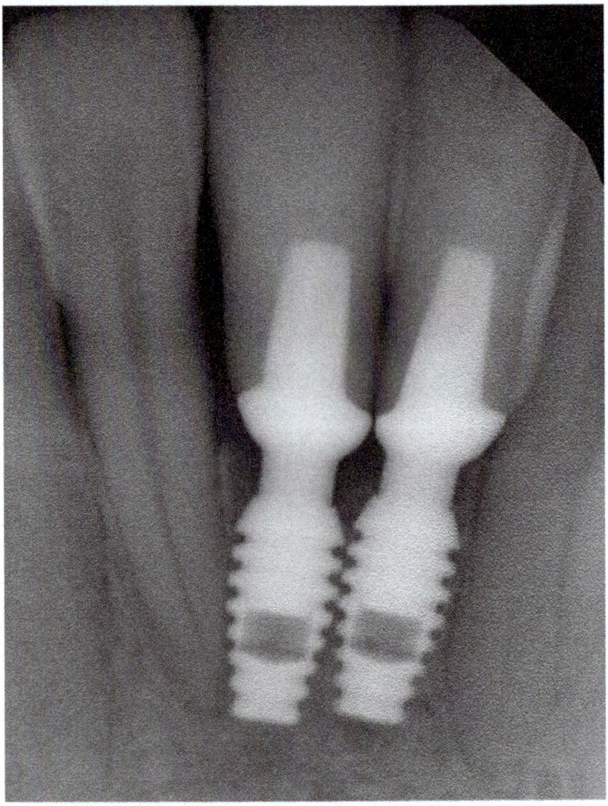

Fig. 13.75 Post-insertion radiograph of two 3.0 × 6.0 mm implants with their seated IACs

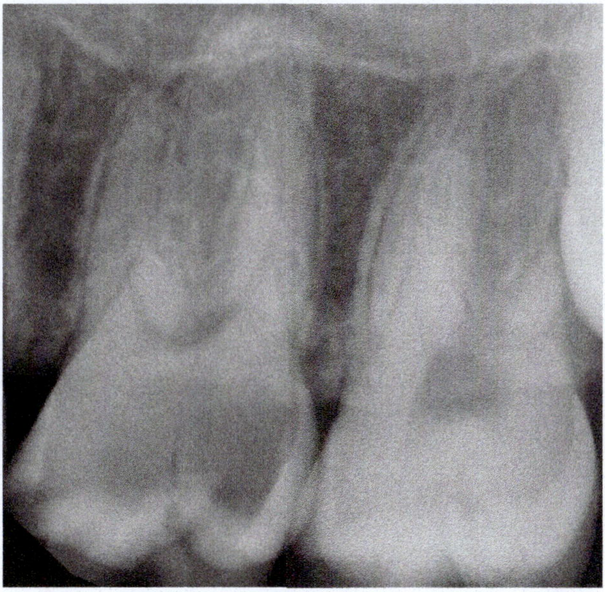

Fig. 13.76 Preoperative radiograph of a non-restorable maxillary left first molar

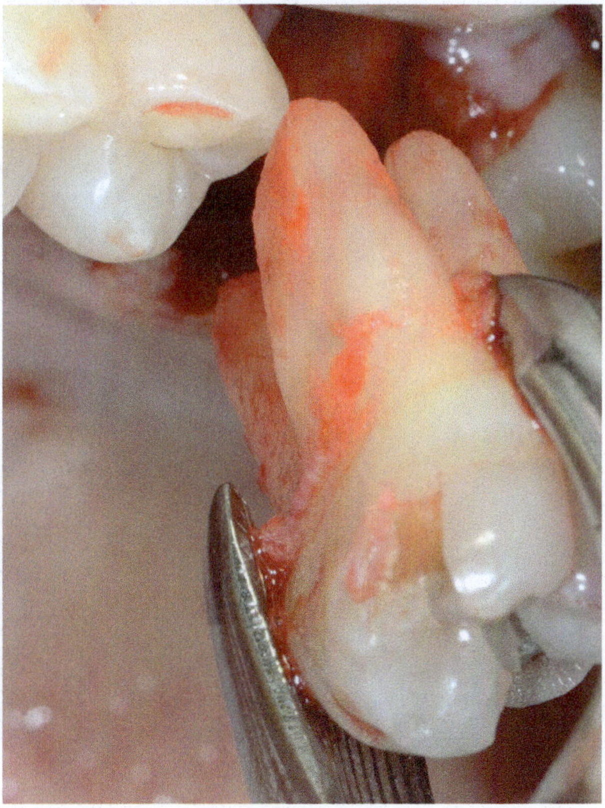

Fig. 13.77 A non-restorable maxillary left first molar is being extracted

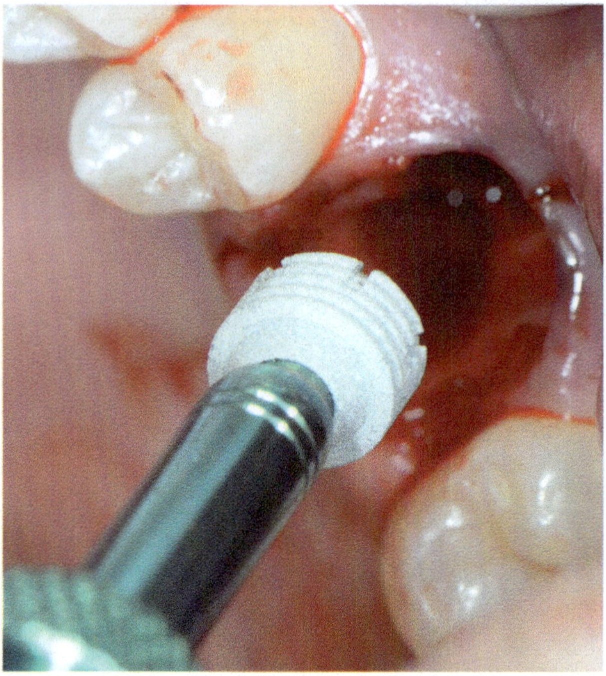

Fig. 13.78 A 6.0 × 6.0 mm implant with a 3.0 mm well is being placed into the extraction socket

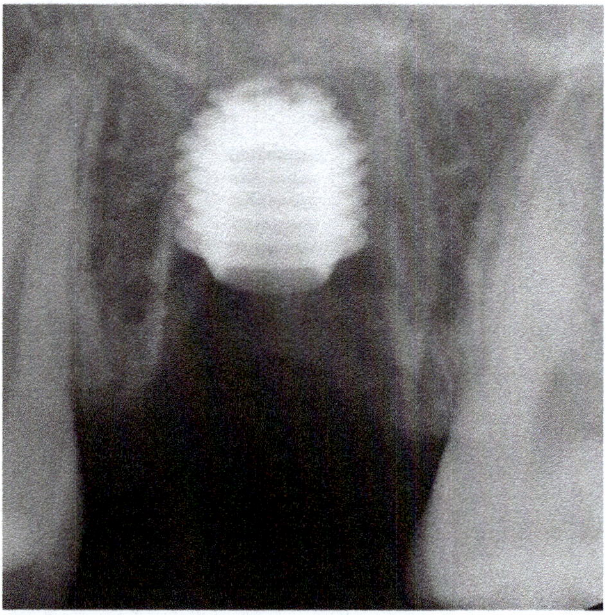

Fig. 13.79 Postoperative radiograph of a 6.0 × 6.0 mm implant

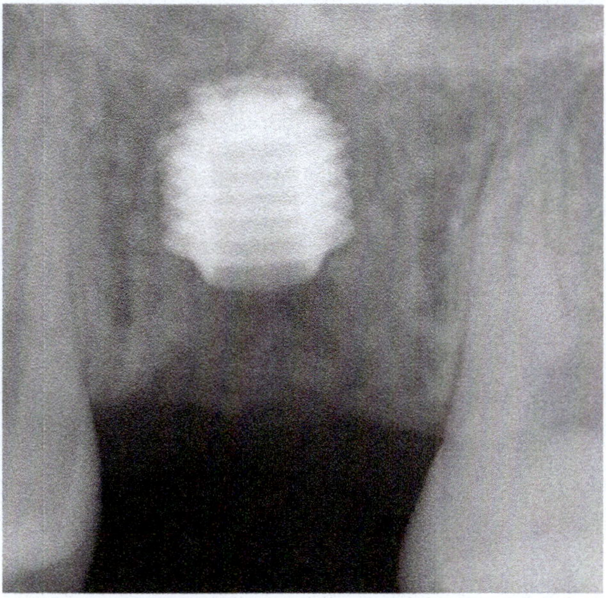

Fig. 13.80 Four-month postoperative radiograph of a 6.0 × 6.0 mm implant prior to its uncovering

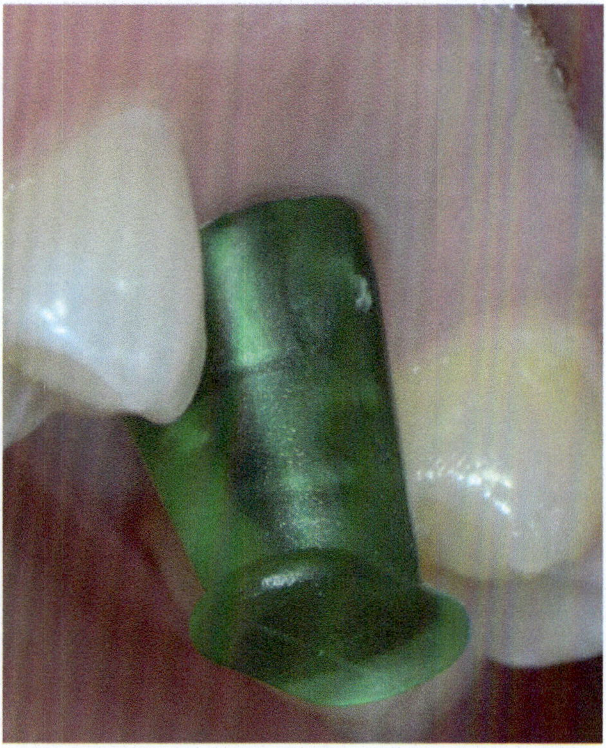

Fig. 13.81 A green 6-6T Universal Abutment impression sleeve is seated on a 6 Standard Profile Universal Abutment

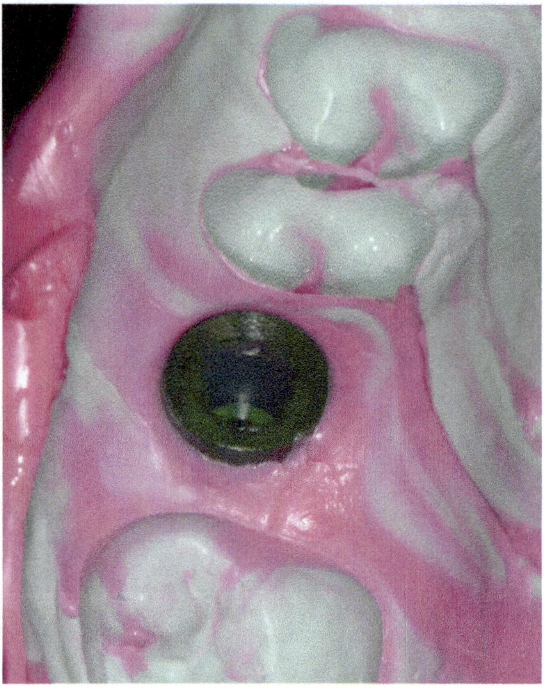

Fig. 13.82 A green Universal Abutment impression sleeve is captured within a full arch indirect abutment-level transfer impression

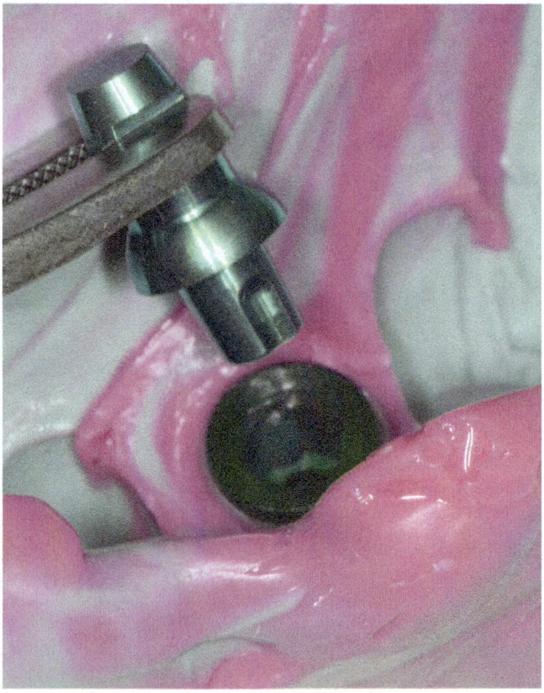

Fig. 13.83 A 6-6T Universal Abutment transfer die is being transferred to the impression sleeve for the laboratory fabrication of a maxillary molar crown

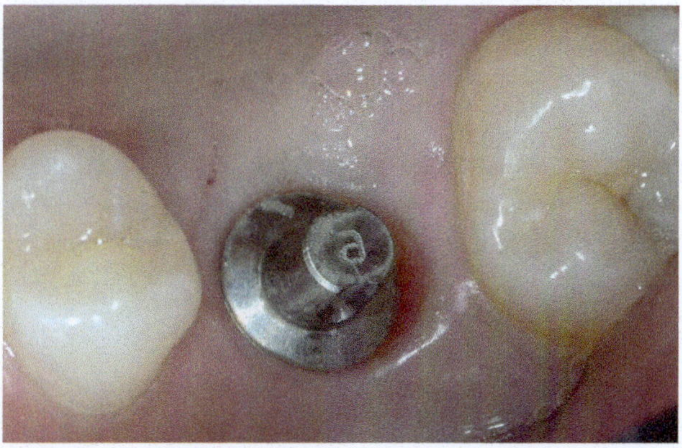

Fig. 13.84 A 6 Standard Profile Universal Abutment is seated in the well of the implant

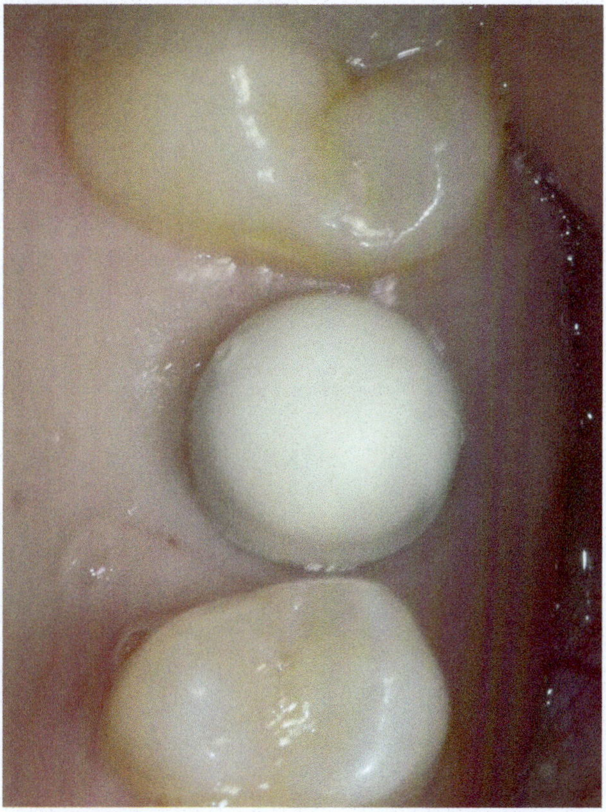

Fig. 13.85 A white healing cap is seated on the Universal Abutment as a temporary crown

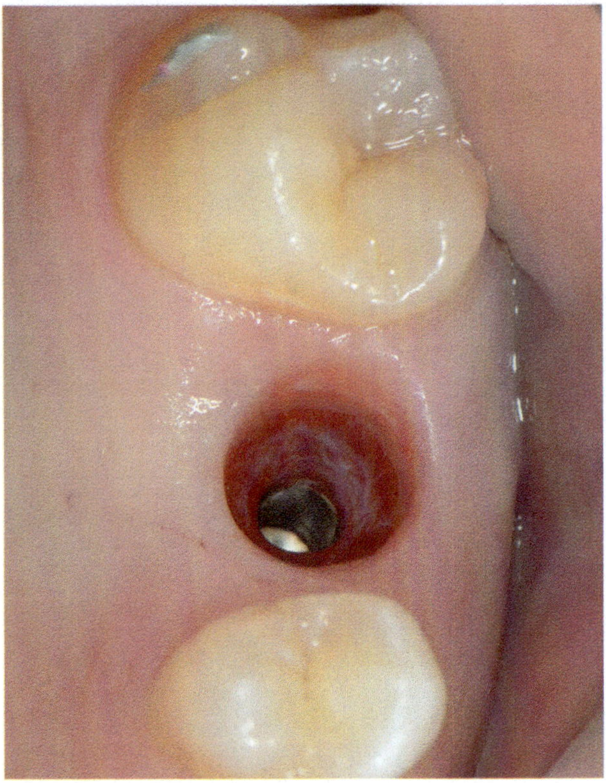

Fig. 13.86 View of an implant well and sulcus

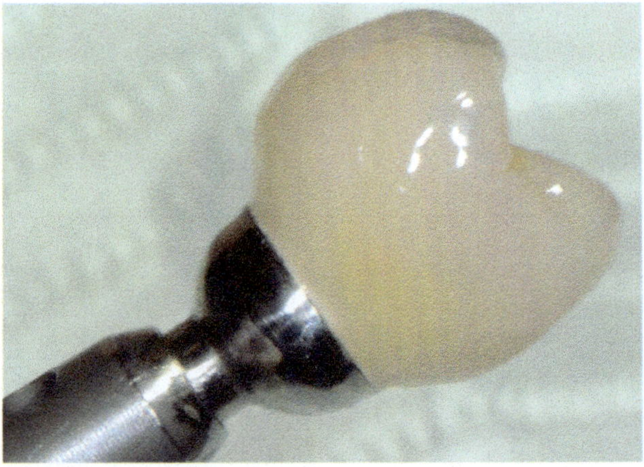

Fig. 13.87 An Integrated Abutment Crown (IAC) prior to its insertion

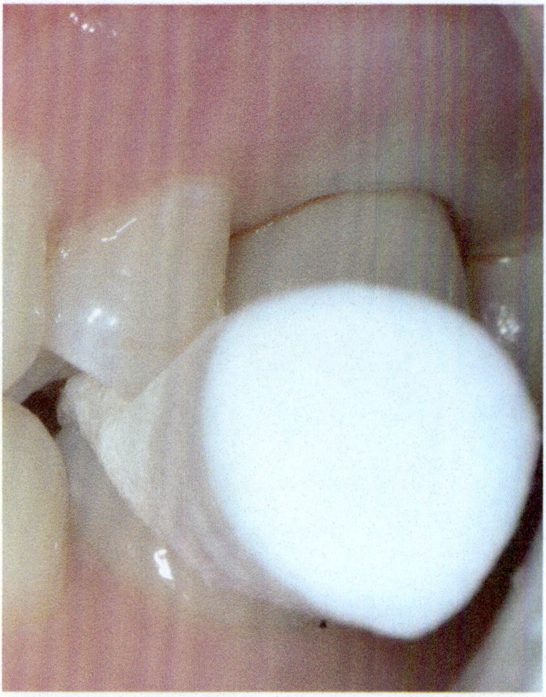

Fig. 13.88 A maxillary molar IAC is being seated with occlusal pressure from a cotton roll

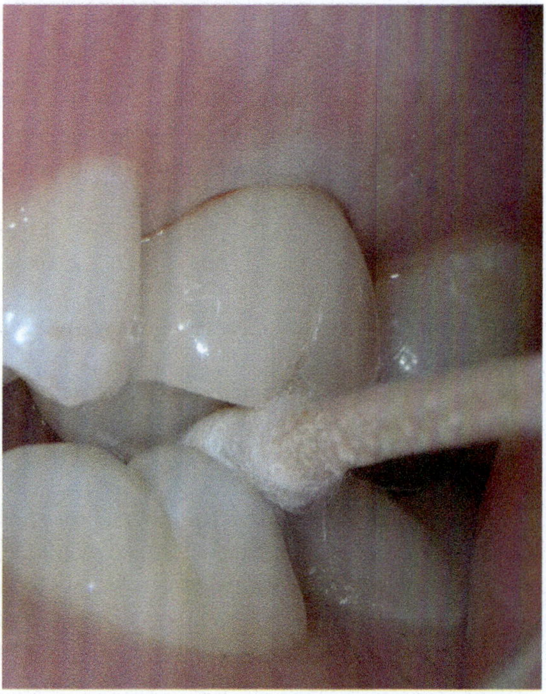

Fig. 13.89 A maxillary molar IAC is being definitively seated with occlusal pressure from a cotton tip applicator

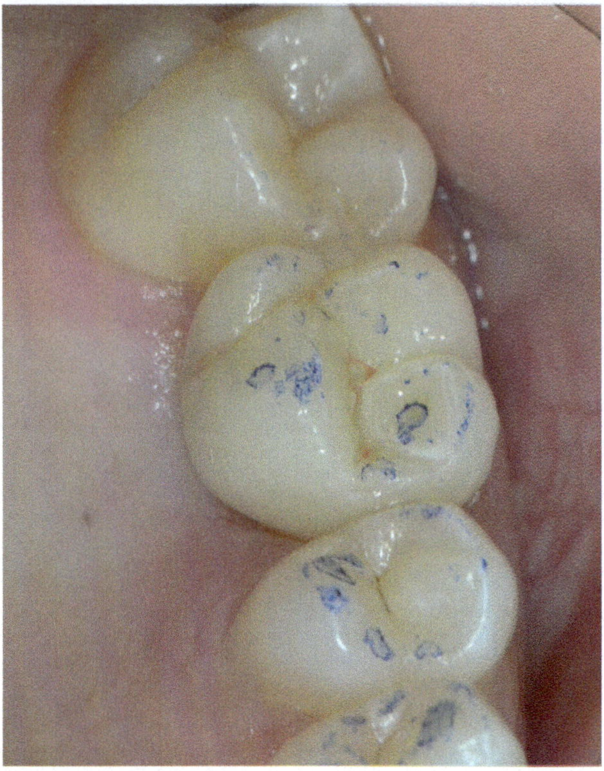

Fig. 13.90 Blue ink marks appropriate occlusal contacts

confirmed complete seating (Figs. 13.90, 13.91, 13.92, and 13.93). If the clinician were to have preferred an alternative crown to the IAC, two other options were prepared to demonstrate the comparison: a lithium disilicate crown and a CAD/CAM polyceramic crown. The extraoral cementation procedure for both crowns is presented in Figs. 13.94, 13.95, 13.96, 13.97, 13.98, 13.99, 13.100, 13.101, 13.102, 13.103, 13.104, 13.105, 13.106, 13.107, 13.108, 13.109, and 13.110.

IAC Case 3: Maxillary Central Incisor IAC with Intraoral Shade Adjustments

A 64-year-old man presented with a non-restorable maxillary right central incisor with a crestal buccal defect, which was extracted and replaced 2 months later with a 4.5 × 8.0 mm implant with a 2.5 mm well (Figs. 13.111 and 13.112). Grafting was also performed with autogenous bone harvested from the osteotomy and with SynthoGraft™, a pure phase beta tricalcium phosphate material. After 5 months of osseointegration, the implant was uncovered and an implant-level impression was taken. Ten days later, the patient returned for the IAC insertion (Figs. 13.113, 13.114, 13.115, and 13.116). At a follow-up visit 1 month after the IAC insertion, intraoral modifications were made to the IAC using a rubber dam, which protected the tissues as well as isolated the anterior teeth. The first step of the adjustment

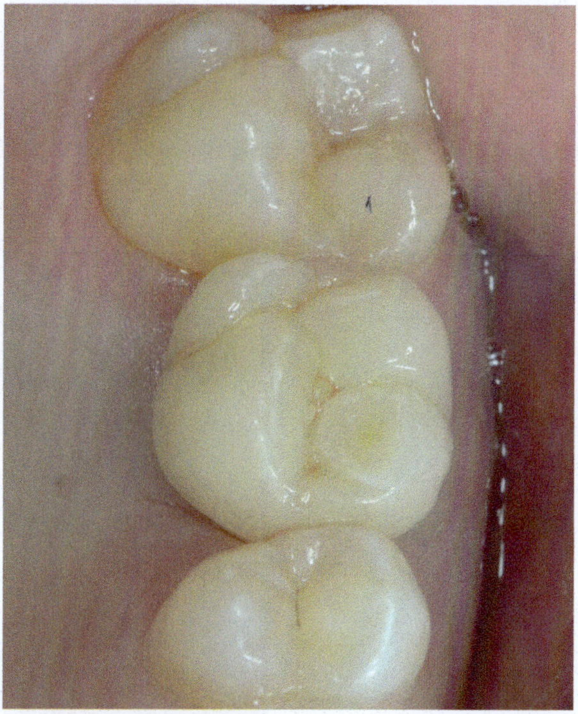

Fig. 13.91 Occlusal view of definitively seated IAC

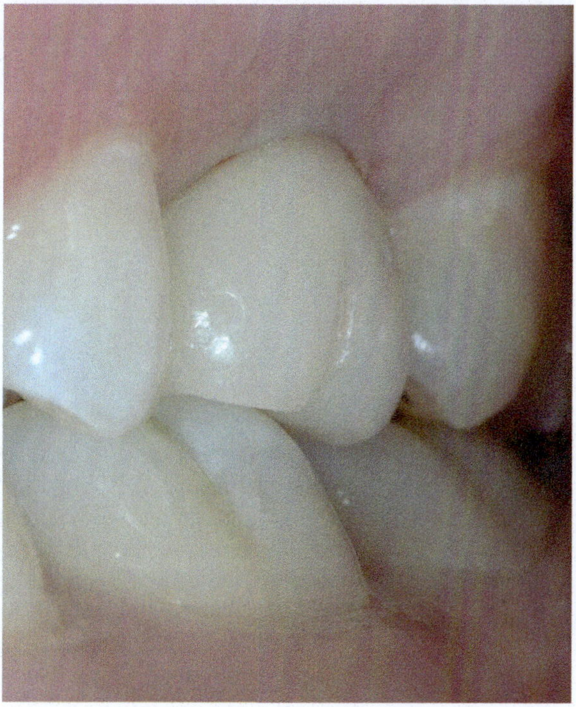

Fig. 13.92 Facial view of definitively seated IAC

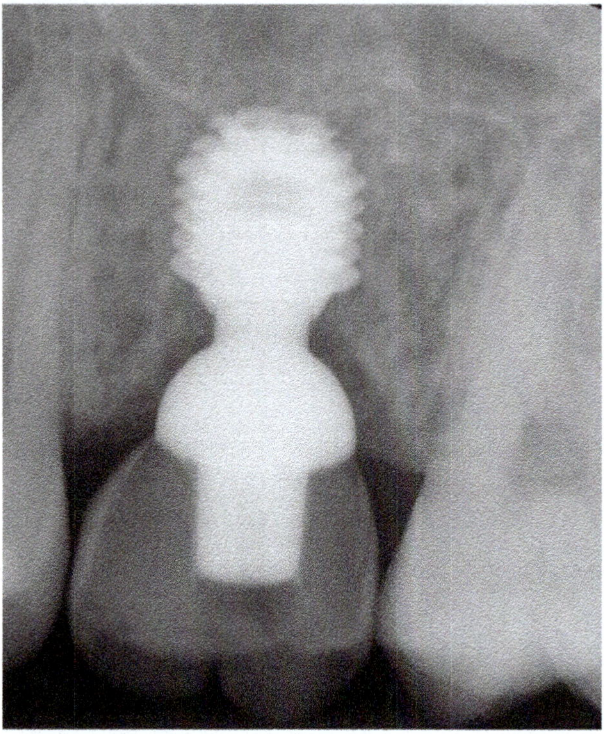

Fig. 13.93 Post-insertion radiograph of a 6.0 x 6.0mm implant with its seated IAC

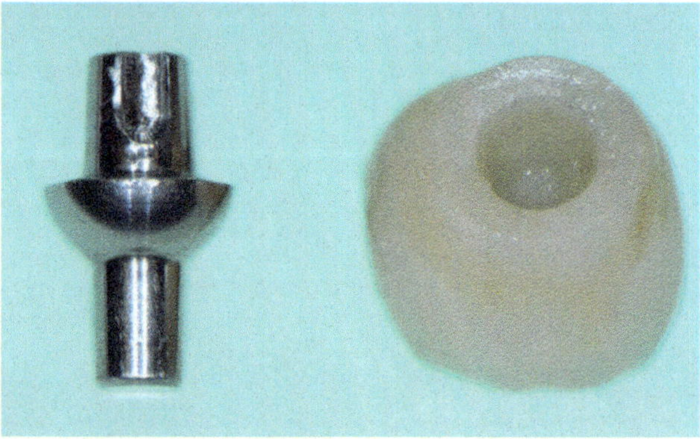

Fig. 13.94 A Universal Abutment and an Emax (lithium disilicate) crown prior to extraoral cementation

process was to add additional polyceramic material of a lighter shade, and light-cure it to the surface of the crown (Figs. 13.117, 13.118, 13.119, 13.120, 13.121, 13.122, and 13.123). After the new layer of material was light-cured, the surface was in need of aesthetic contouring, which was achieved with a pencil and a bur (Figs. 13.124 and 13.125). The surface of the crown was then polished with a series of burs, wheels, and brushes in a progressively softer sequence (Figs. 13.126, 13.127, 13.128, and 13.129). The final result was successful in sharing the aesthetics and colorations of the adjacent natural teeth (Figs. 13.130, 13.131, and 13.132).

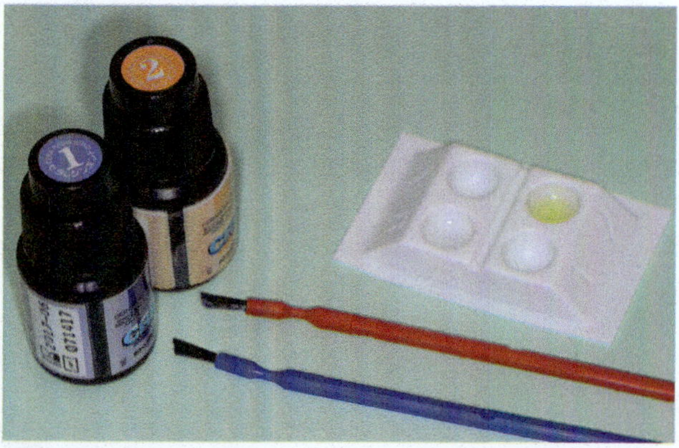

Fig. 13.95 Bonding agents CRB #1 and CRB #2 prior to being applied to the crowns

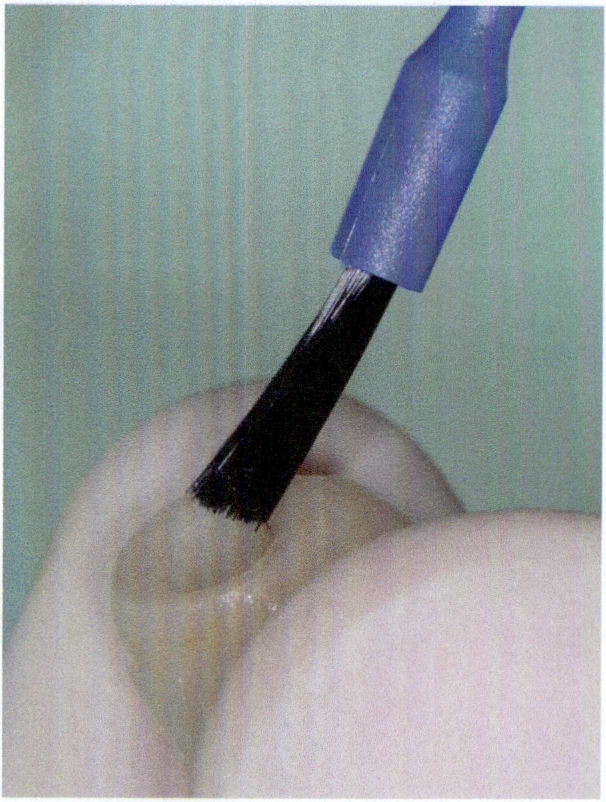

Fig. 13.96 CRB #1 is being applied to the Emax crown

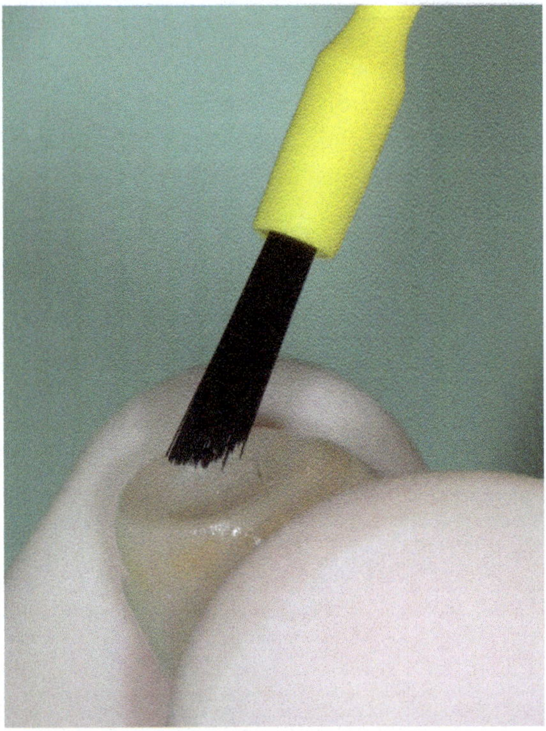

Fig. 13.97 CRB #2 is being applied to the Emax crown

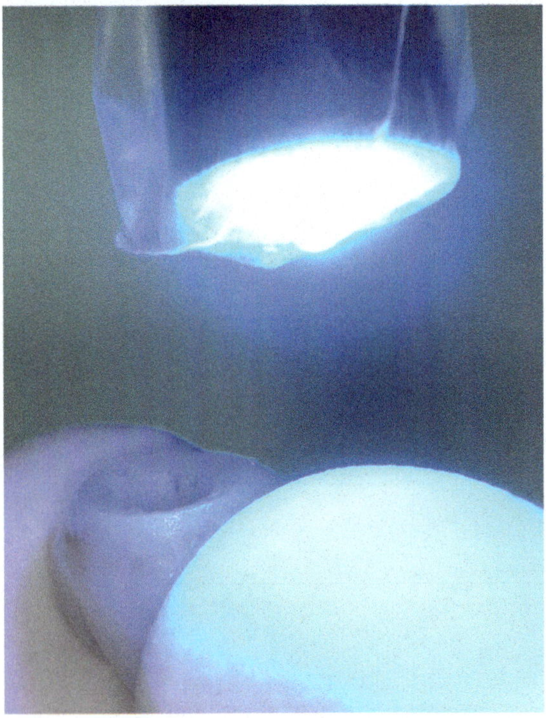

Fig. 13.98 The bonding agents on the Emax crown are being light-cured

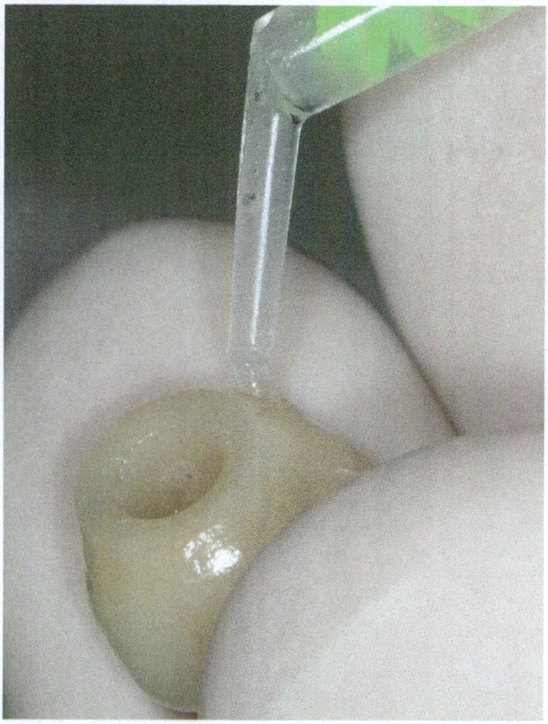

Fig. 13.99 Vaseline is being applied around the Emax crown to facilitate the removal of extraneous cement during cementation of the abutment and crown

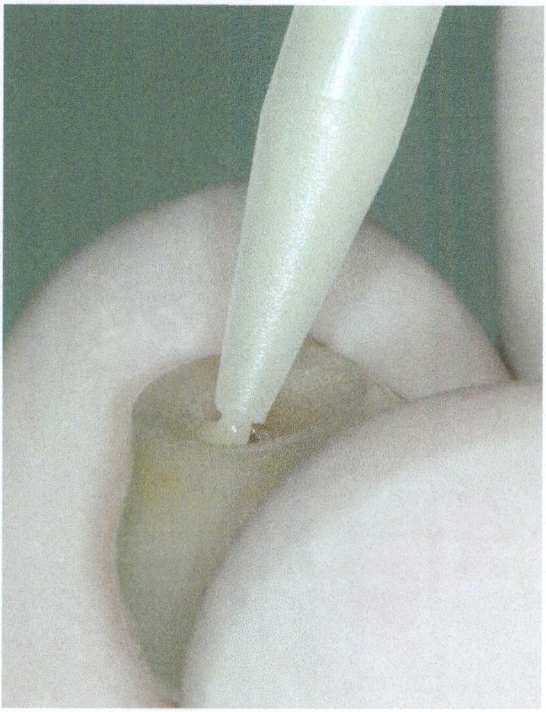

Fig. 13.100 Resin cement is being applied to the bore of the Emax crown

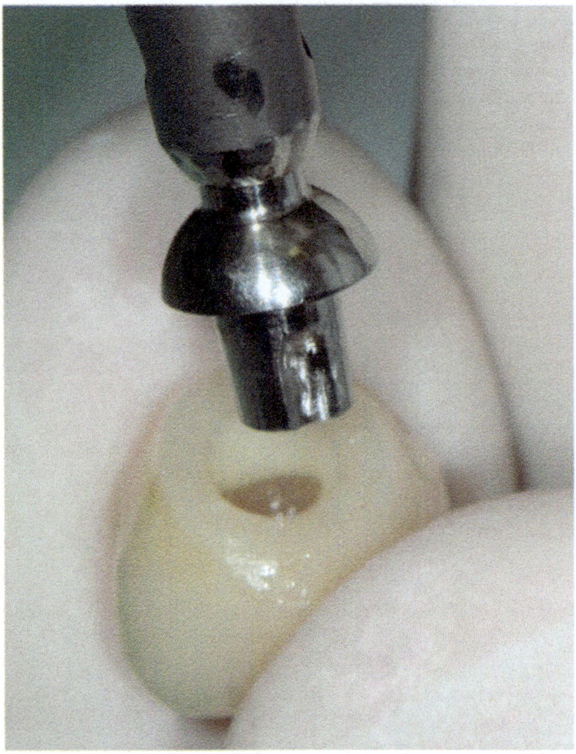

Fig. 13.101 A Universal Abutment is being transported to the cement-filled bore of the Emax crown

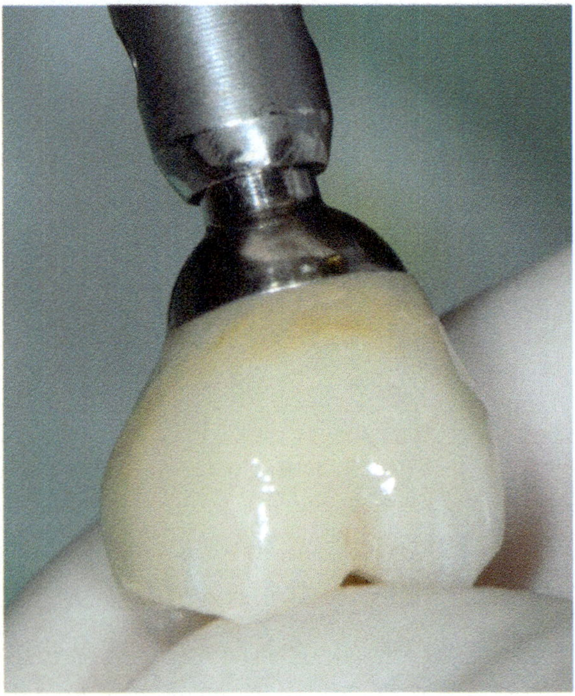

Fig. 13.102 A Universal Abutment is being cemented to the Emax crown

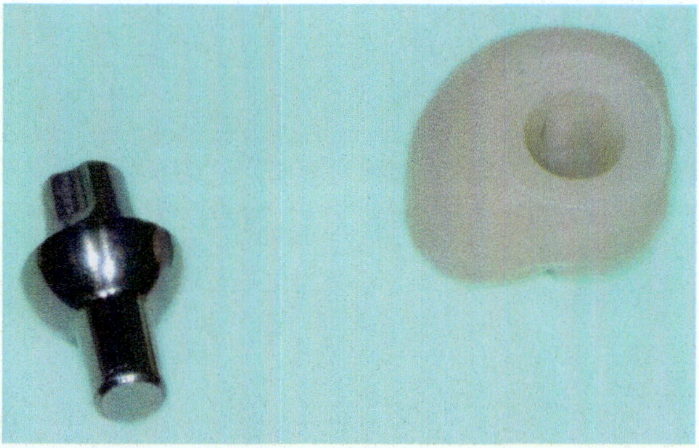

Fig. 13.103 A Universal Abutment and a CAD/CAM crown prior to extraoral cementation

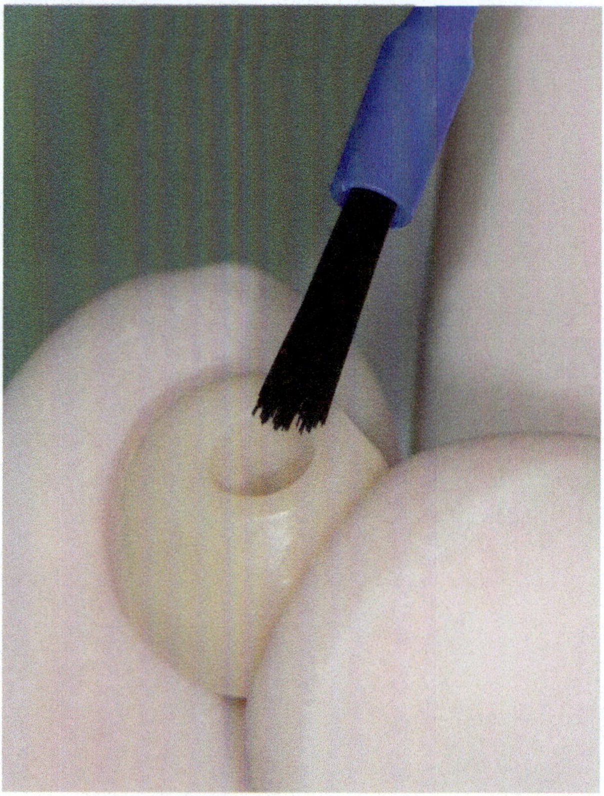

Fig. 13.104 CRB #1 is being applied to the CAD/CAM crown

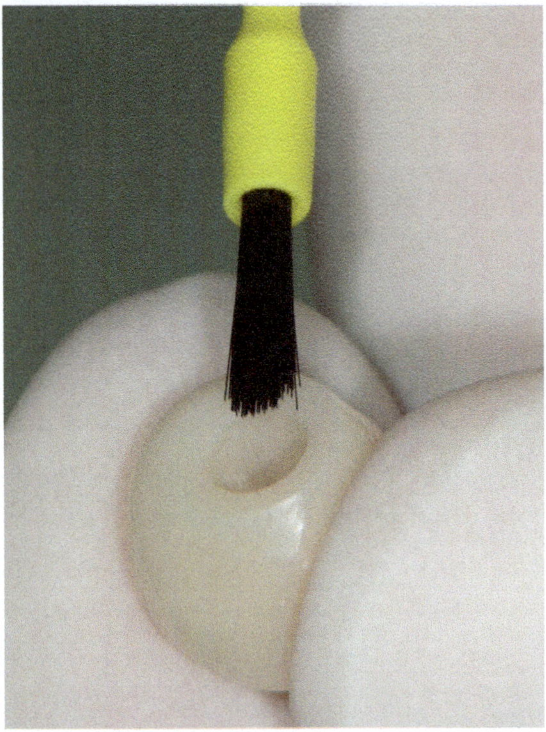

Fig. 13.105 CRB #2 is being applied to the CAD/CAM crown

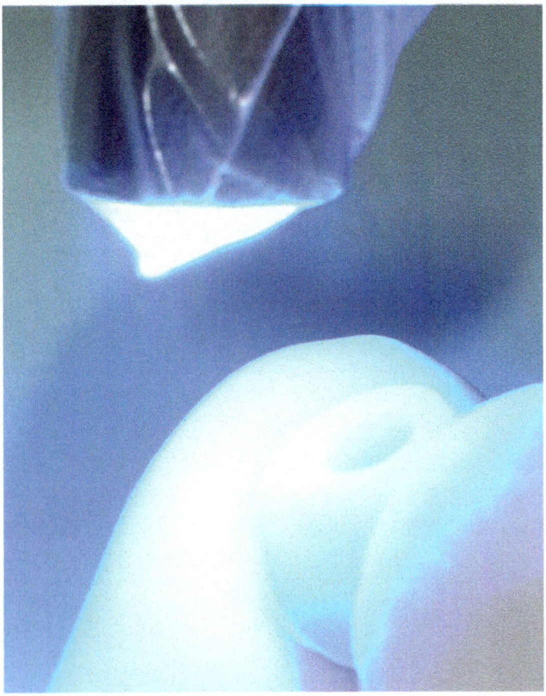

Fig. 13.106 The bonding agents on the CAD/CAM crown are being light-cured

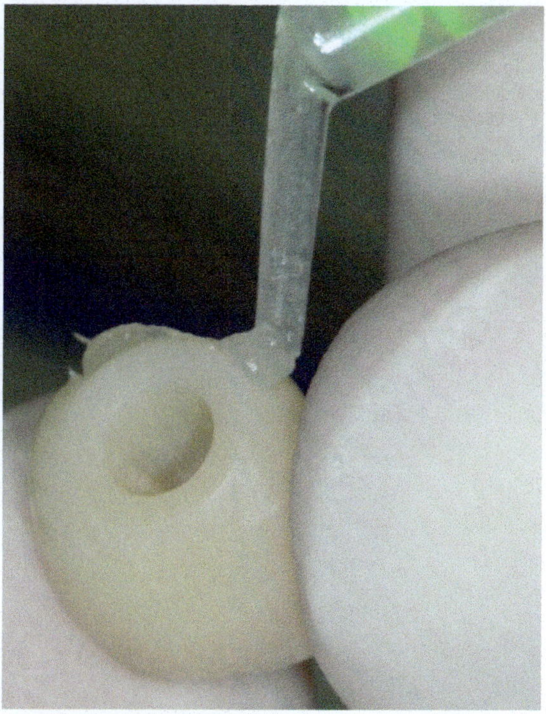

Fig. 13.107 Vaseline is being applied around the CAD/CAM crown to facilitate the removal of extraneous cement during cementation of the abutment and crown

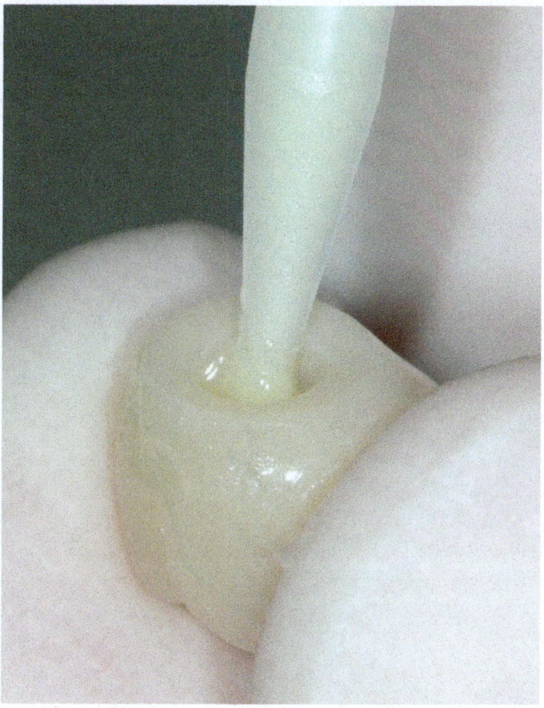

Fig. 13.108 Resin cement is being applied to the bore of the CAD/CAM crown

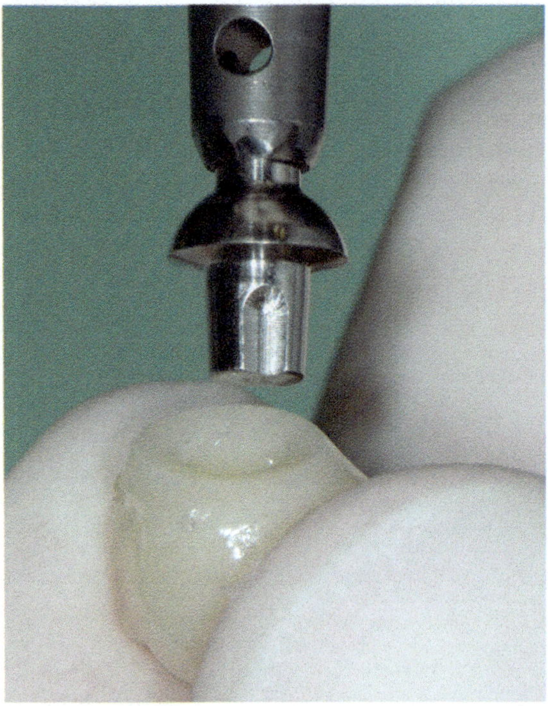

Fig. 13.109 A Universal Abutment is being transported to the cement-filled bore of the CAD/CAM crown

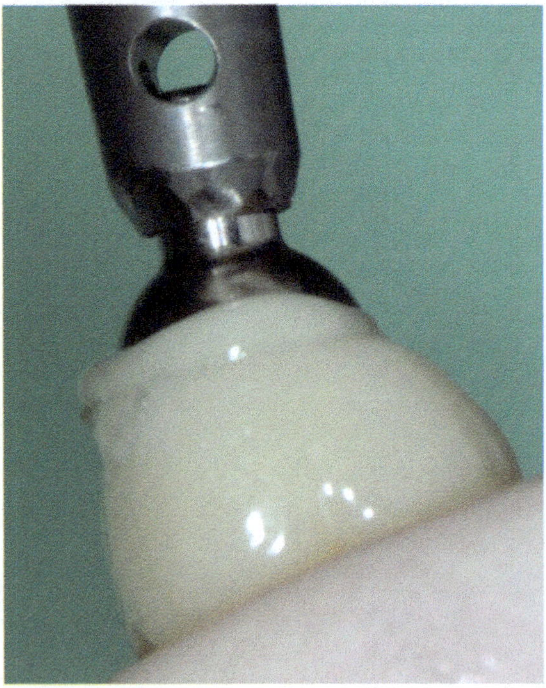

Fig. 13.110 A Universal Abutment is being cemented to the CAD/CAM crown

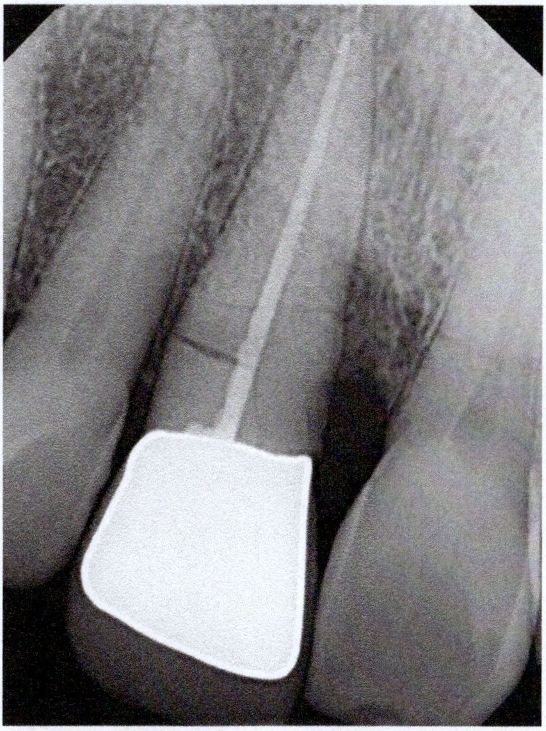

Fig. 13.111 Preoperative radiograph of a non-restorable maxillary right central incisor with a crestal buccal defect

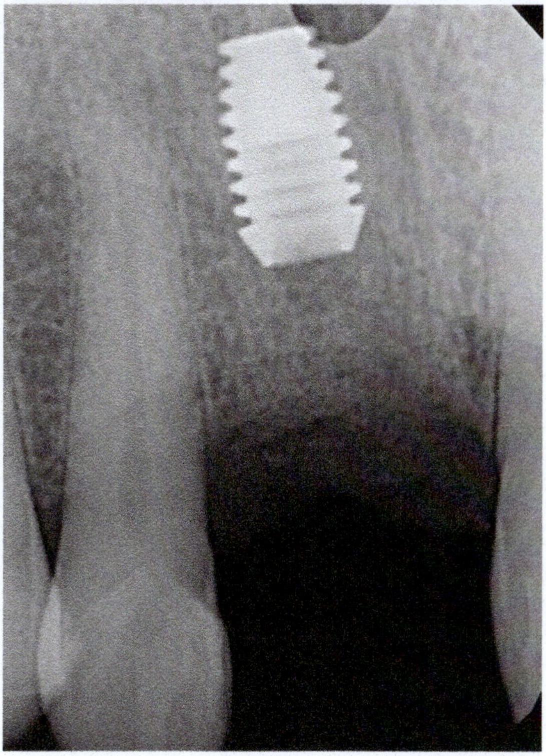

Fig. 13.112 Postoperative radiograph of a 4.5 × 8.0 mm implant with a 2.5 mm well

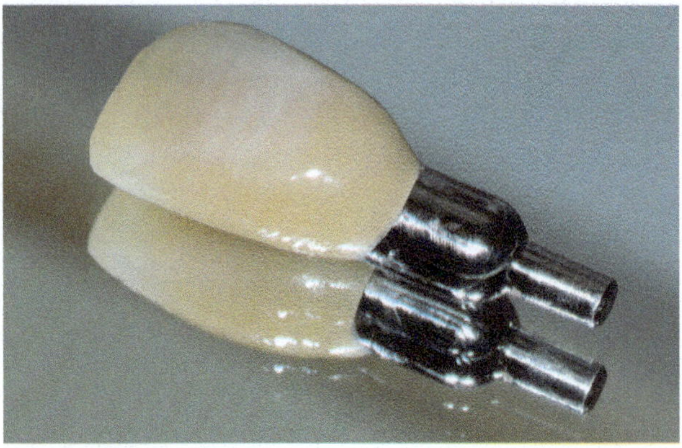

Fig. 13.113 An IAC prior to its insertion

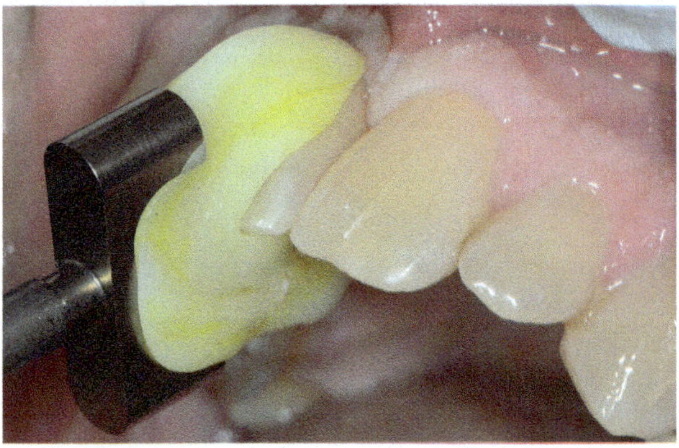

Fig. 13.114 A customized seating jig is being used to definitively seat a maxillary right central incisor IAC

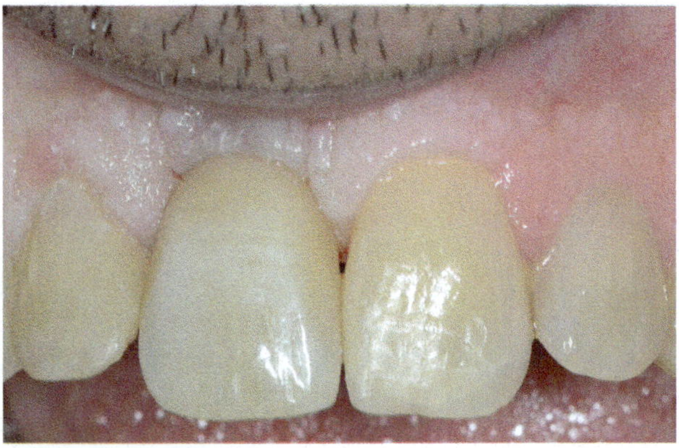

Fig. 13.115 Facial view of a seated maxillary right central incisor IAC

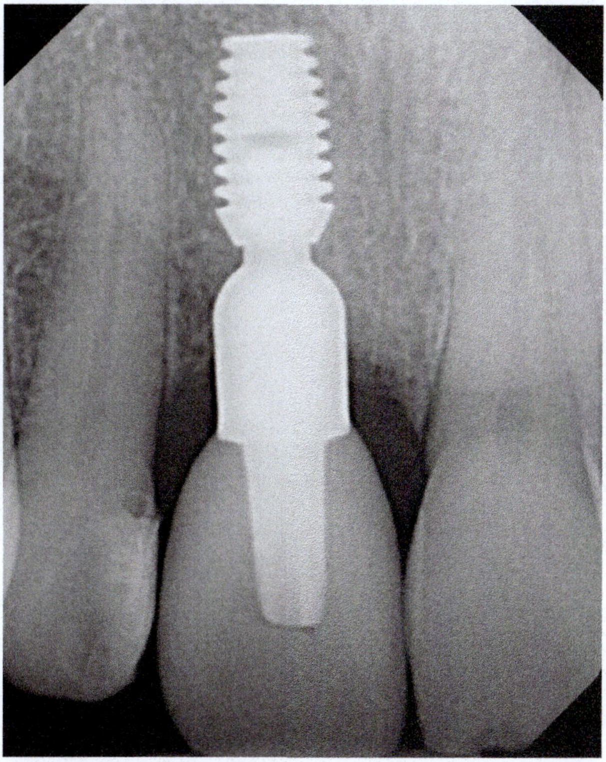

Fig. 13.116 Post-insertion radiograph of a 4.5 × 8.0 mm implant with its seated IAC

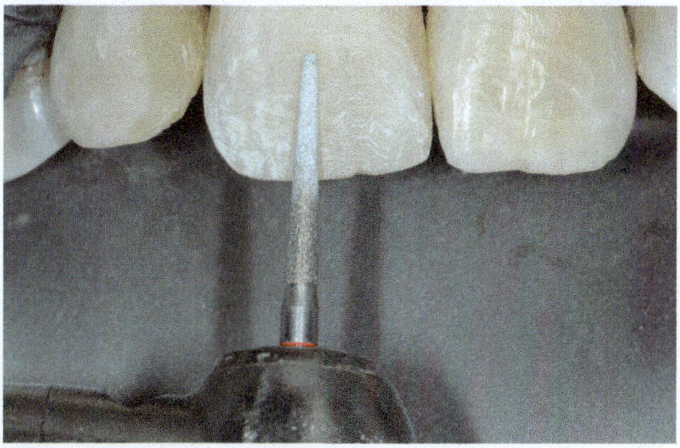

Fig. 13.117 The surface of the IAC is being roughening prior to the application of modeling liquid

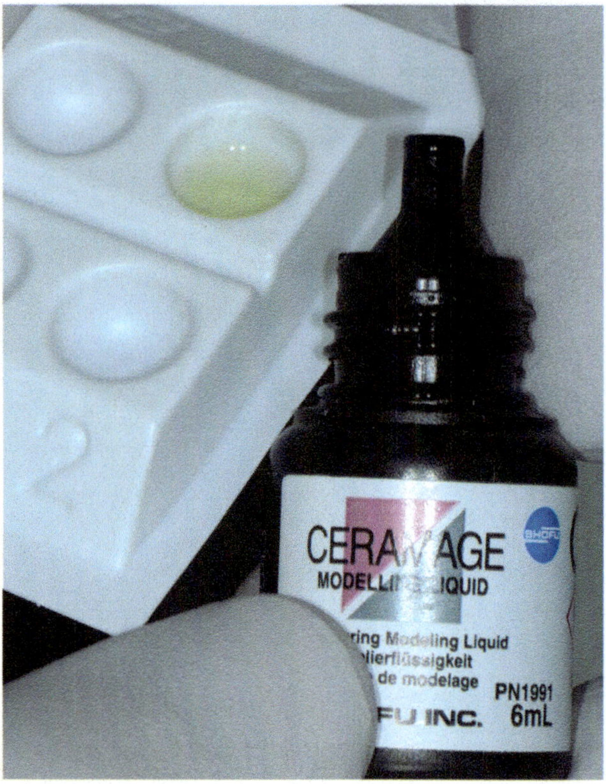

Fig. 13.118 Modeling liquid prior to being applied to the surface of the crown

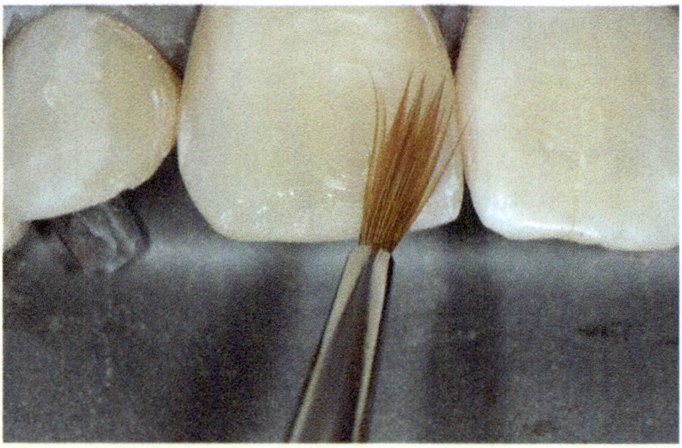

Fig. 13.119 A brush is being used to apply modeling liquid to the surface of the crown

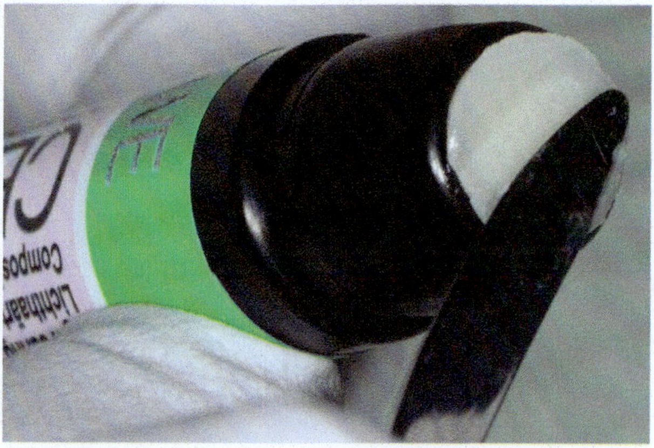

Fig. 13.120 Ceramage, polyceramic material is being applied to a spatula

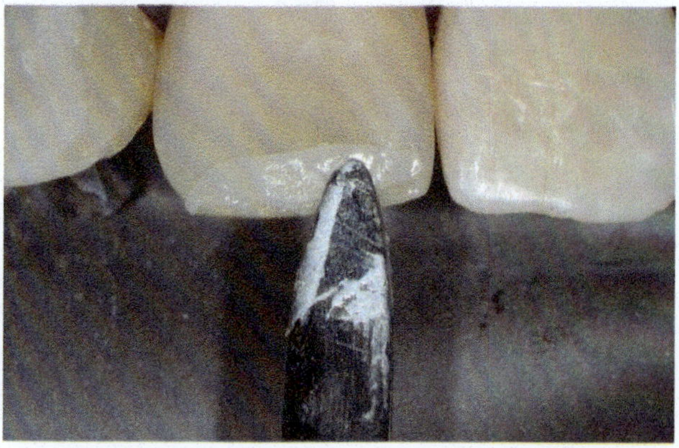

Fig. 13.121 Ceramage, polyceramic material is being added to the surface of the crown

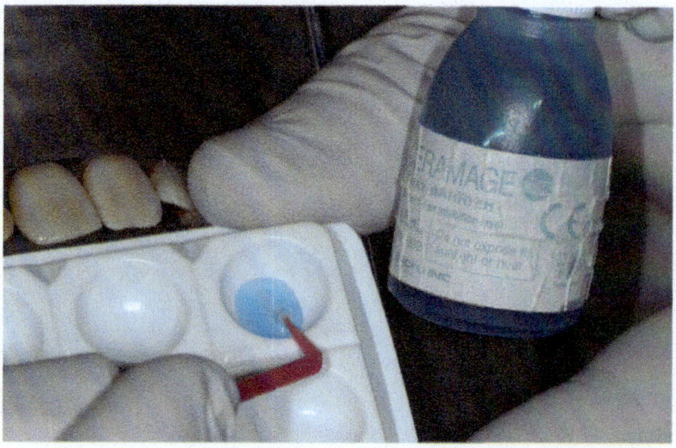

Fig. 13.122 An oxygen barrier prior to being applied to the surface of the crown

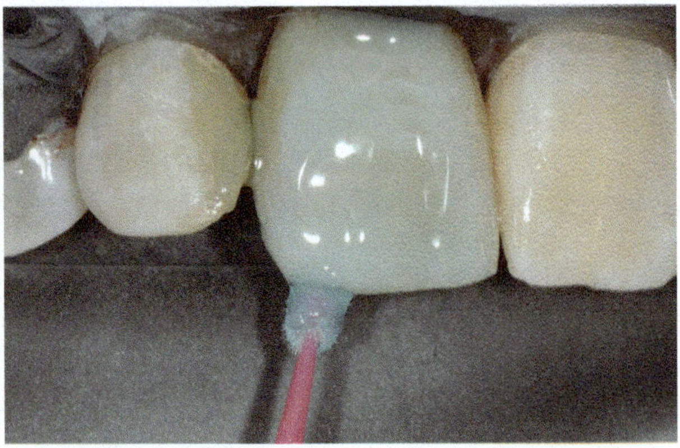

Fig. 13.123 An oxygen barrier is being applied to the surface of the crown for light-curing

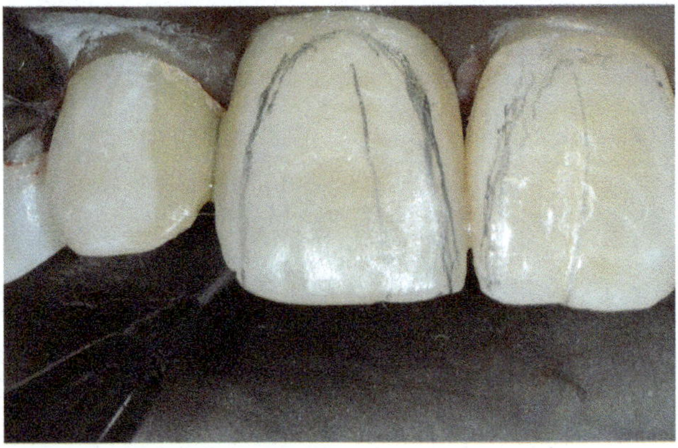

Fig. 13.124 A pencil is being used to mark tracing lines for aesthetic contouring

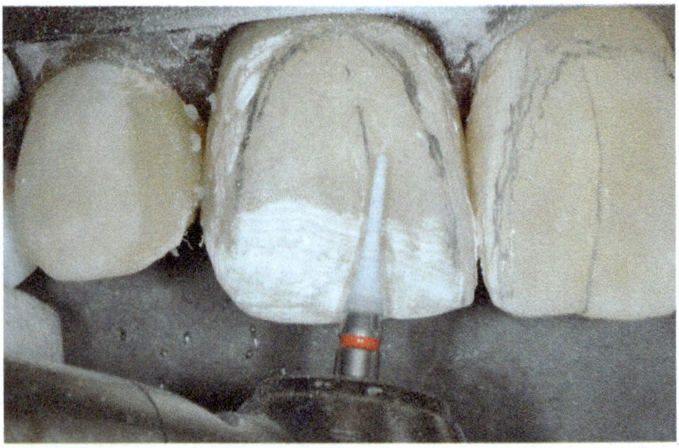

Fig. 13.125 A bur is being used to finalize the crown along the pencil markings for aesthetic contouring

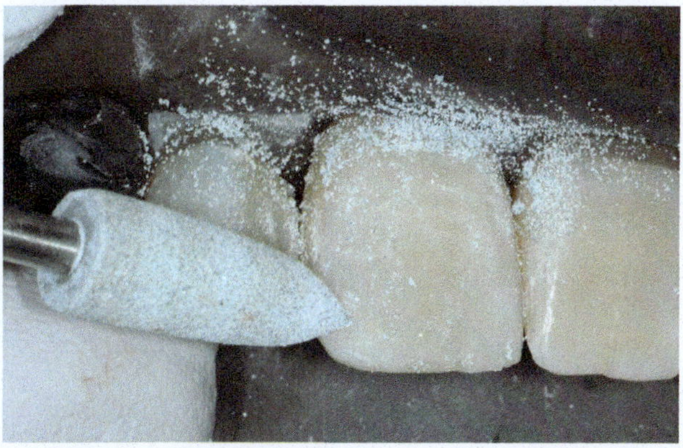

Fig. 13.126 A silicon rubber bur is being used to polish the surface of the modified crown

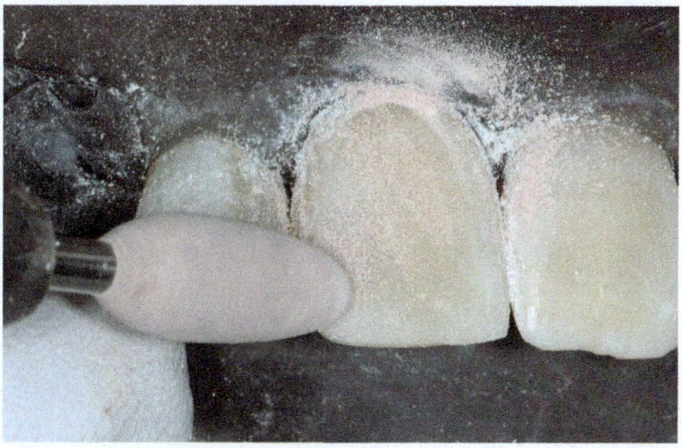

Fig. 13.127 A pink rubber bur is being used to polish the surface of the modified crown

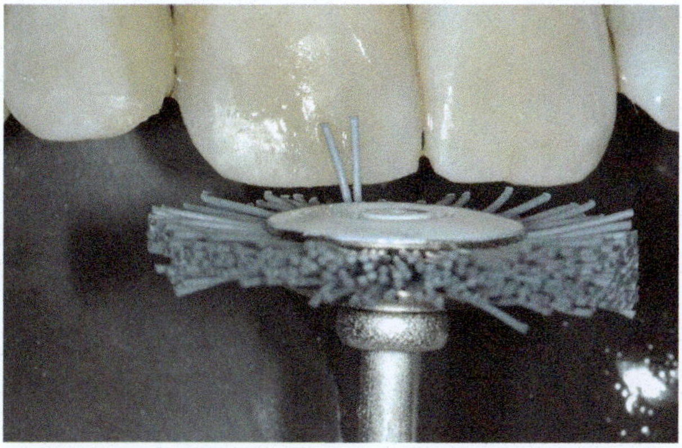

Fig. 13.128 A silicone brush is being used to polish the surface of the modified crown

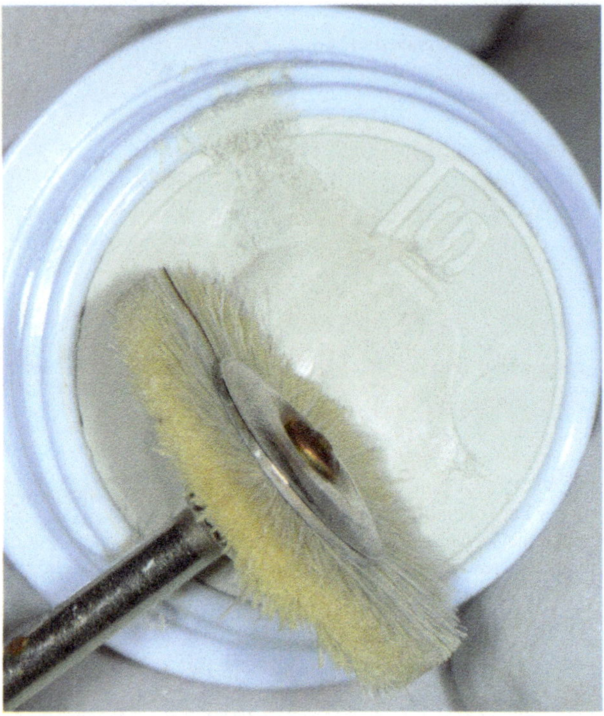

Fig. 13.129 A bristle brush with diamond paste is being used to polish the surface of the modified crown

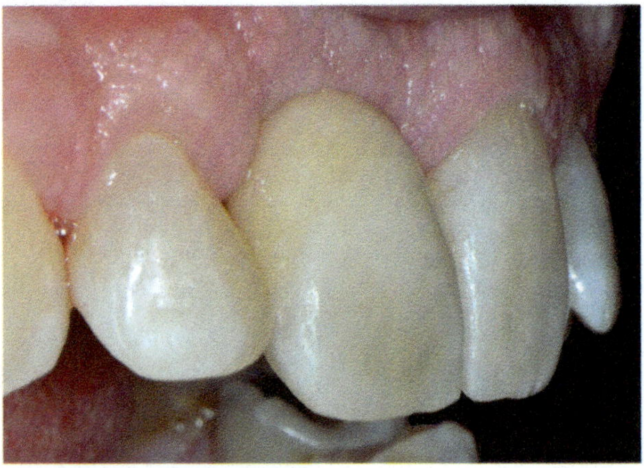

Fig. 13.130 Right profile view of a modified maxillary right central incisor crown

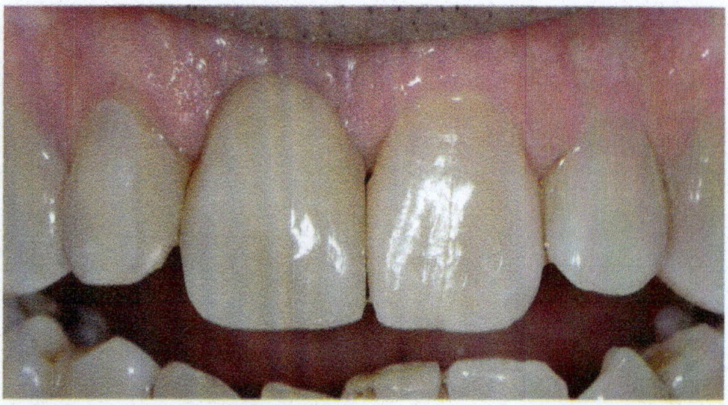

Fig. 13.131 Facial view of a modified maxillary right central incisor crown

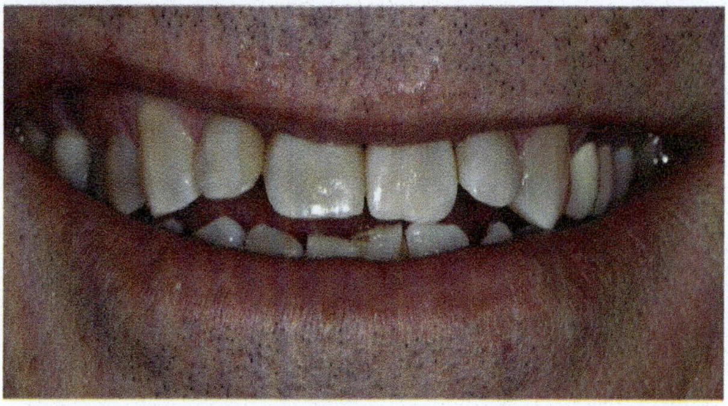

Fig. 13.132 Patient's smile with a modified maxillary right central incisor crown

IAC Case 4: Mandibular Molar IAC

A 44-year-old man presented with a non-restorable deciduous mandibular molar (Tooth K), which was replaced with a 5.0 × 6.0 mm implant with a 3.0 mm well (Fig. 13.133). After 4 months, the implant was uncovered and an implant-level impression was taken (Figs. 13.134, 13.135, and 13.136). A titanium temporary abutment was inserted into the implant well to maintain the implant sulcus for the remainder of the waiting period prior to the fabrication of the IAC (Figs. 13.137 and 13.138). Due to the unseen posterior location of the implant, the temporary abutment sufficed without a crown. At the restorative visit, the implant well was cleaned prior to the insertion of the IAC (Figs. 13.139, 13.140, and 13.141). The interproximal and occlusal contacts were checked with blue ink on floss and articulating paper (Figs. 13.142 and 13.143). Once the contacts were verified, a radiograph confirmed the complete seating of the IAC (Fig. 13.144).

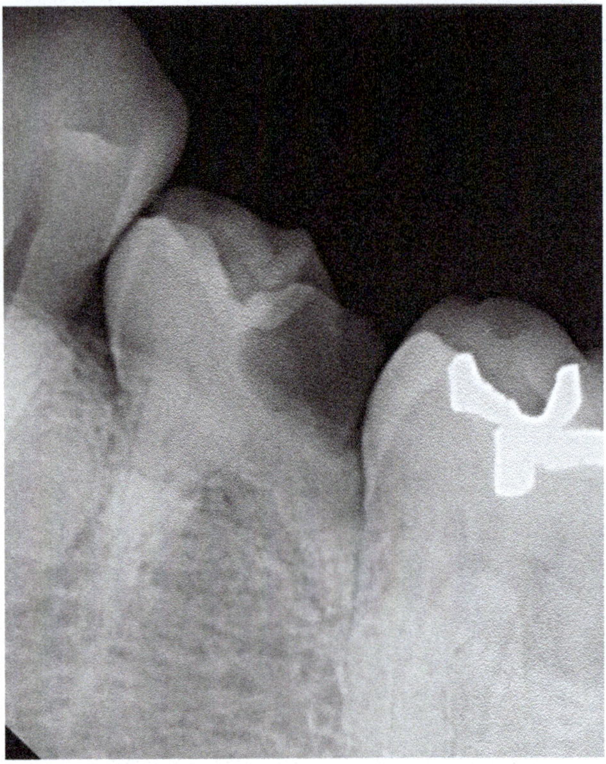

Fig. 13.133 Preoperative radiograph of a non-restorable deciduous mandibular molar (Tooth K)

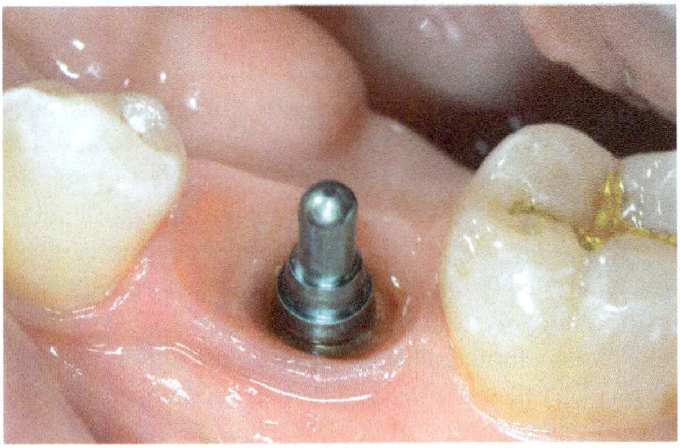

Fig. 13.134 A green 3.0 mm titanium impression post is seated in the well of an implant for the fabrication of an implant-level impression

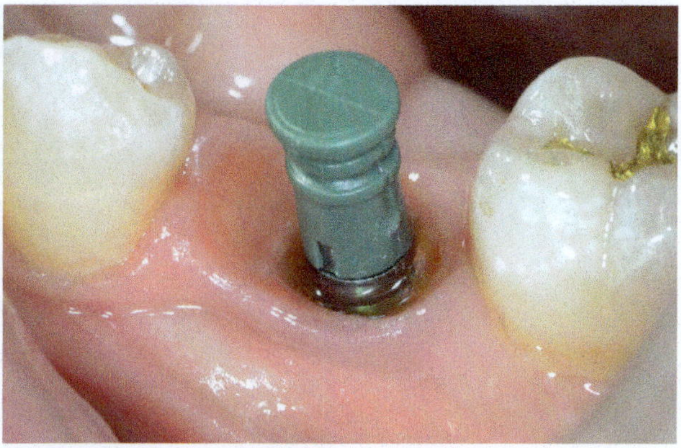

Fig. 13.135 A green acrylic impression sleeve is seated on its impression post

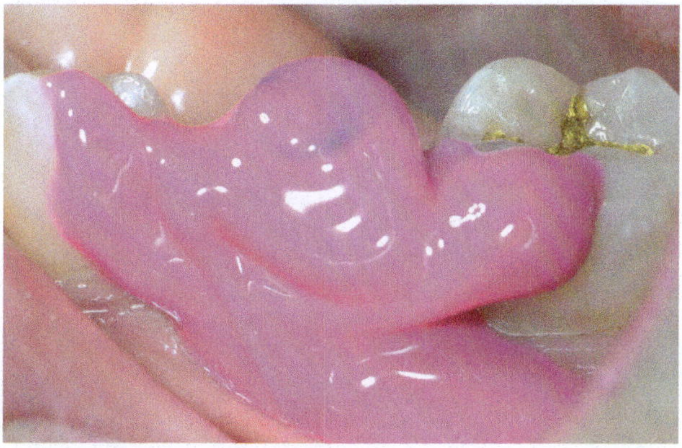

Fig. 13.136 Impression material is being applied around the impression sleeve

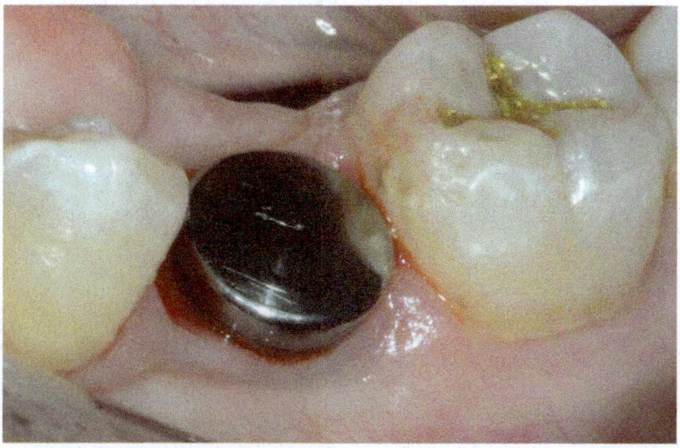

Fig. 13.137 A titanium temporary abutment is seated in an implant for the remainder of the waiting period prior to the fabrication of the IAC

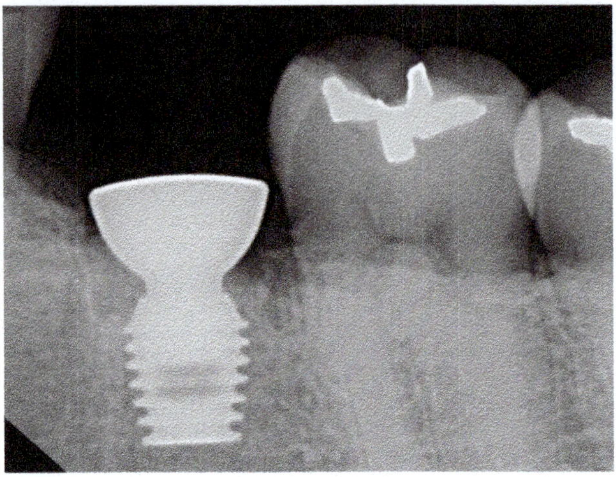

Fig. 13.138 Postoperative radiograph of a 5.0 × 6.0 mm implant with its temporary abutment

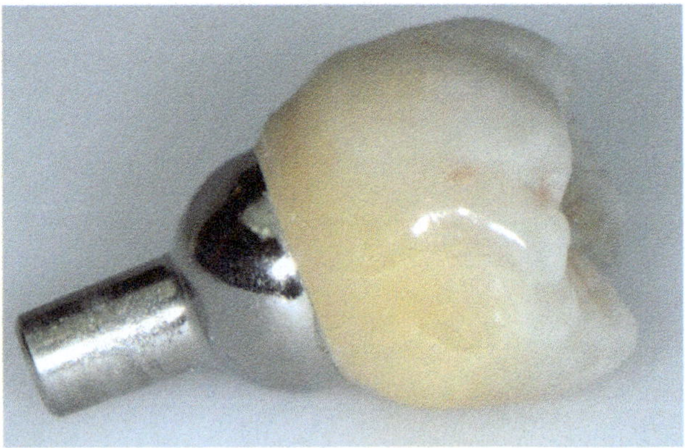

Fig. 13.139 An IAC prior to its insertion

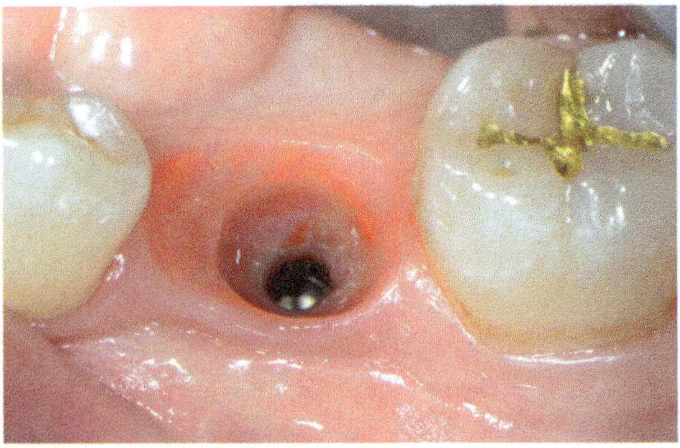

Fig. 13.140 View of a cleaned implant well and sulcus

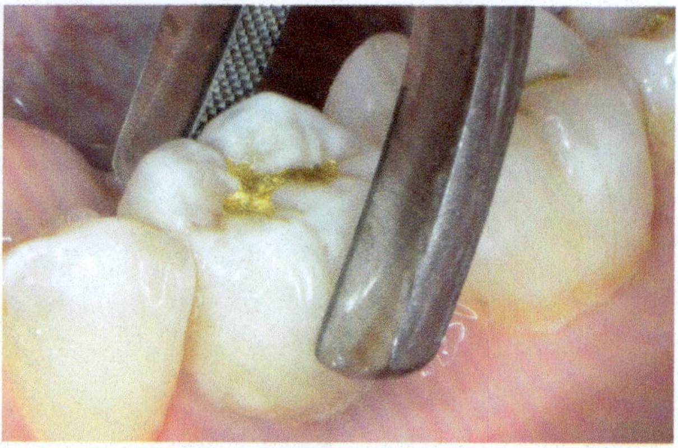

Fig. 13.141 An IAC with gold sealants is being transported to its implant well with forceps

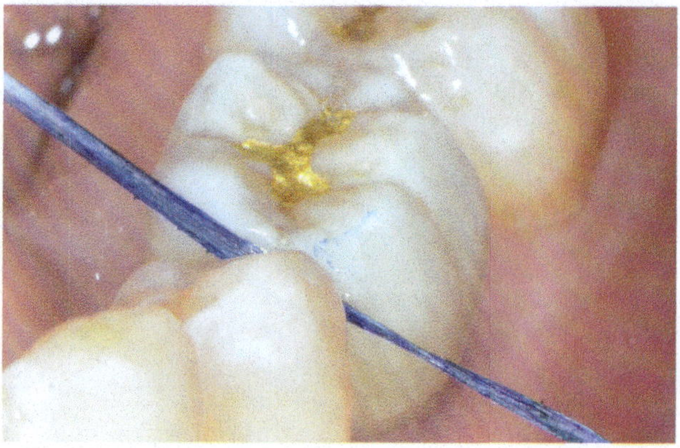

Fig. 13.142 Floss marked with blue ink is being used to check the interproximal contacts

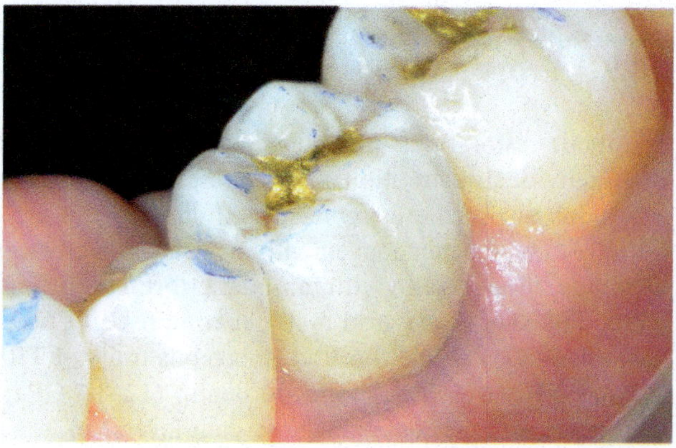

Fig. 13.143 Blue ink from articulating paper marks the occlusal contacts

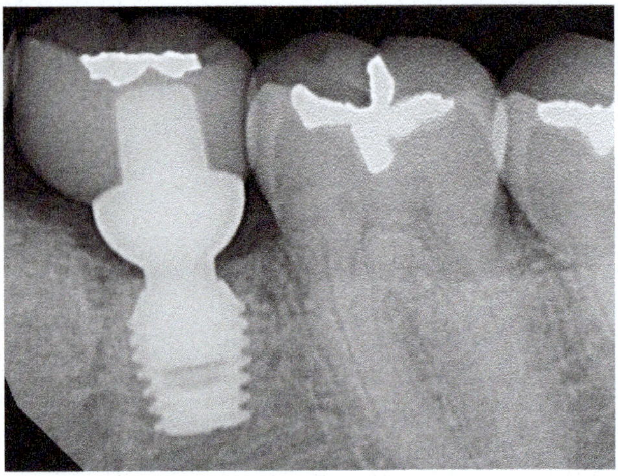

Fig. 13.144 Post-insertion radiograph of a 5.0 × 6.0 mm implant with its seated IAC

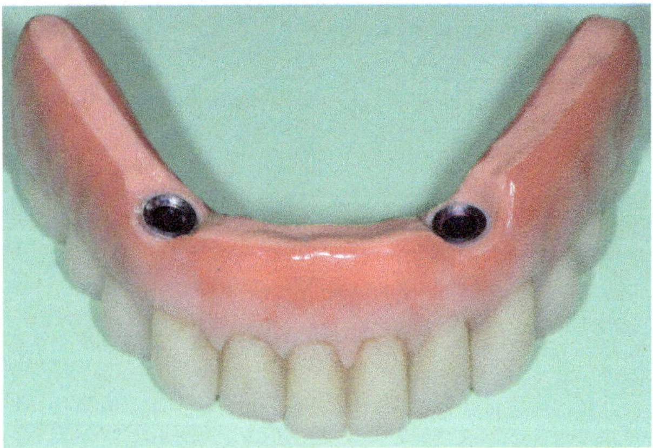

Fig. 13.145 A mandibular two-unit TRINIA prosthesis with cantilevers up to 24 mm long

13.5 Prosthetic Restorations and TRINIA®

Prosthetic restorations often demand arduous procedures that take much more time than individual restorations, but there are certain techniques that can facilitate the insertions of prostheses. One such strategy is the use of the CAD/CAM material, TRINIA®, which can conveniently be used with any implant, and it can be modified chairside, if necessary, with minimal effort. Utilized as a restorative material since 2010, TRINIA is a hybrid material composed of 60% filaments of fiberglass and 40% resin. One of the most advantageous traits of TRINIA is its flexural modulus of 18.8 GPa, which is similar to dentin (12–14 GPa). This elasticity enables the prosthesis to function with large cantilevers, in some cases up to 24 mm long (Figs. 13.145, 13.146, and 13.147). Another benefit of the material is its bond strength, which is compatible with any polyceramic material of similar bond

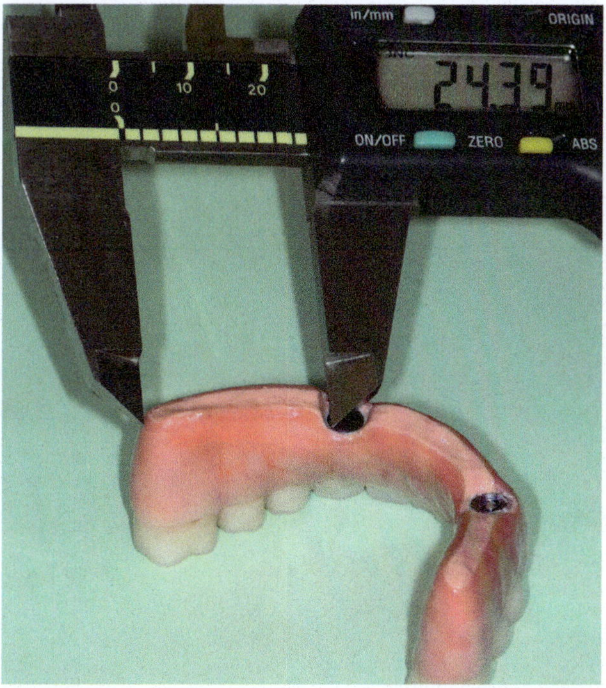

Fig. 13.146 Cantilever of a two-unit TRINIA prosthesis is being measured with a calibration device at 24.39 mm

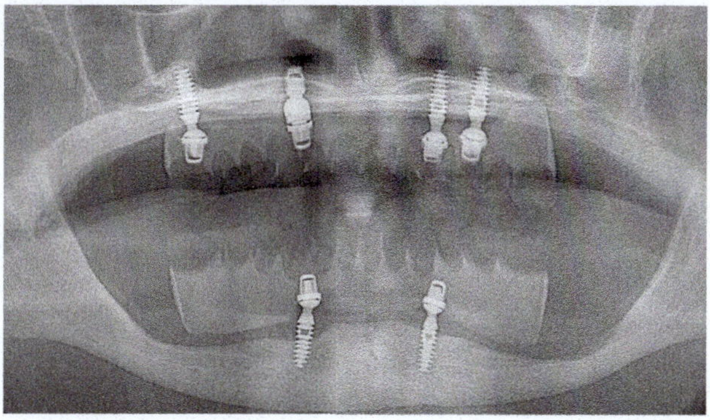

Fig. 13.147 Panoramic radiograph of a two-unit TRINIA prosthesis with large cantilevers

strength, and is capable of withstanding a high range of temperatures [14]. It is light in weight and available in either a pink or cream color, and in the shape of a disc or block (Figs. 13.148, 13.49, and 13.150). TRINIA can be used to mill prosthetic substructures or abutment copings, and since it does not require curing or sintering, the processing is cost-effective in comparison to other restorative materials. The following cases demonstrate the versatility of TRINIA and the efficiency of fabricating and inserting these multi-unit restorations.

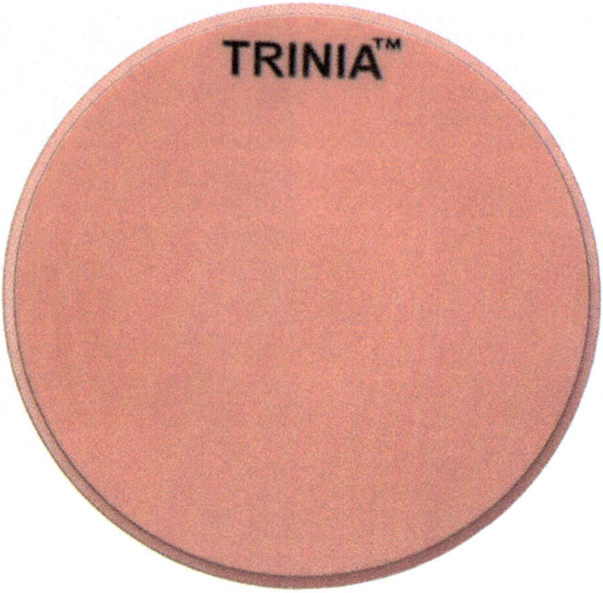

Fig. 13.148 A pink TRINIA disc

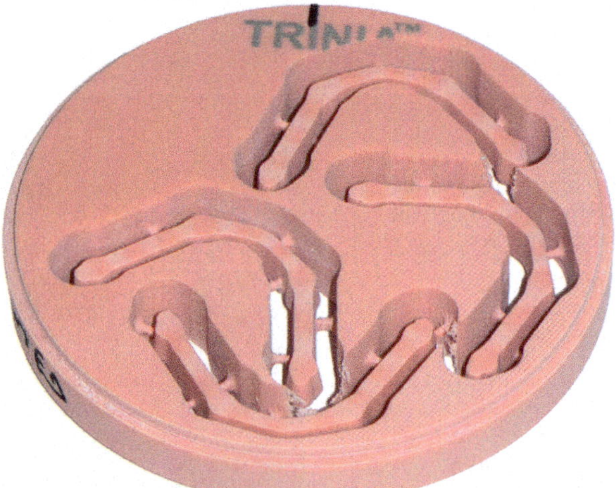

Fig. 13.149 A pink TRINIA disc with four milled prosthetic substructures

TRINIA Case 1: Four-Unit TRINIA Bridge for the Anterior Maxilla

A 47-year-old woman presented with non-restorable maxillary lateral incisors and severely compromised bone in the area of her maxillary central incisors due to a car accident 6 months previously. The four teeth were extracted and two 4.5 × 8.0 mm implants with 2.5 mm wells were placed into the areas of the lateral incisors using the Bicon two-stage technique (Figs. 13.151 and 13.152); at the second stage, 4 months later, the implants were uncovered an implant-level impression was made. The four-unit bridge was fabricated with a TRINIA substructure and layers of poly-ceramic buildup (Figs. 13.153, 13.154, 13.155, 13.156, and 13.157). At the

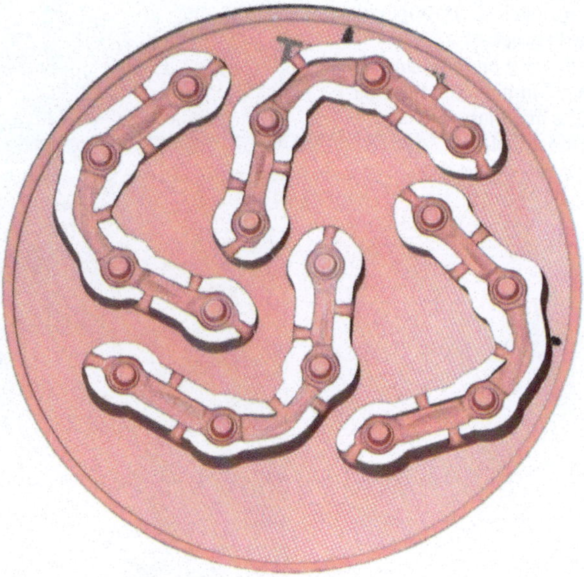

Fig. 13.150 A pink TRINIA disc with four milled prosthetic substructures

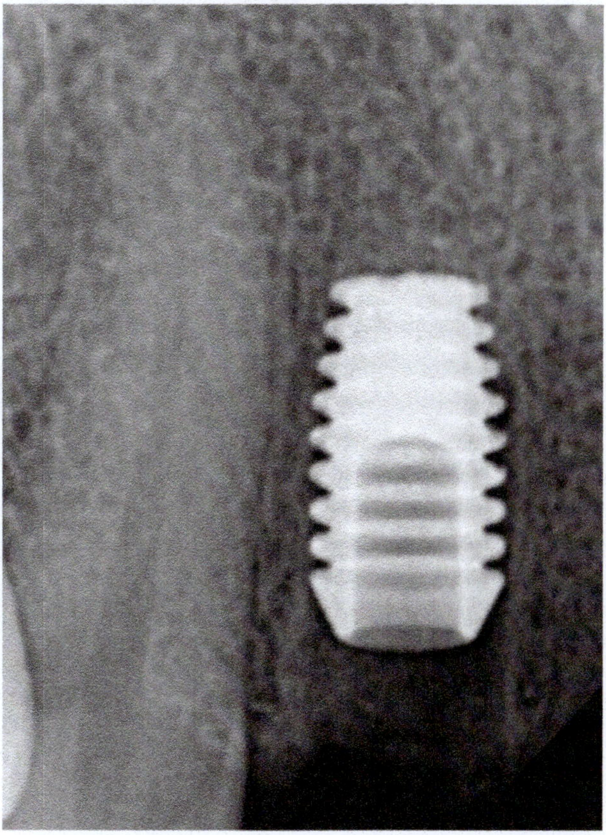

Fig. 13.151 Postoperative radiograph of a 4.5 × 8.0 mm implant with a 2.5 mm well in the area of a maxillary right lateral incisor

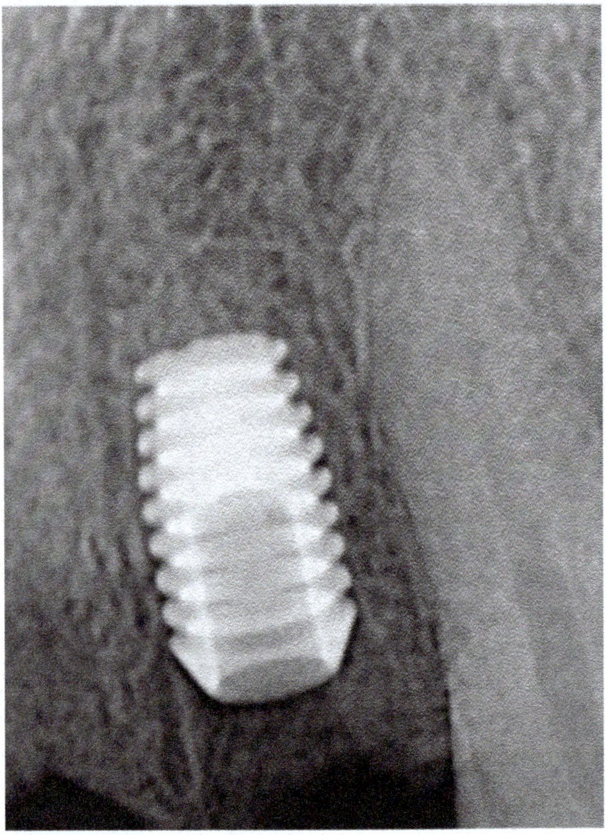

Fig. 13.152 Postoperative radiograph of a 4.5 × 8.0 mm implant with a 2.5 mm well in the area of a maxillary left lateral incisor

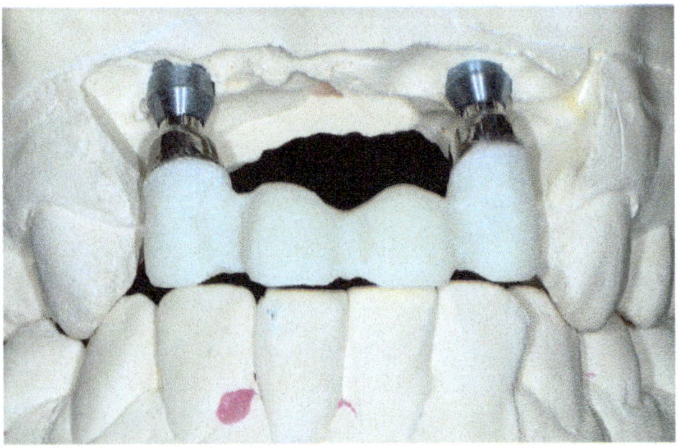

Fig. 13.153 A four-unit TRINIA substructure is seated on two abutments in a stone model

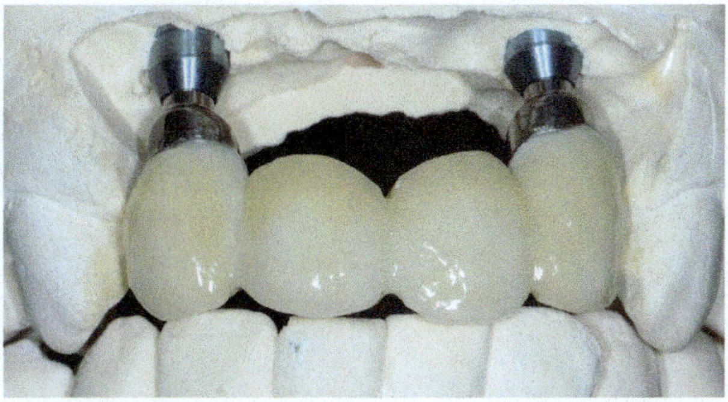

Fig. 13.154 View after first layers of polyceramic material have been added to the TRINIA substructure

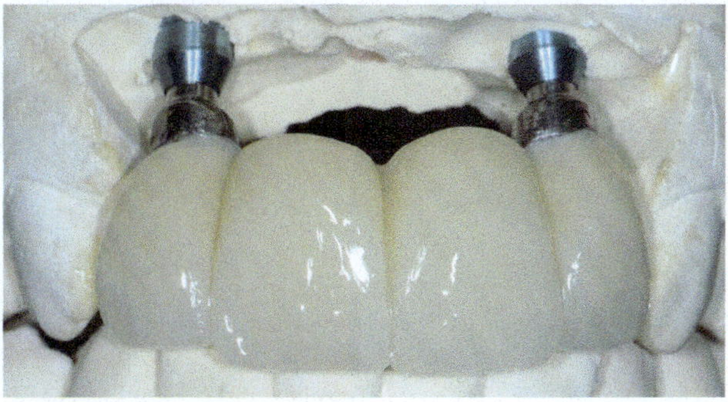

Fig. 13.155 View after final layers of polyceramic material have been added to the TRINIA substructure

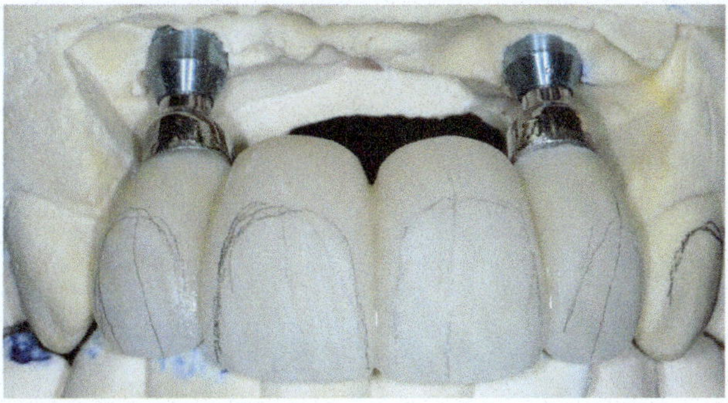

Fig. 13.156 Pencil lines mark the surface of the bridge for guidance during aesthetic contouring

restorative visit, the two sandblasted abutments were inserted into their respective implant wells with an orientation and seating jig, and subsequently tapped for definitive seating (Figs. 13.158, 13.159, and 13.160). The bridge was then inserted onto the abutments without cement so as to give the gingival tissues time to form papillae prior to the permanent seating. One week later, the gingival tissues presented a healthy response to the bridge, thus the bridge was permanently cemented onto the abutments (Figs. 13.161, 13.162, 13.163, and 13.164). The patient was instructed on two methods of cleaning underneath the fixed bridge: the use of a proxy brush, and

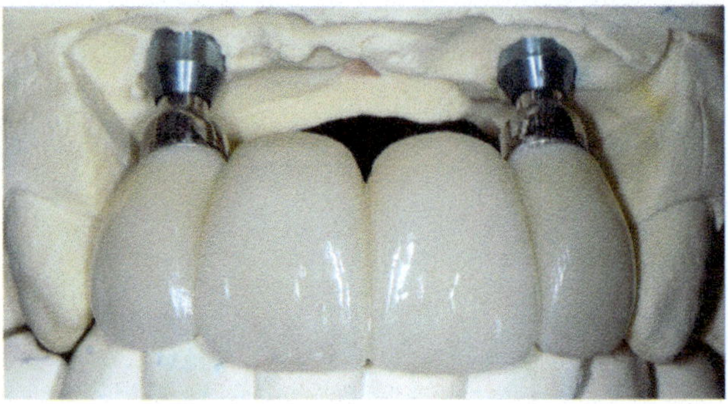

Fig. 13.157 A finished four-unit TRINIA bridge is seated on two abutments in a stone model

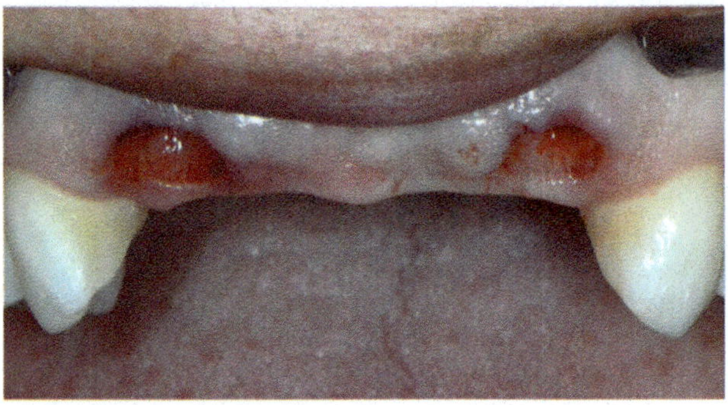

Fig. 13.158 Facial view of two sulci prior to the insertion of two sandblasted abutments

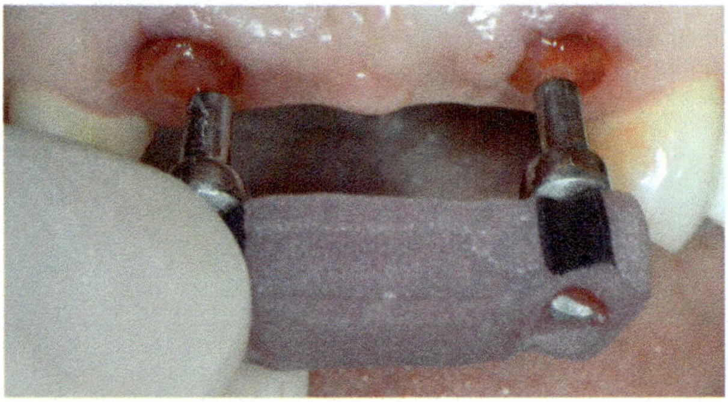

Fig. 13.159 Two abutments are being transported to their respective sulci with an orientation and seating jig

the use of a floss threader (Figs. 13.165 and 13.166). The complete seating of the fixed bridge was confirmed with radiographs (Figs. 13.167, 13.168, 13.169, and 13.170).

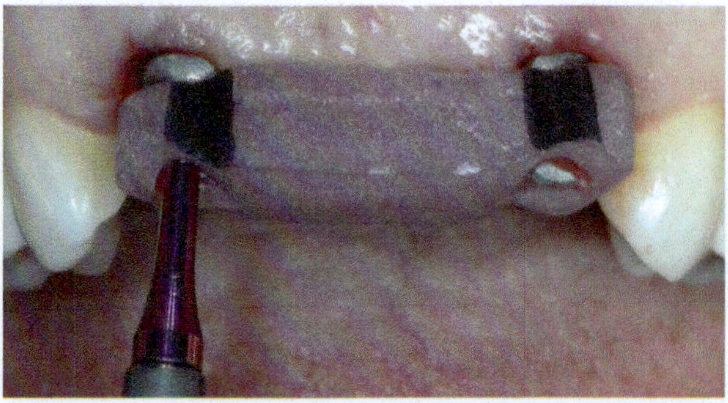

Fig. 13.160 An implant seating tip is being used to tap the two abutments as they are being positioned with the orientation and seating jig

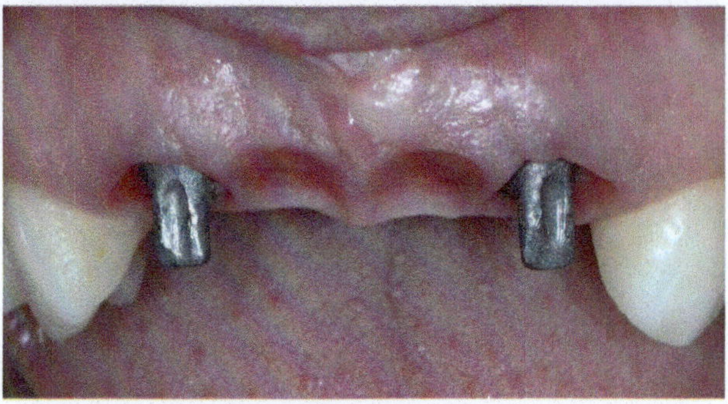

Fig. 13.161 One-week post-insertion view of healthy gingival tissues and papilla beginning to form

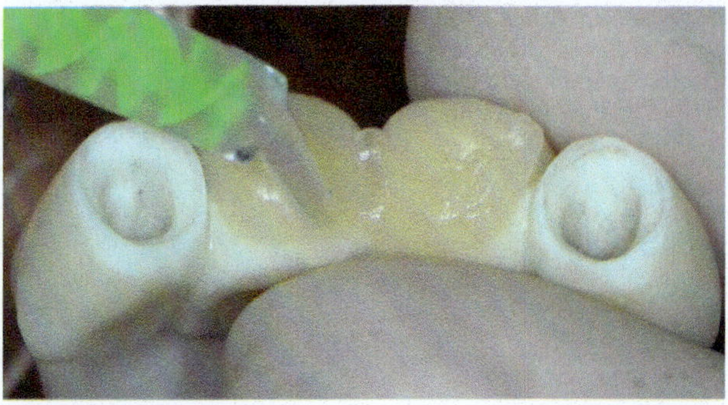

Fig. 13.162 Vaseline is being applied around a bridge to facilitate the removal of extraneous cement

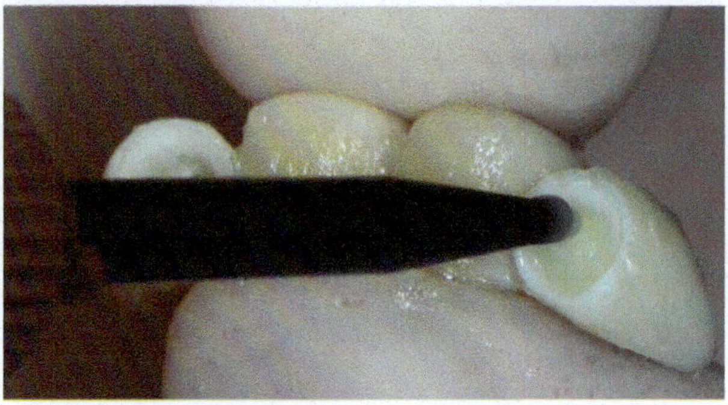

Fig. 13.163 Resin cement is being applied to the bores of a bridge

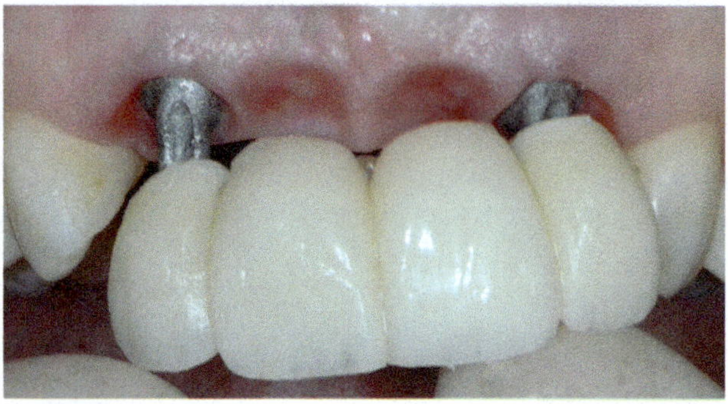

Fig. 13.164 A four-unit TRINIA bridge is being cemented onto two sandblasted abutments

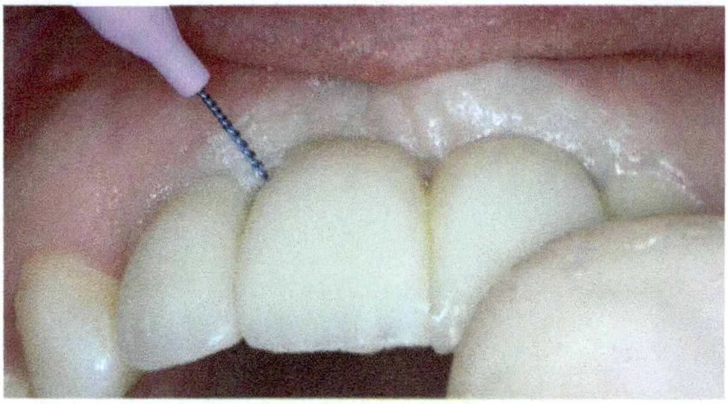

Fig. 13.165 A proxy brush is being used to floss between the gingival tissues and the fixed bridge

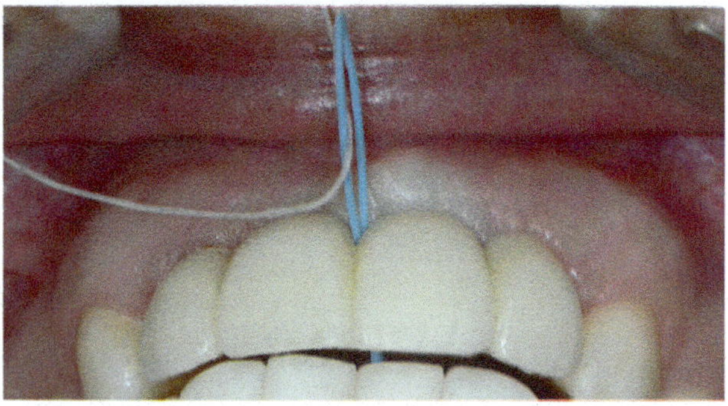

Fig. 13.166 A floss threader is being used to floss between the gingival tissues and the fixed bridge

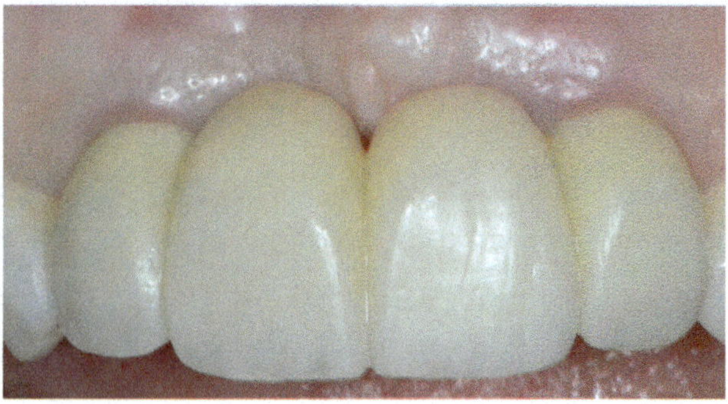

Fig. 13.167 Facial view of a definitively seated four-unit TRINIA bridge in the anterior maxilla

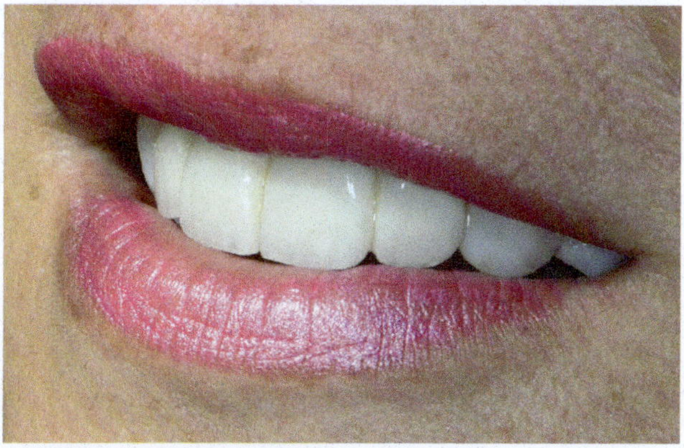

Fig. 13.168 Patient's smile with a four-unit TRINIA bridge in the anterior maxilla

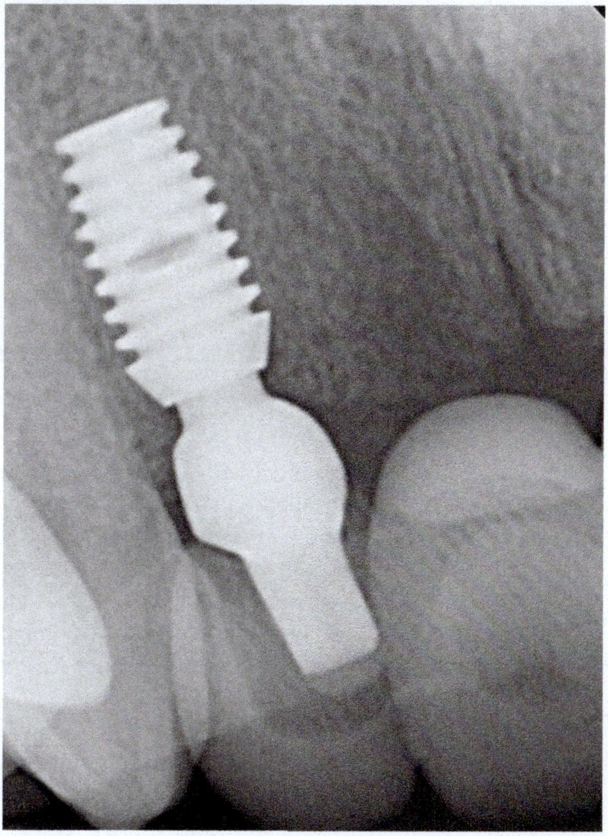

Fig. 13.169 Post-insertion radiograph of a 4.5 × 8.0 mm implant with its seated TRINIA bridge in the area of a maxillary right lateral incisor

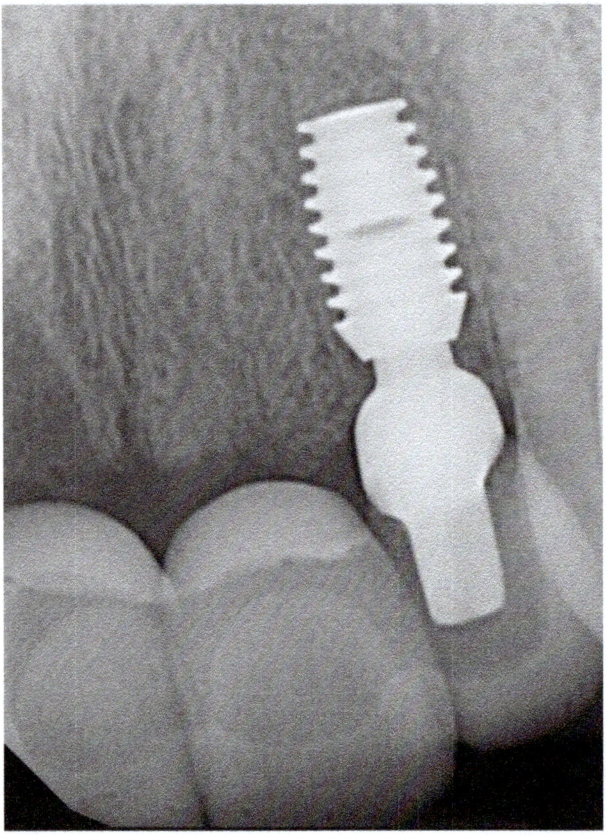

Fig. 13.170 Post-insertion radiograph of a 4.5 × 8.0 mm implant with its seated TRINIA bridge in the area of a maxillary left lateral incisor

TRINIA Case 2: Three-Unit TRINIA Bridge for the Posterior Mandible

A 60-year-old woman presented with a non-restorable mandibular right first premolar and a non-restorable mandibular right first molar, which were treated with a 4.5 × 6.0 mm and a 5.0 × 6.0 mm implant, respectively (Fig. 13.171). Four months later, the implants were uncovered, at which time the adjacent second molar was extracted due to advanced dental caries to the root and periapical pathology. The laboratory fabricated two types of bridges for comparison: one bridge was composed of a hybrid of materials (first milled from a Shofu HC disc and then layered with polyceramic material); the other bridge was handcrafted with a buildup of polyceramic material (Figs. 13.172, 13.173, 13.174, 13.175, and 13.176). Despite the differing superstructures, a TRINIA bar comprised both substructures. At the restorative visit, the titanium temporary abutments were removed for the insertion of two permanent sandblasted abutments (Figs. 13.177, 13.178, and 13.179). Upon insertion of the two TRINIA bridges, the one with the hybrid material teeth was found to be less aesthetic than the bridge with the handcrafted polyceramic teeth, so it was the latter that was chosen for cementation (Figs. 13.180 and 13.181). It is worth noting that although the bridge with the hybrid material teeth is less aesthetic,

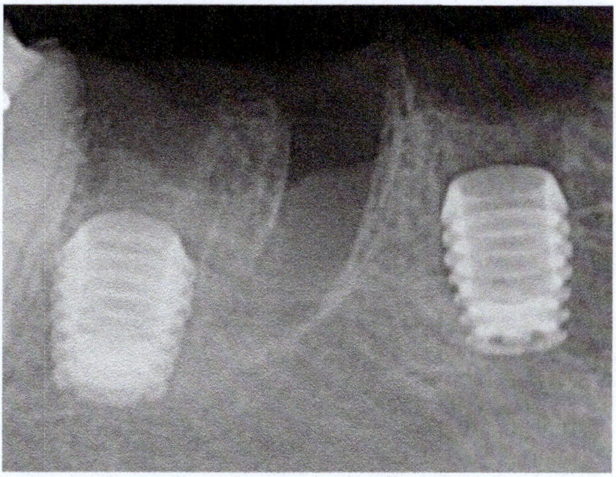

Fig. 13.171 Postoperative radiograph of a 4.5 × 6.0 mm and a 5.0 × 6.0 mm implant in the posterior mandible

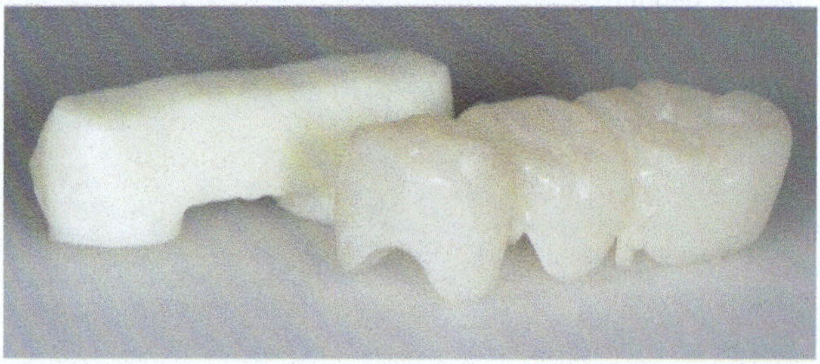

Fig. 13.172 A milled TRINIA bar and milled Shofu HC teeth prior to their fusion as the substructure and superstructure for a hybrid material bridge

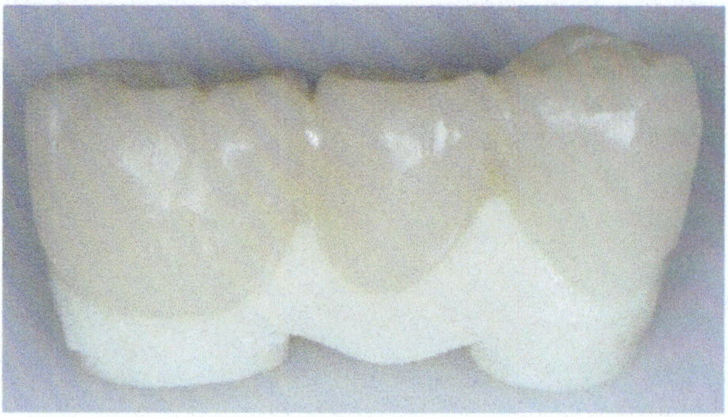

Fig. 13.173 Milled Shofu HC teeth seated on a milled TRINIA bar prior to their fusion as the substructure and superstructure for a hybrid material bridge

it provides a cost-effective option for the patient and laboratory alike. The cementation process began with the application of Vaseline around the ridge side of the bridge to facilitate the removal of extraneous cement (Fig. 13.182). Once the bores were filled with resin cement, the bridge was transported to the two abutments where it received occlusal pressure from the patient biting down on a cotton roll (Figs. 13.183 and 13.184). After the cementation, the interproximal contacts were

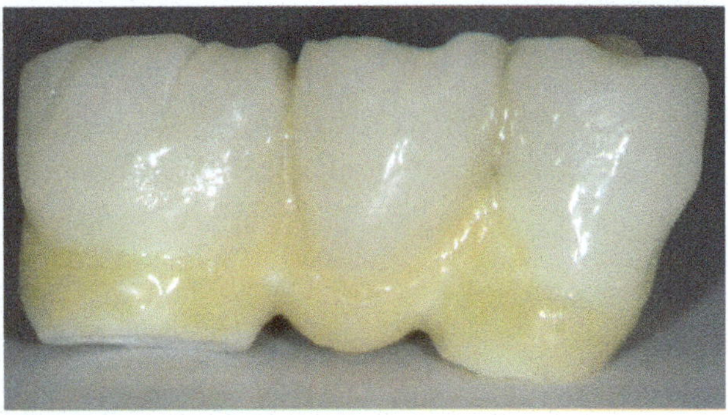

Fig. 13.174 A finished hybrid material bridge after the fusion of the TRINIA substructure and HC superstructure, and a coating of polyceramic material

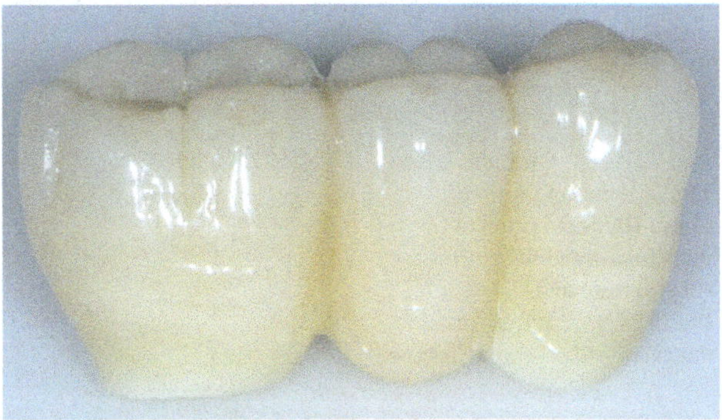

Fig. 13.175 A finished bridge composed of a TRINIA substructure and a handcrafted polyceramic material buildup superstructure

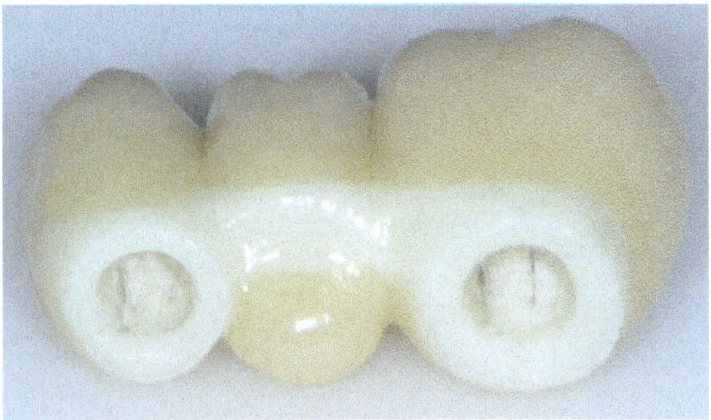

Fig. 13.176 A ridge-side view of a finished bridge composed of a TRINIA substructure and a handcrafted polyceramic material buildup

checked with floss, and the occlusal contacts were checked with articulating paper (Figs. 13.185 and 13.186). The blue ink marked points of contact that were too high, so a series of polishing burs and brushes were used to adjust the bridge until appropriate occlusal contacts were achieved (Figs. 13.187 and 13.188). A post-insertion radiograph revealed complete seating of the fixed three-unit bridge (Fig. 13.189).

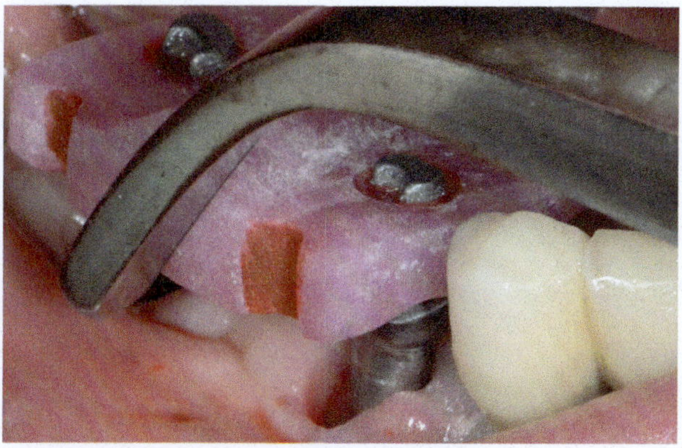

Fig. 13.177 Two sandblasted abutments are being transported to their implants with an orientation and seating jig

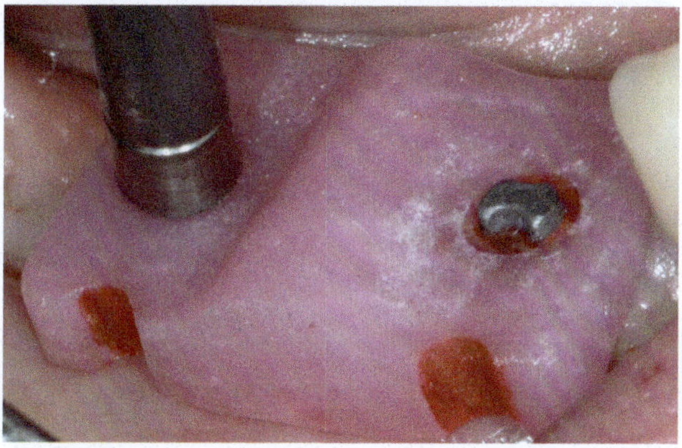

Fig. 13.178 A standard seating tip on a threaded handle is being used to tap the abutments while they are positioned in the orientation and seating jig

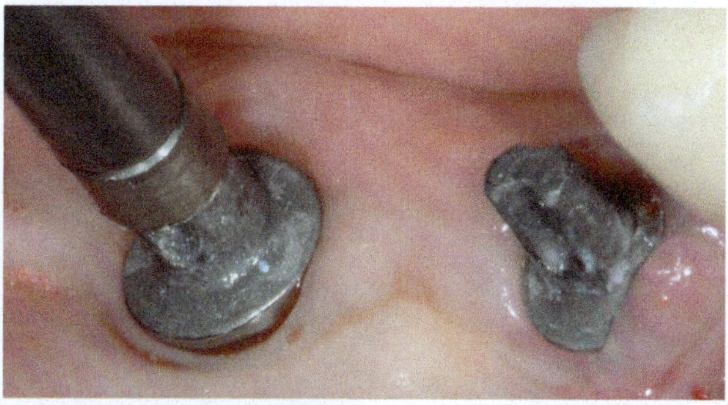

Fig. 13.179 A standard seating tip on a threaded handle is being used to definitively tap the abutments

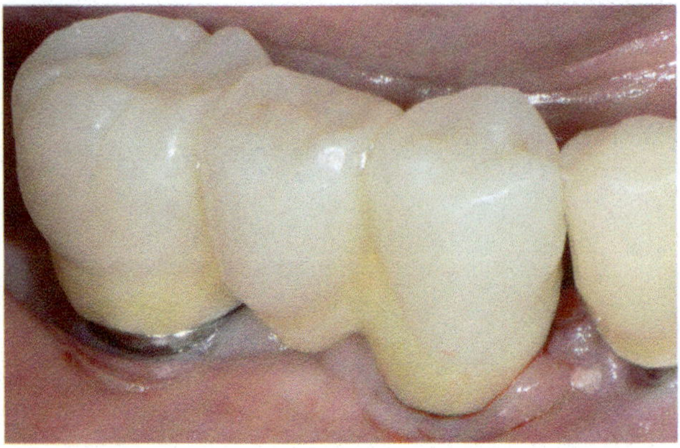

Fig. 13.180 Intraoral view of a TRINIA bridge with hybrid material teeth

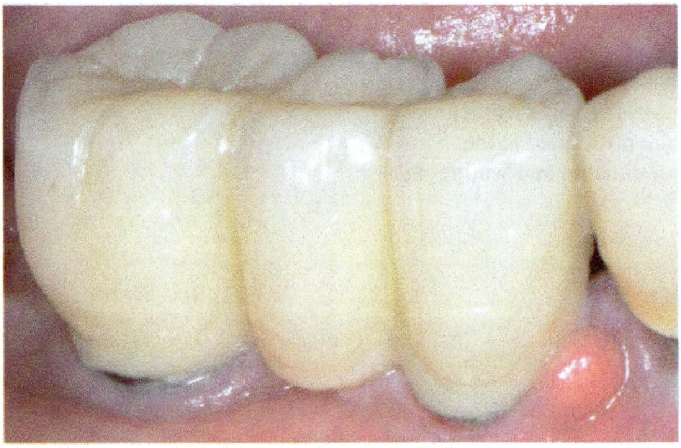

Fig. 13.181 Intraoral view a TRINIA bridge with handcrafted teeth of polyceramic material buildup

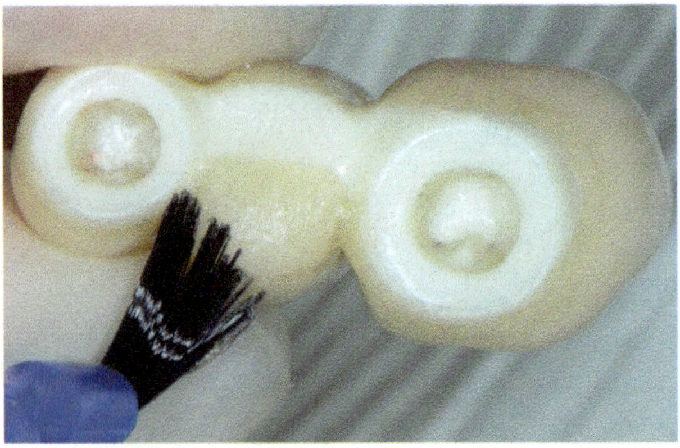

Fig. 13.182 Vaseline is being applied to the TRINIA bridge to facilitate the removal of extraneous cement during cementation

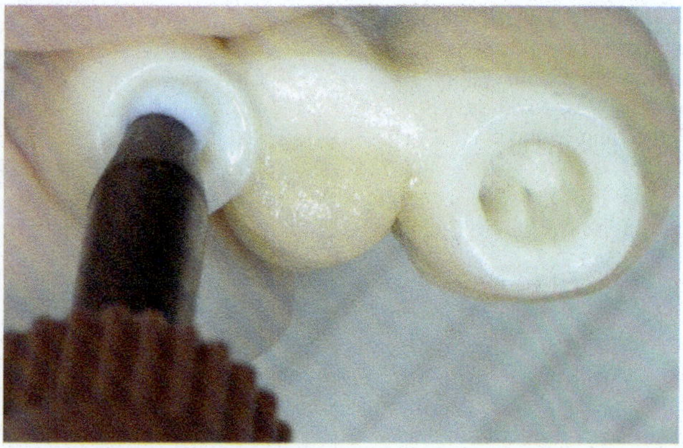

Fig. 13.183 Resin cement is being applied to the bores of the TRINIA bridge

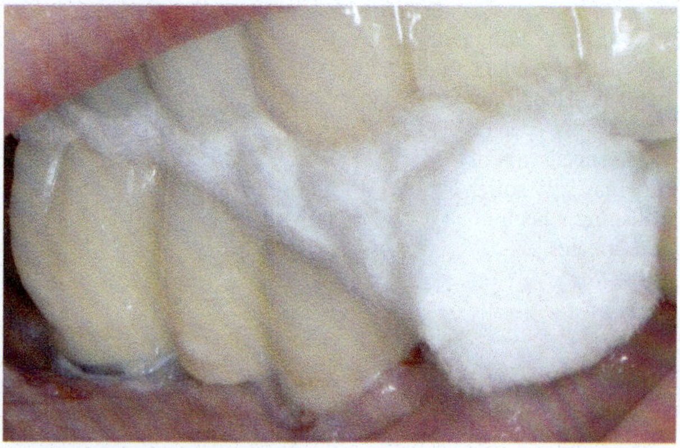

Fig. 13.184 A three-unit TRINIA bridge is being seated with occlusal pressure from a cotton roll

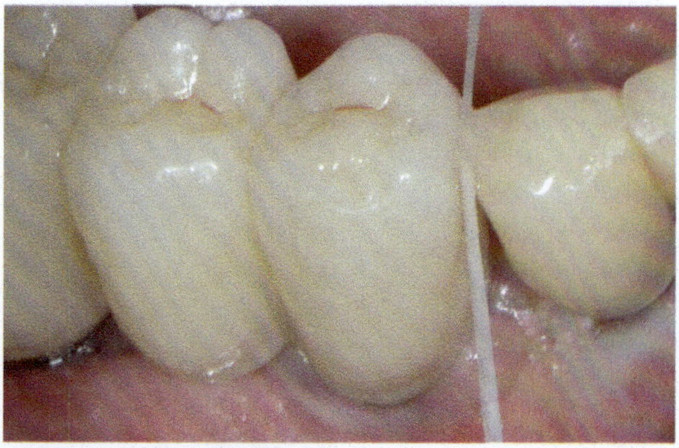

Fig. 13.185 Floss is being used to check the interproximal contacts of the bridge and the adjacent teeth

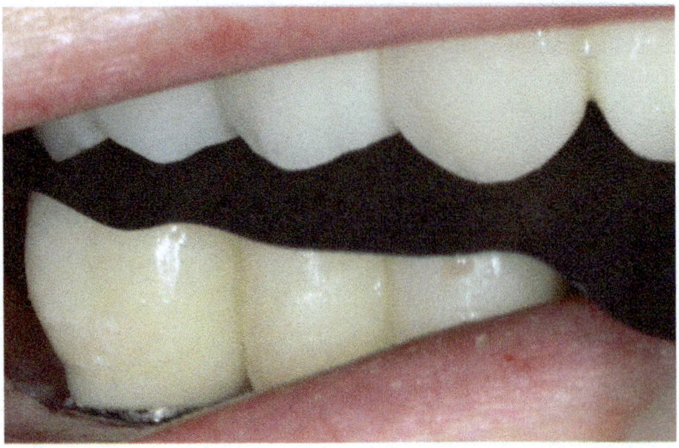

Fig. 13.186 Articulating paper is being used to check the occlusal contacts of the bridge and the opposing teeth

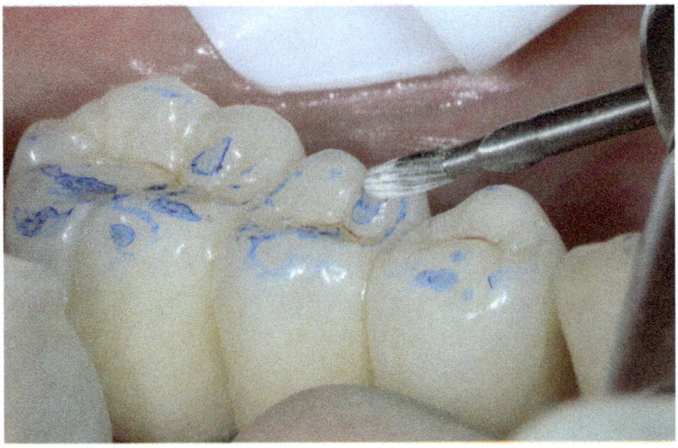

Fig. 13.187 Points of high occlusal contact are being polished intraorally with a slow-speed bur prior to the succession of progressively softer polishing wheels and brushes

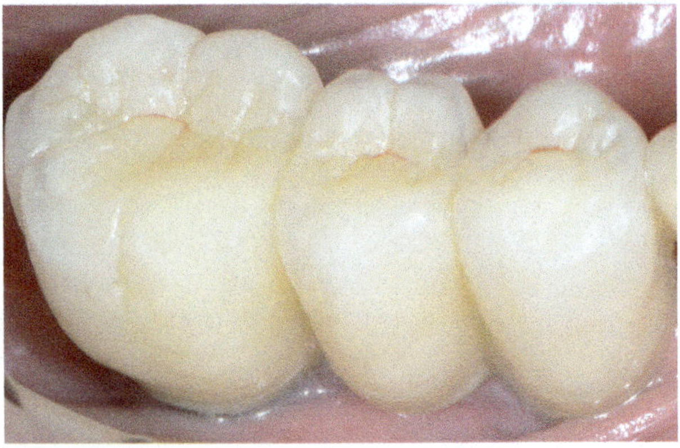

Fig. 13.188 Intraoral view of a definitively seated three-unit TRINIA bridge in the posterior mandible

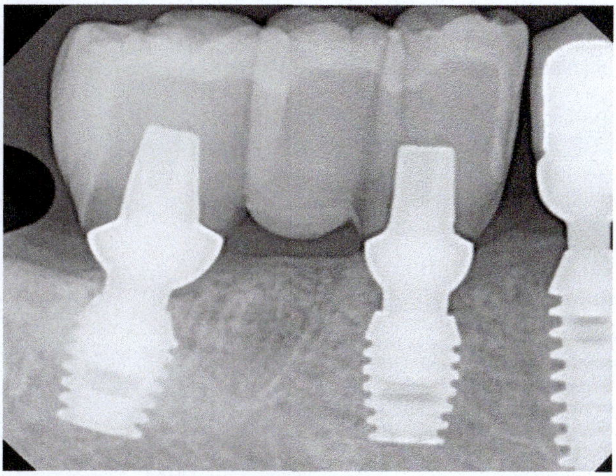

Fig. 13.189 Post-insertion radiograph of a 4.5 × 6.0 mm and a 5.0 × 6.0 mm implant with their seated three-unit TRINIA bridge in the posterior mandible

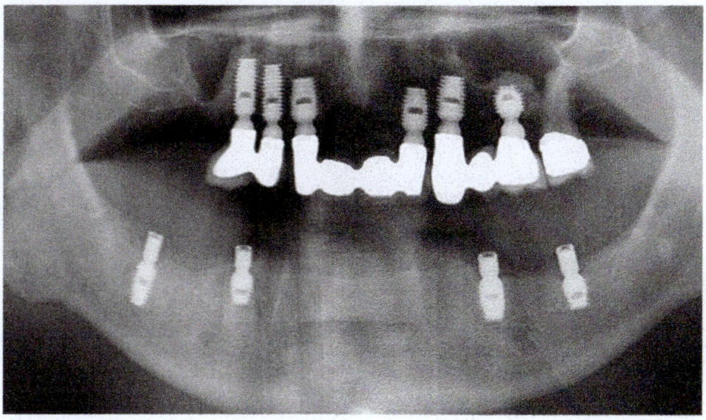

Fig. 13.190 Preoperative radiograph of four implants with Locator Abutments

TRINIA Case 3: Full Arch Telescopic TRINIA Mandibular Prosthesis with Gothic Arch Technique

An 82-year-old man presented with a full arch mandibular overdenture on four Locator Abutments, which he wanted to replace (Figs. 13.190, 13.191, and 13.192). A telescopic TRINIA prosthesis was chosen as the course of treatment due to its versatility as a retentive permanent prosthesis, which can also be removed when desired. The entire treatment took place within 2 weeks, beginning at the consultation with an occlusal registration and an implant-level transfer impression (Figs. 13.193, 13.194, 13.195, and 13.196). The impression was sent to the laboratory where the technicians used it to create stone master models, which were then used to fabricate the resin plates for the Gothic arch tracing (Figs. 13.197, 13.198, 13.199, and 13.200). Gothic arch tracing is a precise technique for recording at a given vertical dimension and centric relation of occlusion. A metal tracing plate attached to a wax and resin rim was blackened with ink prior to being inserted onto the mandibular arch (Fig. 13.201). A single post on the ridge side of the wax and resin rim was inserted into one of the implants to facilitate stability of the Gothic

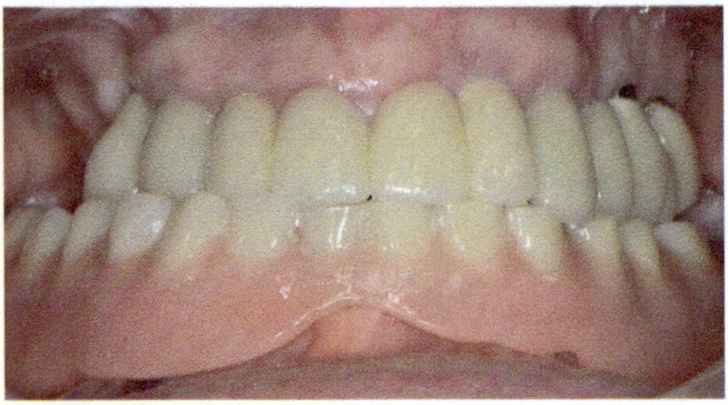

Fig. 13.191 Preoperative clinical view of a mandibular overdenture

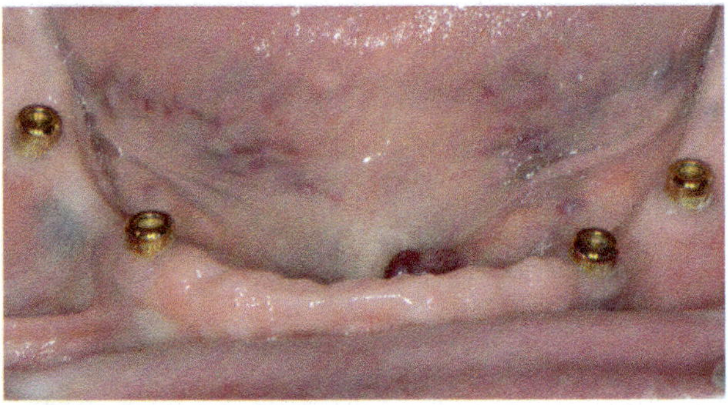

Fig. 13.192 Preoperative clinical view of four mandibular Locator Abutments

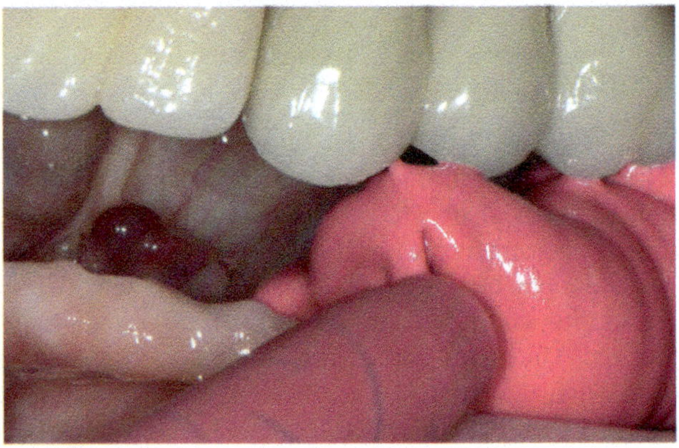

Fig. 13.193 Occlusal registration material is being applied around impression sleeves

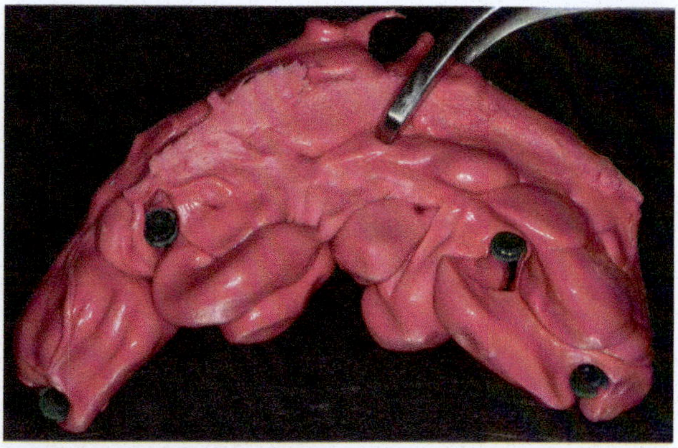

Fig. 13.194 View of impression sleeves captured in an occlusal registration

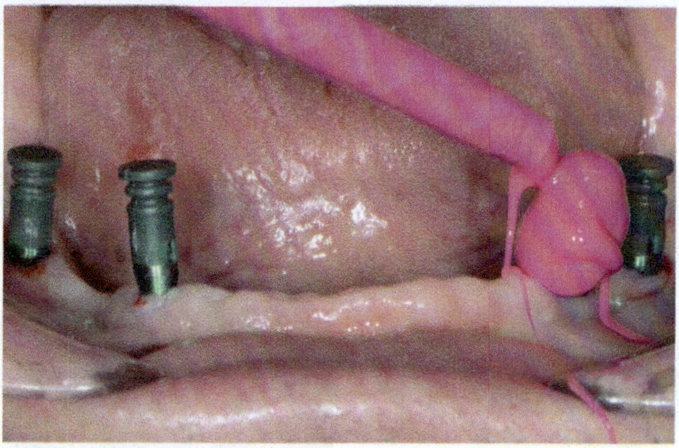

Fig. 13.195 Impression material is being applied around four impression sleeves

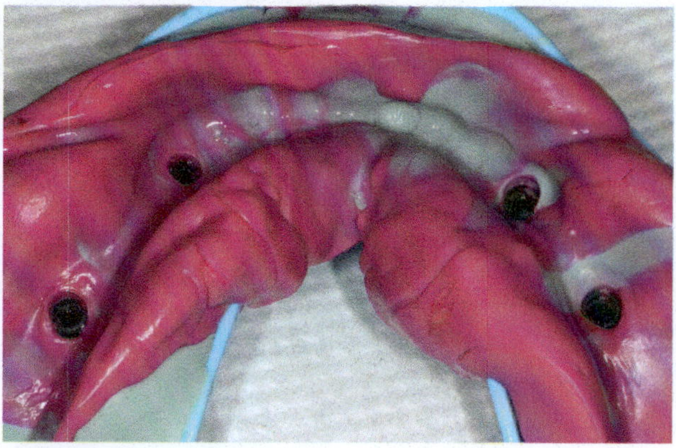

Fig. 13.196 View of four impression sleeves captured in a full arch implant-level impression

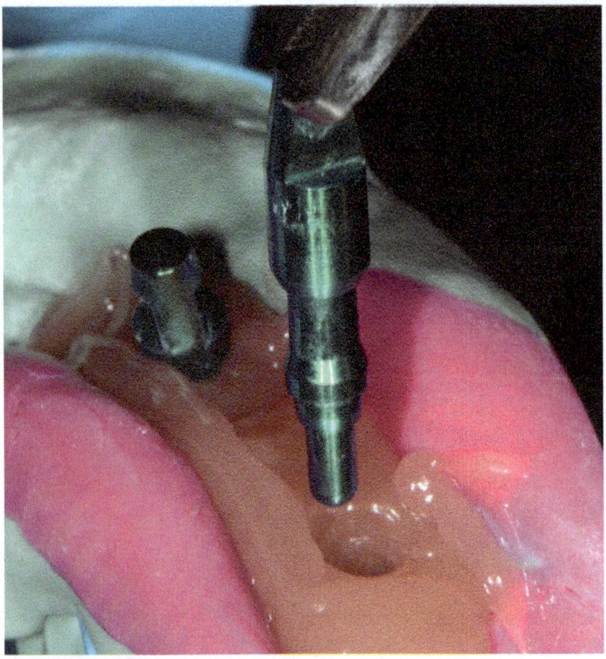

Fig. 13.197 An impression post attached to an implant analog is being inserted into the captured sleeve within the impression

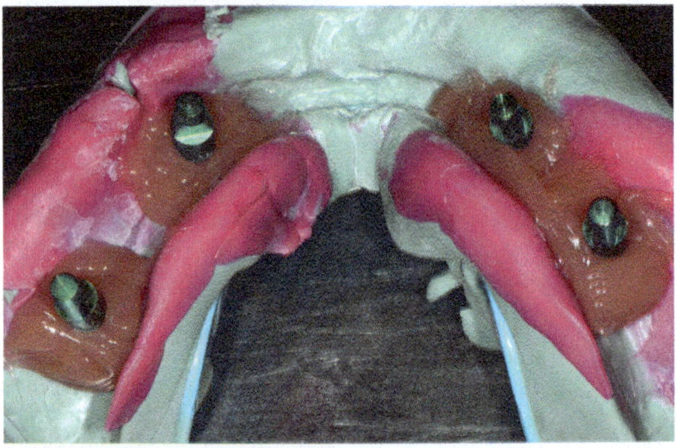

Fig. 13.198 Four implant analogs seated in a full arch impression with soft tissue moulage

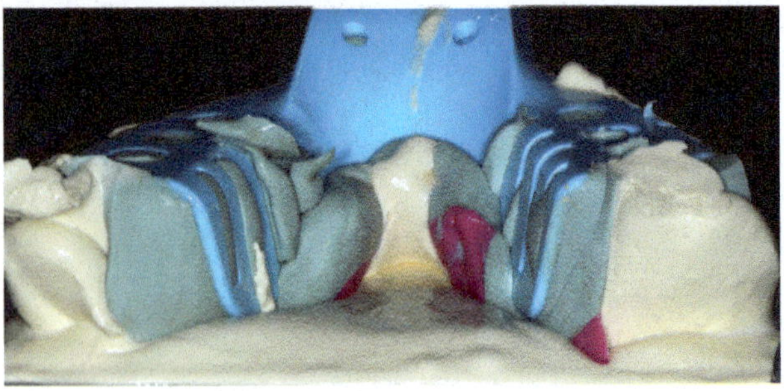

Fig. 13.199 A full arch impression is being used to fabricate a stone master model

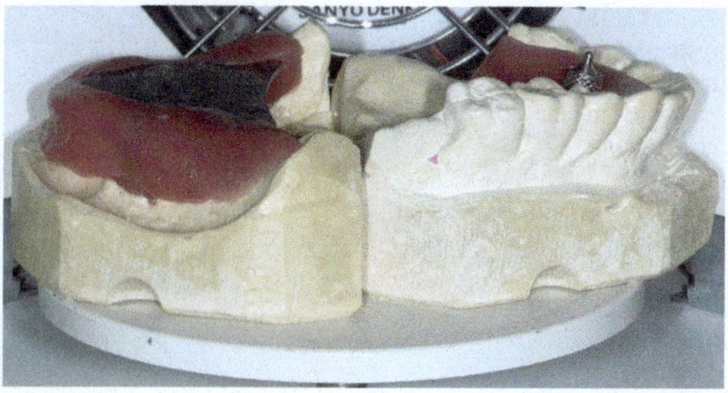

Fig. 13.200 Stone master models with resin plates fabricated for Gothic arch tracing

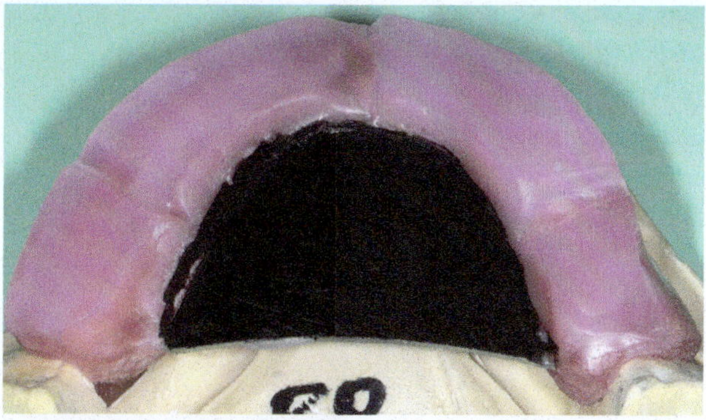

Fig. 13.201 A metal tracing plate attached to a wax and resin rim is blackened with ink for the Gothic arch tracing

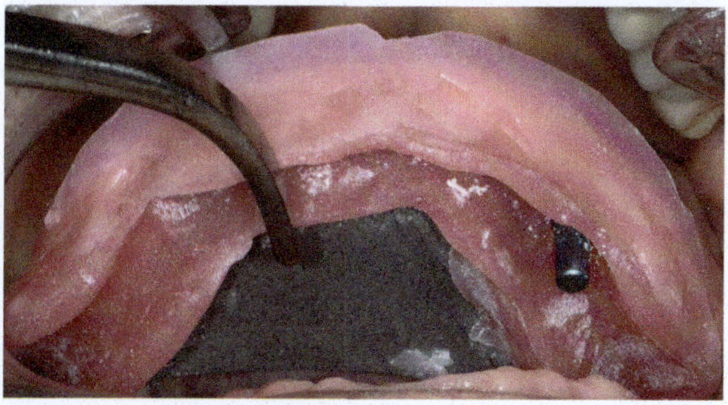

Fig. 13.202 A single post on the ridge side of the wax and resin rim is being inserted into an implant well to facilitate stability during the Gothic arch tracing

arch device during tracing (Fig. 13.202). On the maxillary arch, a resin plate with a stylus was inserted (Fig. 13.203). The patient was instructed to move his jaw around at random while keeping his mouth closed so that the maxillary stylus could maintain contact on the mandibular tracing plate (Fig. 13.204). Once the Gothic arch was clearly visible, a plastic disc was luted with sticky wax to the tracing plate, its hole centered on the apex of the Gothic arch (Fig. 13.205). The plate was then re-inserted, and the patient was asked to close until the maxillary stylus fell into position with the hole of the disc. Occlusal registration material was injected between the two

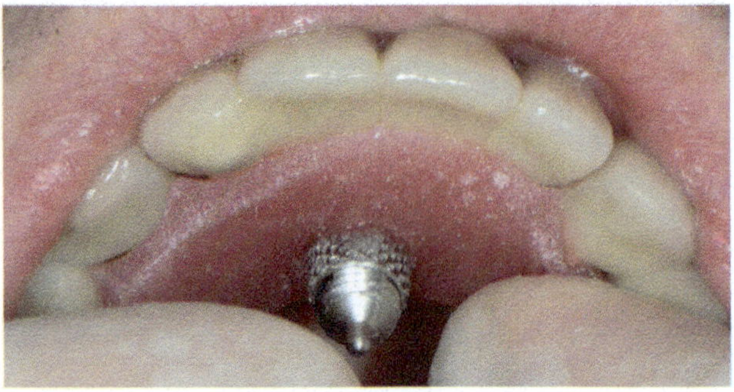

Fig. 13.203 A maxillary resin plate with a stylus is being inserted onto the palate for the Gothic arch tracing

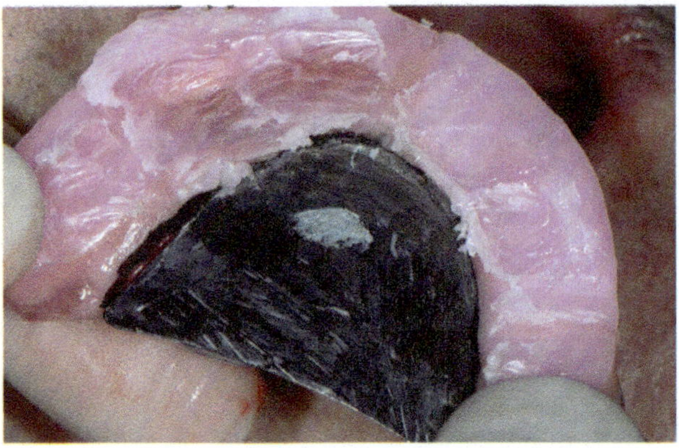

Fig. 13.204 A Gothic arch drawn on the blackened tracing plate by the stylus during random movements of the patient's mandible

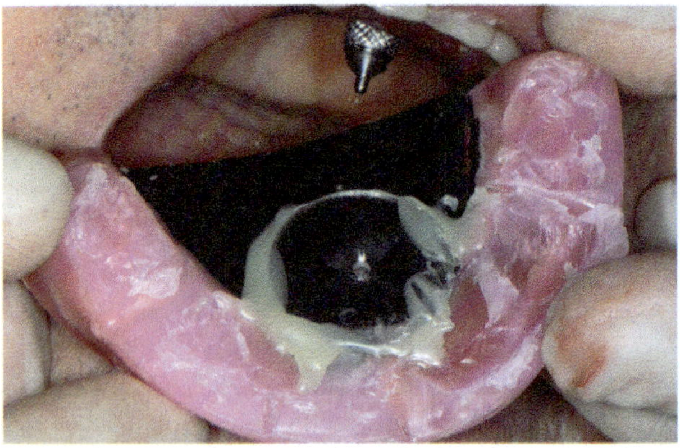

Fig. 13.205 A plastic disc is luted to the tracing plate with sticky wax so that its hole is centered on the apex of the Gothic arch

connected resin plates to capture and record a centric occlusal relationship (Fig. 13.206). The assembled Gothic arch device was sent to the laboratory to be used for the CAD/CAM design of the TRINIA prosthesis (Figs. 13.207, 13.208,

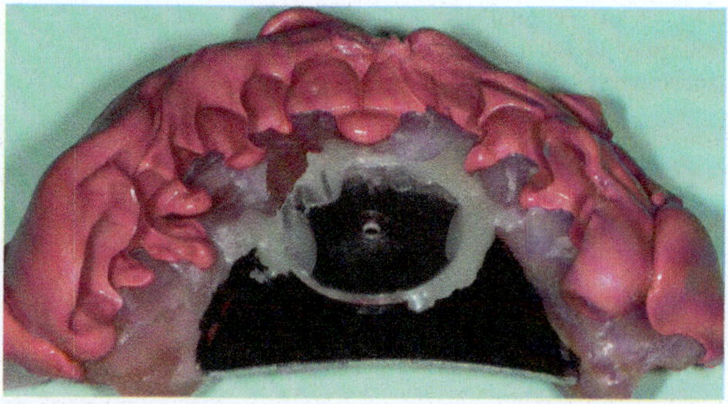

Fig. 13.206 An occlusal registration while the stylus was positioned in the plastic disc of the tracing plate is captured with material

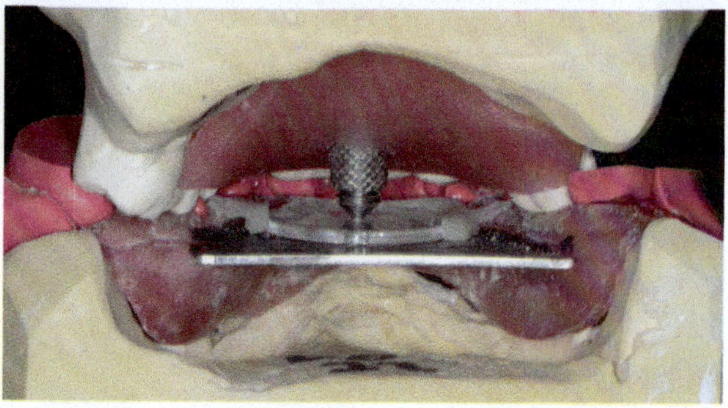

Fig. 13.207 View of an assembled Gothic arch device, with the stylus positioned in the plastic disc of the tracing plate

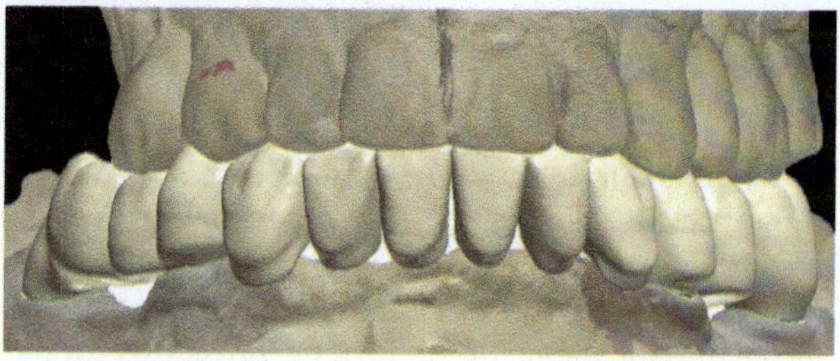

Fig. 13.208 A digital image of a designed mandibular prosthesis

13.209, 13.210, and 13.211). The laboratory technician layered the TRINIA substructure with a buildup of the polyceramic material, Ceramage, to handcraft the teeth of the prosthesis (Figs. 13.212 and 13.213). At the restorative visit, the Universal Abutments were transported to their implants by two Vaseline-lined orientation and seating jigs. The abutments were initially seated and tapped with the jig prior to being definitively tapped without the jig. The retentive copings were then seated and gently tapped onto the abutments, with Vaseline inside their bores to facilitate their removal from the abutments during their cementation to the

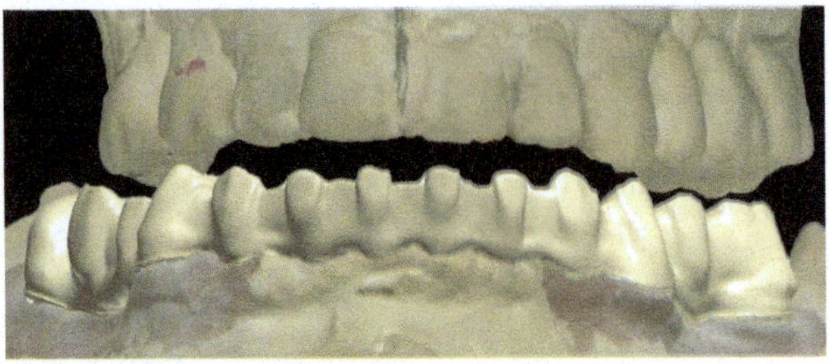

Fig. 13.209 Digital design of TRINIA substructure

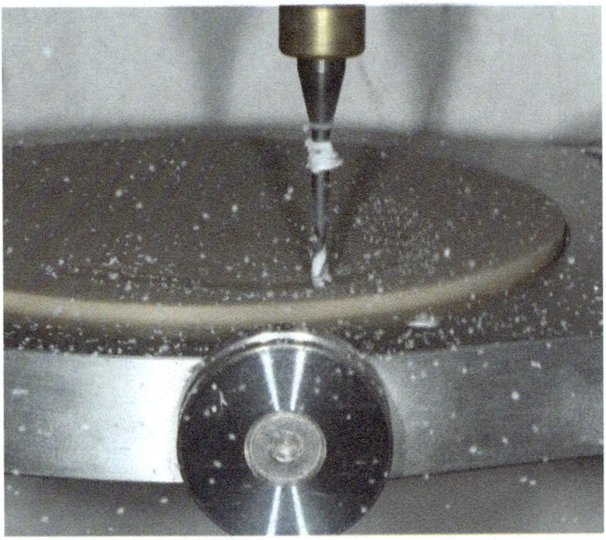

Fig. 13.210 A TRINIA disc in a milling machine is being used to fabricate a mandibular framework

prosthesis. During the cementation process, cotton rolls applied occlusal pressure (Figs. 13.214 and 13.215). Once the copings were cemented to the bores of the prosthesis, Vaseline was injected into the copings to facilitate the patient's initial removal of the prosthesis for cleaning (Figs. 13.216 and 13.217). It was recommended to the patient to remove the prosthesis for hygienic purposes. For patients uncomfortable removing their telescopic prostheses, proxy brushes, toothbrushes and toothpaste, and water picks are all suggested modes of cleaning, as well as hygiene appointments every 6 months. The final radiographic and clinical views of the full arch telescopic TRINIA mandibular prosthesis presented satisfactory results (Figs. 13.218, 13.219, and 13.220).

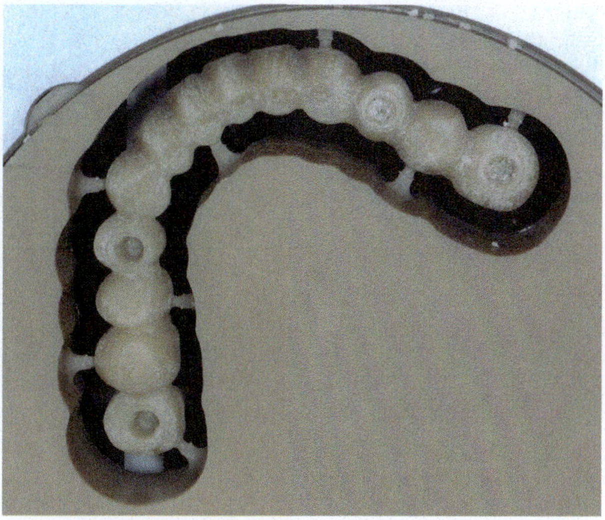

Fig. 13.211 View of a mandibular framework milled in a TRINIA disc

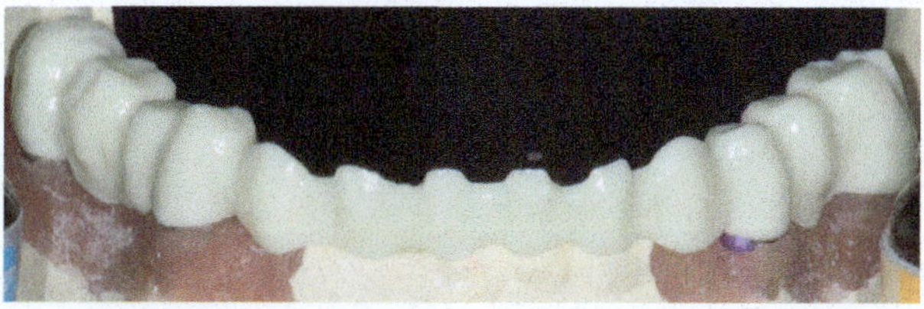

Fig. 13.212 A mandibular TRINIA framework on a stone model prior to the application of polyceramic material

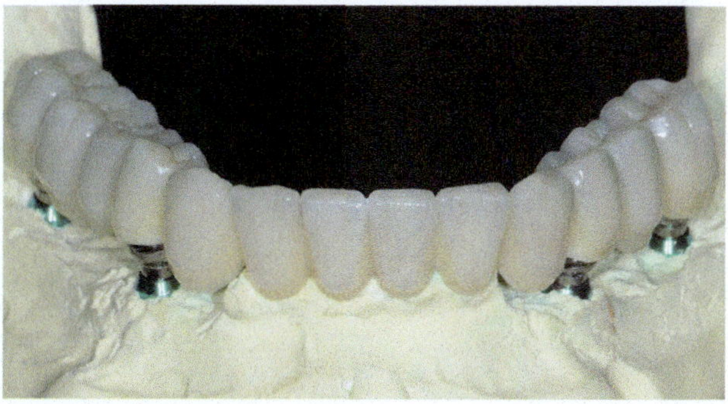

Fig. 13.213 A mandibular TRINIA prosthesis on a stone model

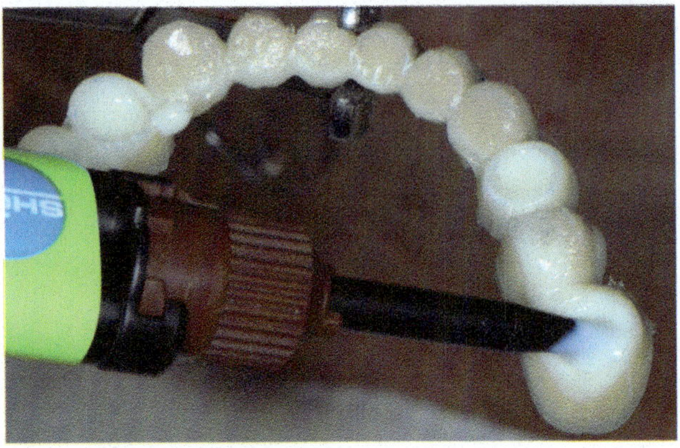

Fig. 13.214 Resin cement is being applied to the bores of the TRINIA prosthesis

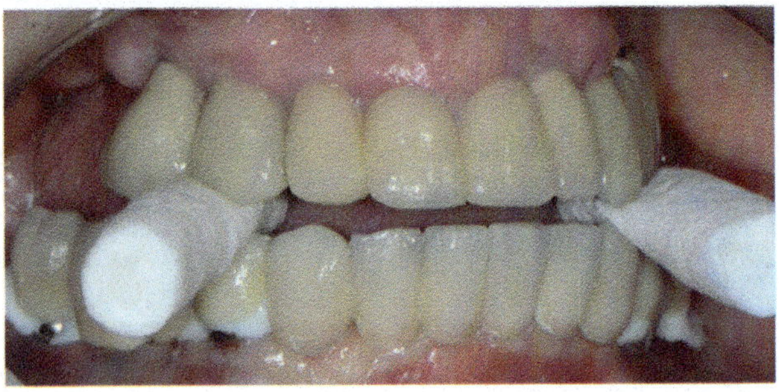

Fig. 13.215 Cotton rolls are being used to apply occlusal pressure to the TRINIA prosthesis during cementation

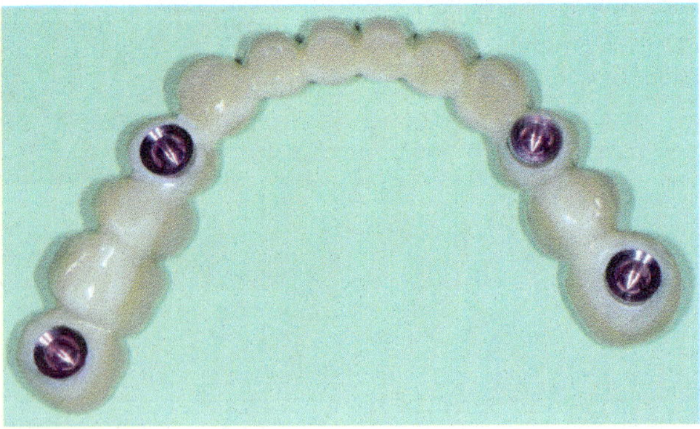

Fig. 13.216 View of four retentive copings cemented to the bores of the TRINIA prosthesis

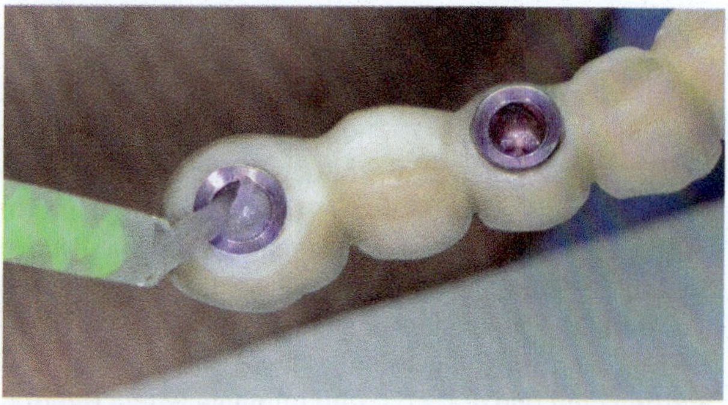

Fig. 13.217 Vaseline is being applied to the bores of the copings to facilitate the patient's initial removal of the prosthesis for cleaning

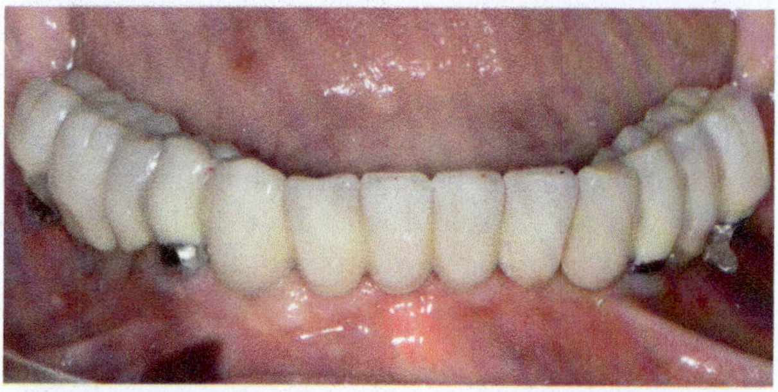

Fig. 13.218 Intraoral view of a telescopic TRINIA mandibular prosthesis

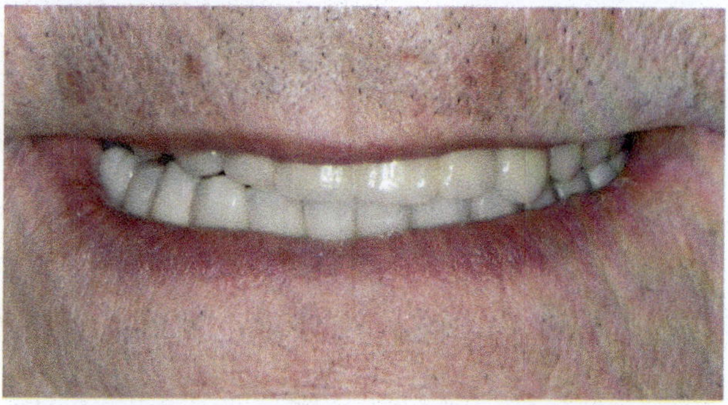

Fig. 13.219 Patient's smile with a telescopic TRINIA mandibular prosthesis

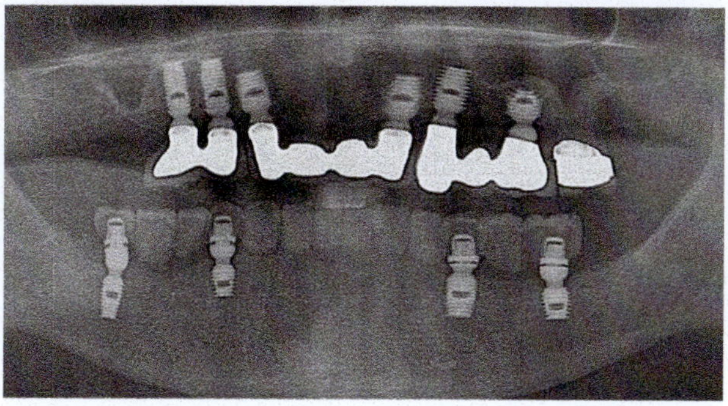

Fig. 13.220 Post-insertion radiograph of four implants with their seated telescopic TRINIA mandibular prosthesis

TRINIA Case 4: Full Arch Telescopic TRIO-TRINIA® Maxillary Prosthesis with Hybrid Material

An 83-year-old woman presented with a failed maxillary prosthesis supported by five screw-retained IMZ implants, which had fractured or had been lost (Figs. 13.221 and 13.222). At first, new screws were inserted to replace the broken and lost screws, and the patient's prosthesis was tightened for the interim before a new denture could be fabricated. Upon closer examination, it was discovered that only one screw was holding the entire appliance together; thus, it was removed and a new treatment plan was formed. Three new Bicon implants were placed: a 4.0 × 6.0 mm implant with a 2.5 mm well was placed in the area of the maxillary right central incisor with bone grafting, and two 4.5 × 6.0 mm implants with 3.0 mm wells were placed in the areas of the maxillary second premolars with internal sinus lifts. The grafting procedure consisted of SynthoGraft material mixed with the patient's blood, layered over harvested autogenous bone that was placed over the exposed buccal surface of the implant at the crest. A collagen membrane was also placed over the anterior implant to cover the palatal defect. To facilitate healing of the internal sinus lifts, 2.0 × 10 cc of blood were drawn and put in a centrifuge for 12 min at 2400 RPM to fabricate Leukocyte- and Platelet-Rich Fibrin (L-PRF) plugs, which were placed into the osteotomies prior to the insertion of the posterior implants. Six months later, the implants were uncovered for an implant-level impression, a Gothic arch tracing, and

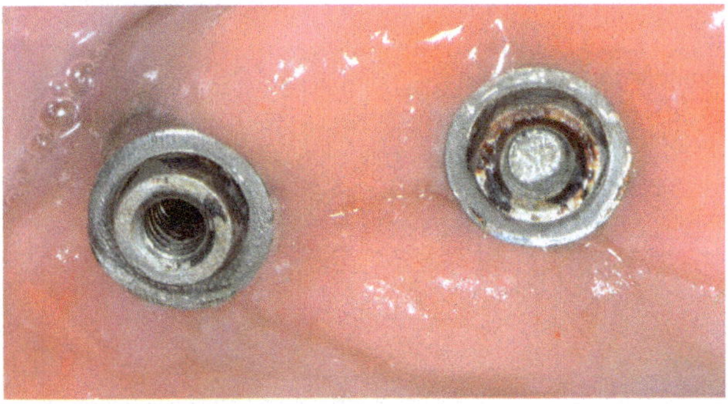

Fig. 13.221 Two broken screw-retained implants in the maxilla

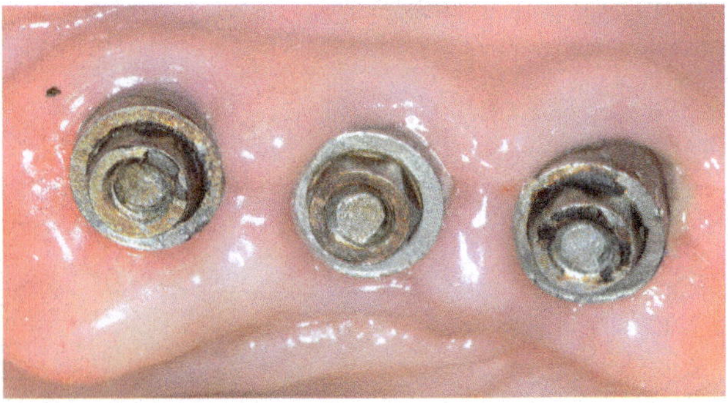

Fig. 13.222 Three broken screw-retained implants in the maxilla

an occlusal registration to be taken (Fig. 13.223). The assembled Gothic arch device was sent to the laboratory to fabricate a wax rim with a composite teeth arrangement, which was used to determine the lip-line, mid-line, and smile-line, and to take a second occlusal registration (Figs. 13.224 and 13.225). The laboratory then designed the telescopic TRINIA substructure, and a separate superstructure of teeth milled from a Shofu HC disc using CAD/CAM software (Figs. 13.226, 13.227, 13.228, 13.229, 13.230, and 13.231). A resin orientation and seating jig and a verification jig were fabricated to facilitate the insertion of the Universal Abutments and to verify the fit of the copings in the seated prosthesis (Figs. 13.232 and 13.233). At the restorative visit, the titanium temporary abutments were removed and replaced with the three permanent Universal Abutments, which were seated using the numerically marked sequence of the orientation and seating jig (Figs. 13.234 and 13.235). Vaseline was then applied to the inside of the retentive copings and to the ridge side of the prosthesis to facilitate the removal of extraneous resin cement during the

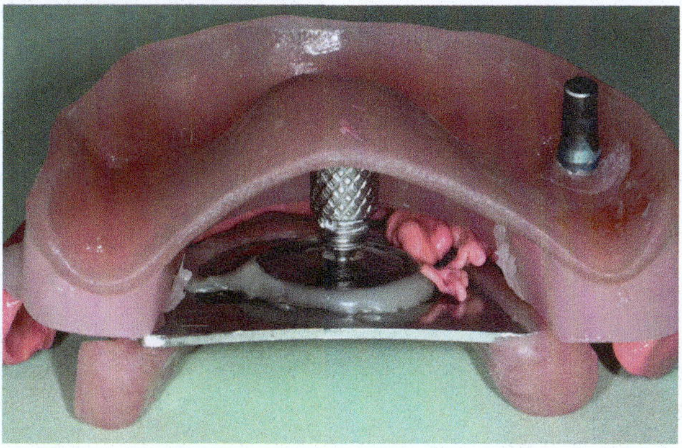

Fig. 13.223 An occlusal registration while the stylus was positioned in the plastic disc of the tracing plate is captured with material

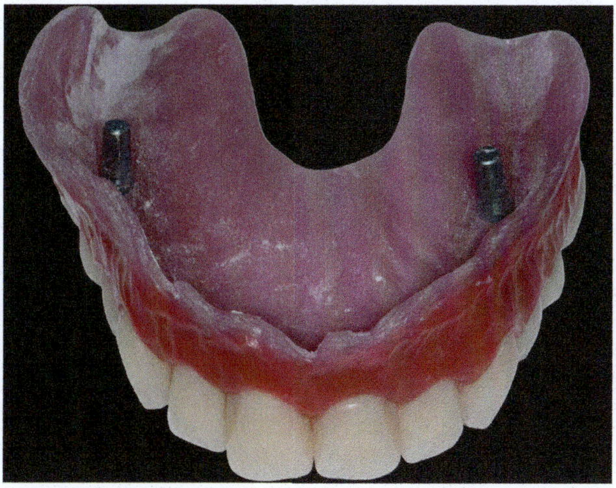

Fig. 13.224 A wax rim with a composite teeth arrangement prior to its insertion for a second occlusal registration

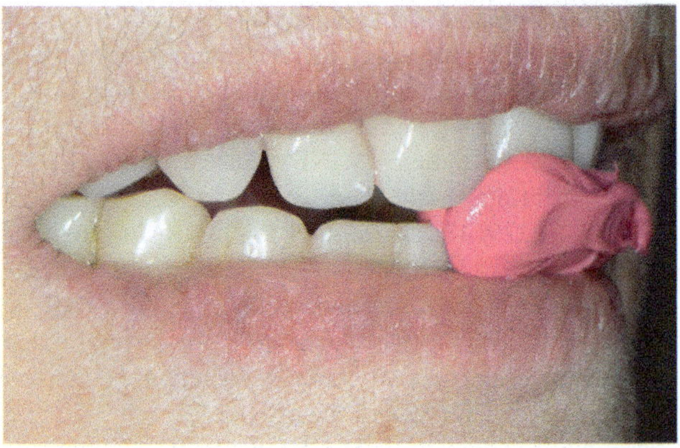

Fig. 13.225 A wax rim with a composite teeth arrangement is being used to record a second occlusal registration

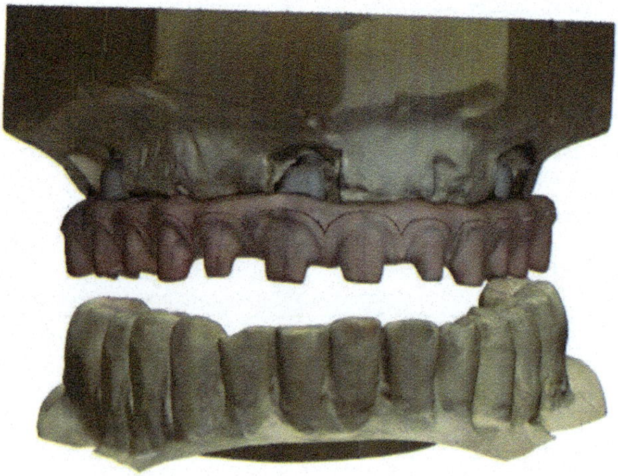

Fig. 13.226 A digital design for a maxillary framework

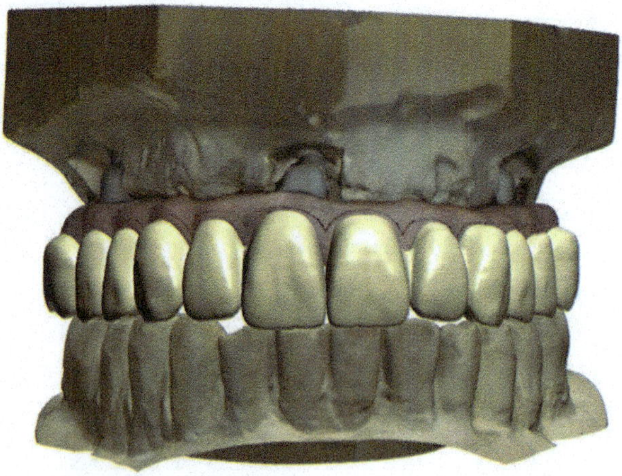

Fig. 13.227 A digital image of a designed maxillary prosthesis with a TRINIA substructure and a separate superstructure of teeth milled from a Shofu HC disc

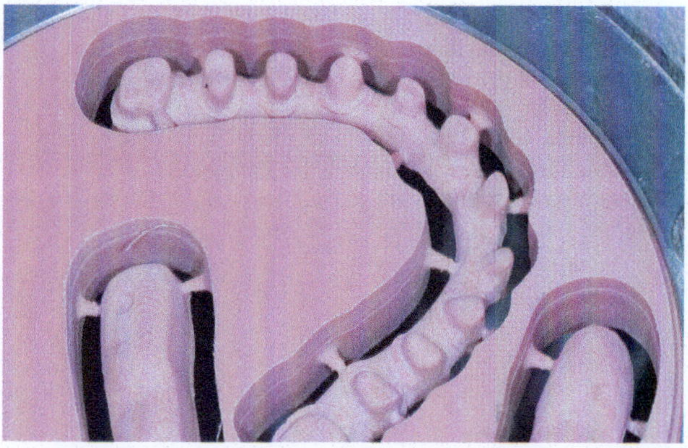

Fig. 13.228 View of a maxillary framework milled in a TRINIA disc

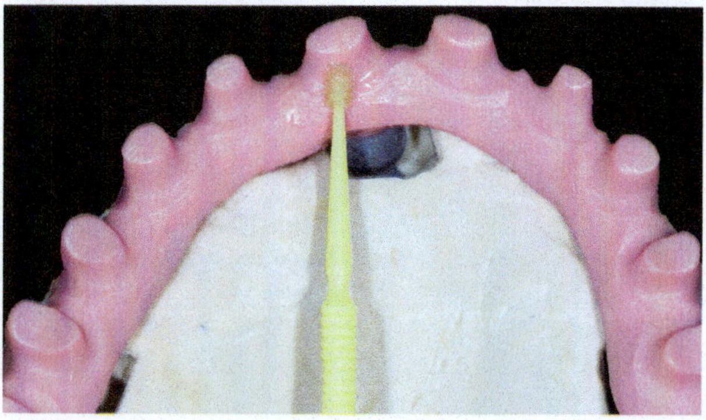

Fig. 13.229 Bonding agent is being applied to the TRINIA framework prior to the insertion of its superstructure

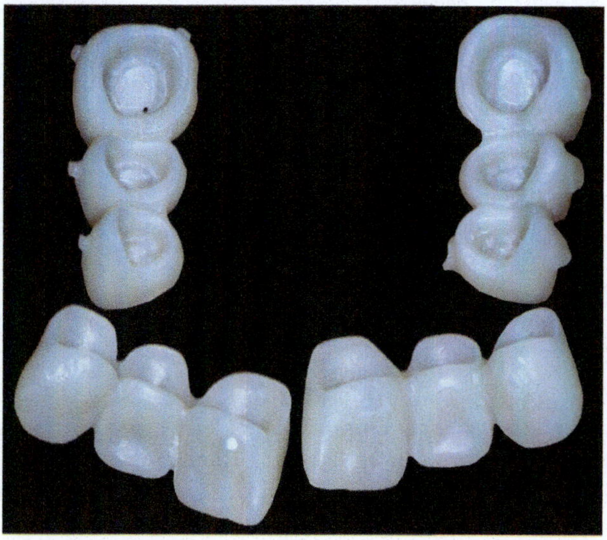

Fig. 13.230 View of teeth milled from a Shofu HC disc prior to their insertion onto a TRINIA framework

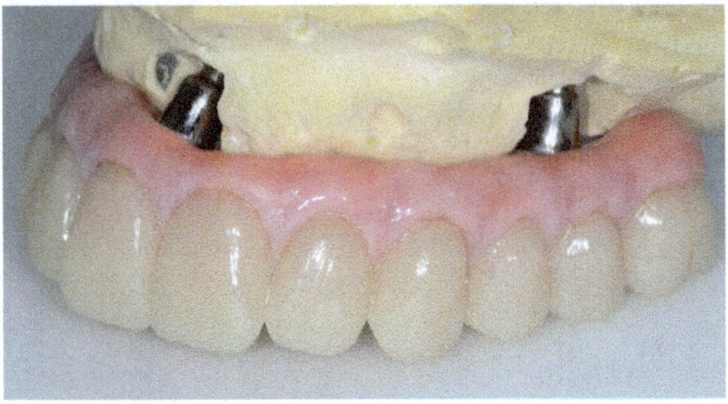

Fig. 13.231 A finished hybrid material maxillary prosthesis after the fusion of the TRINIA substructure and HC superstructure, and a coating of polyceramic material

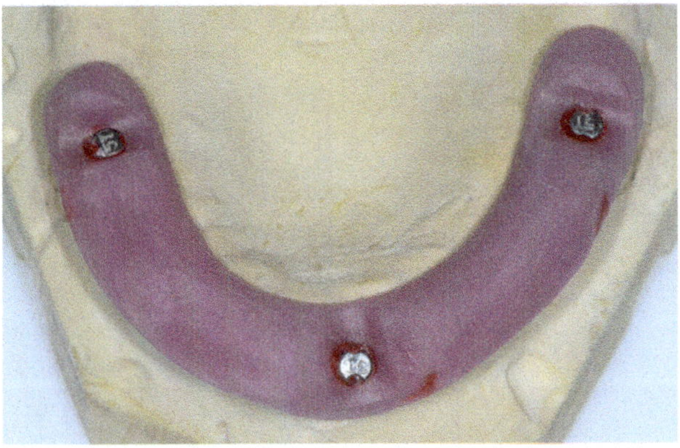

Fig. 13.232 An orientation and seating jig is seated on Universal Abutments prior to their insertion

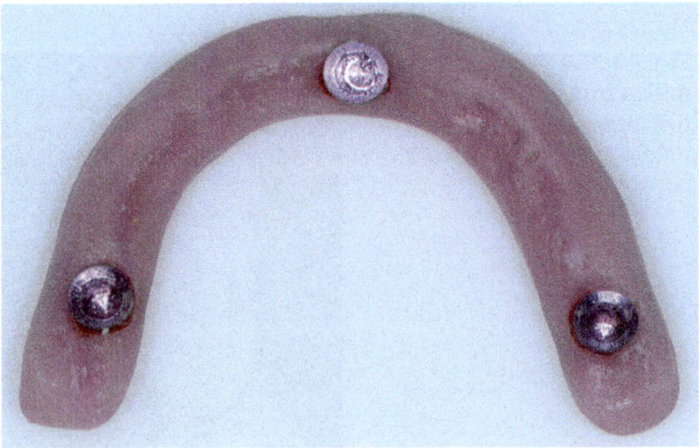

Fig. 13.233 A verification jig with three retentive copings prior to its insertion onto the seated Universal Abutments to verify the fit of the copings in the prosthesis

copings' cementation to the bores of the prosthesis (Figs. 13.236, 13.237, 13.238, 13.239, 13.240, and 13.241). Articulating paper was used to verify appropriate occlusal contacts, and a radiograph was taken to confirm the complete seating of the telescopic TRIO-TRINIA prosthesis (Figs. 13.242, 13.243, 13.244, and 13.245).

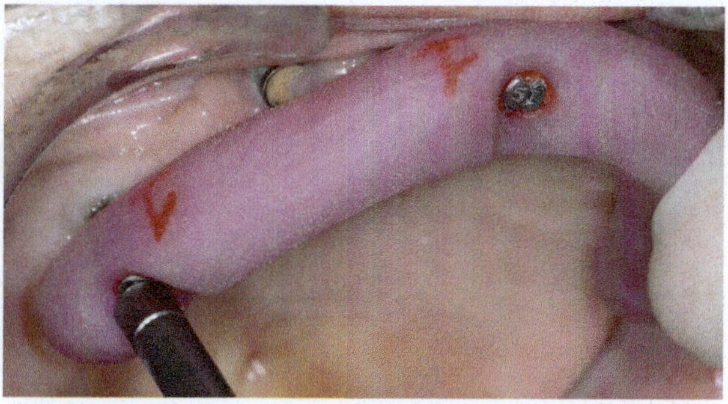

Fig. 13.234 Universal Abutments are being tapped with a standard seating tip while being positioned with an orientation and seating jig

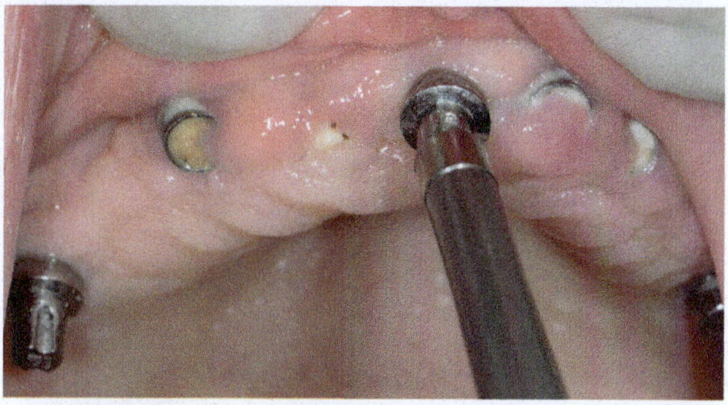

Fig. 13.235 Universal Abutments are being definitively tapped without the orientation and seating jig

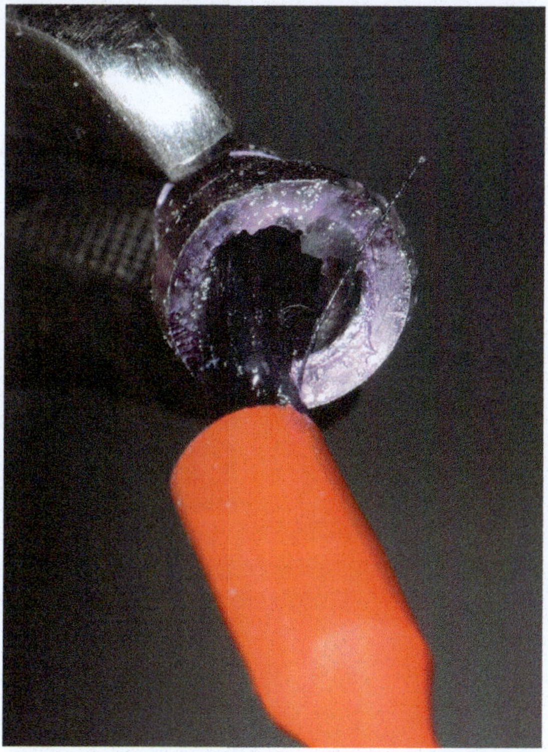

Fig. 13.236 Vaseline is being applied to the bore of a retentive coping to facilitate its removal from the abutment during its cementation to the prosthesis

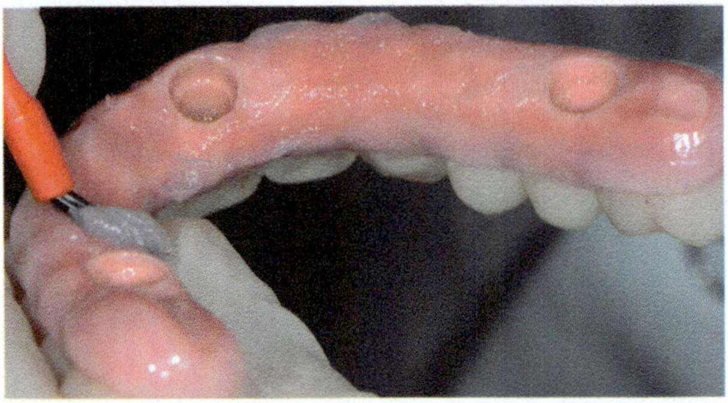

Fig. 13.237 Vaseline is being applied around the prosthesis to facilitate the removal of extraneous cement

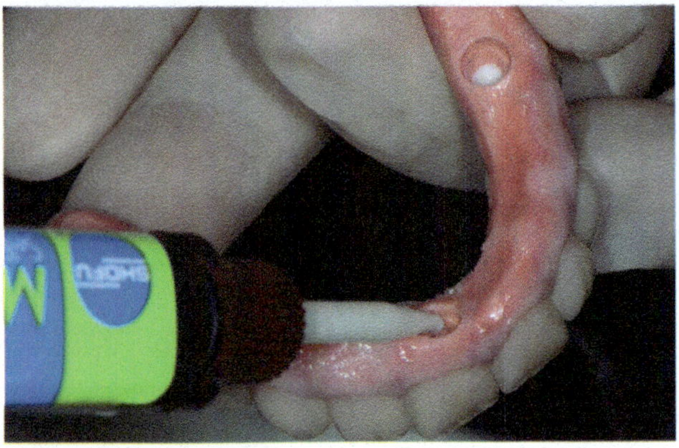

Fig. 13.238 Resin cement is being applied to the bores of the TRINIA prosthesis

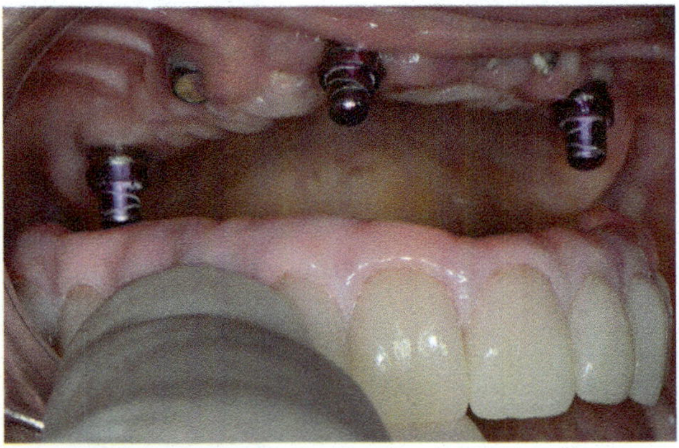

Fig. 13.239 A maxillary TRINIA prosthesis is being seated onto three retentive copings for cementation

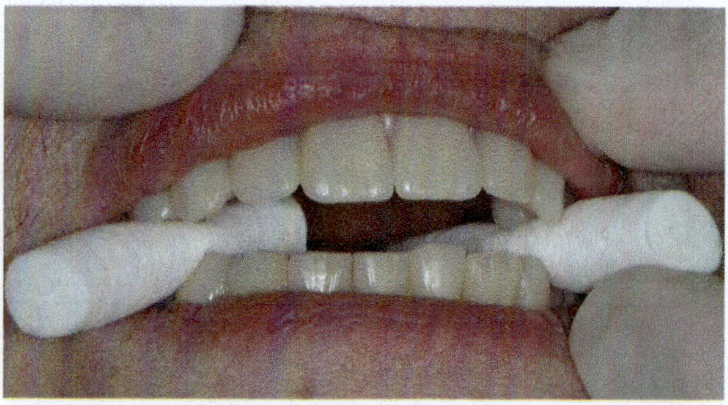

Fig. 13.240 Cotton rolls are being used to apply occlusal pressure to the TRINIA prosthesis during cementation

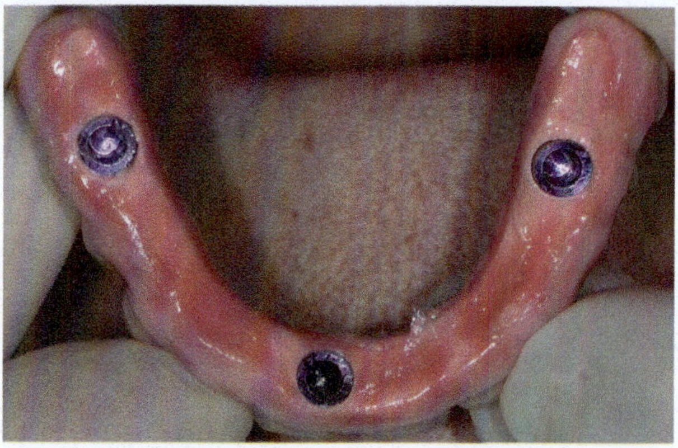

Fig. 13.241 View of three retentive copings cemented to the bores of the TRINIA prosthesis

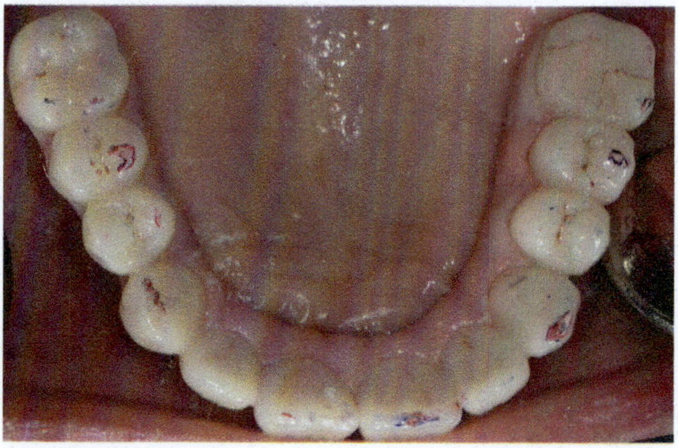

Fig. 13.242 Ink from articulating paper marks appropriate occlusal contacts

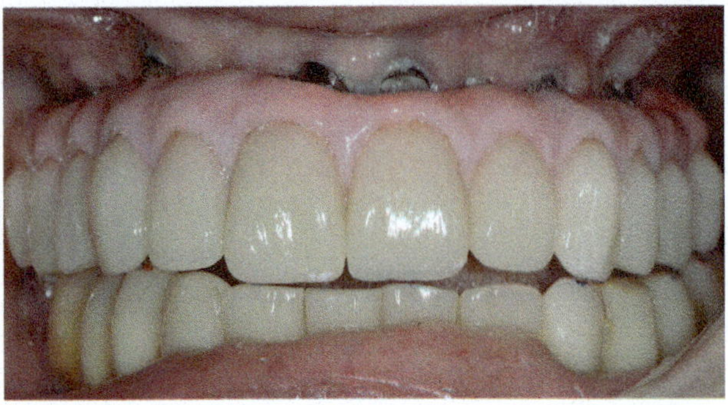

Fig. 13.243 Facial view of a telescopic TRIO-TRINIA prosthesis

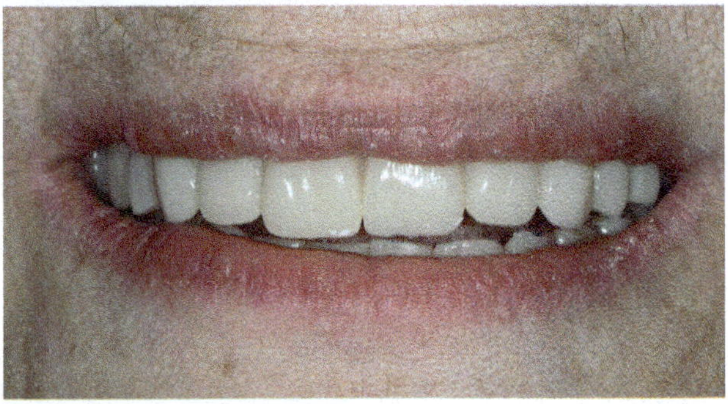

Fig. 13.244 Patient's smile with a telescopic TRIO-TRINIA prosthesis

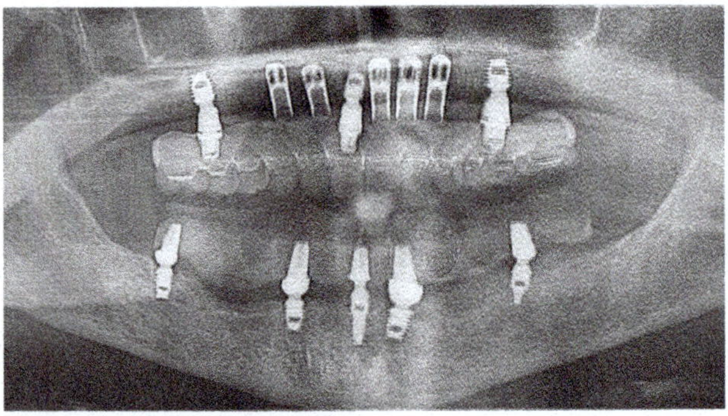

Fig. 13.245 Post-insertion radiograph of three implants with their telescopic TRIO-TRINIA maxillary prosthesis

13.6 Conclusion

Gathering what we've learned about short implants from historical studies to multivariate analyses, it is fair to say that restorations with large crown-to-implant ratios are not detrimental to bone and, quite conversely, can lead to bone gain. A combination of factors including restoration material, size of the implant, and location in the mouth can all affect the surrounding bone of the implant. Additionally, the techniques used during the fabrication, insertion, and maintenance of a prosthesis can also determine the success or failure of the restoration, and should be performed with knowledge and care.

Bicon restorative techniques simplify prosthetic insertions through the use of a design that allows for 360° of Universal Abutment positioning and for modifications to be made intraorally at any time. The Bicon implant-to-abutment connection also eliminates the need for screws, torque drivers, and cement, which can lead to bacterial contamination and infection, or the loosening and fracture of the restoration. The Bicon system is versatile, and its restorations can vary to accommodate a patient's needs, from a full arch of Individual Abutment Crowns, to a full arch prosthesis on a minimal number of implants or a prosthesis supported by implants of a different system altogether (Figs. 13.246, 13.247, and 13.248). If respect for the restorative steps and techniques are followed, even the most extreme clinical situations can yield successful results.

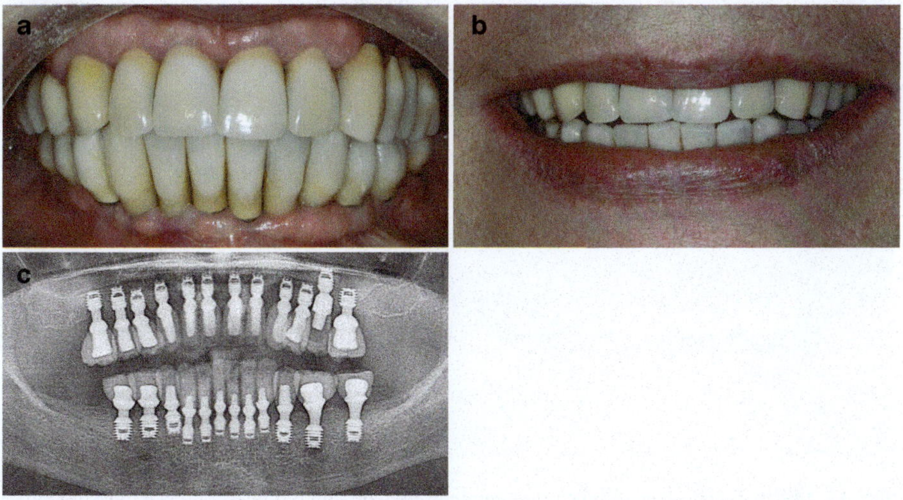

Fig. 13.246 Clinical and radiographic views of 24 maxillary and mandibular Integrated Abutment Crowns over 10 years old, shown in a facial view (**a**), a view of the patient's smile (**b**), and a panoramic radiographic view (**c**)

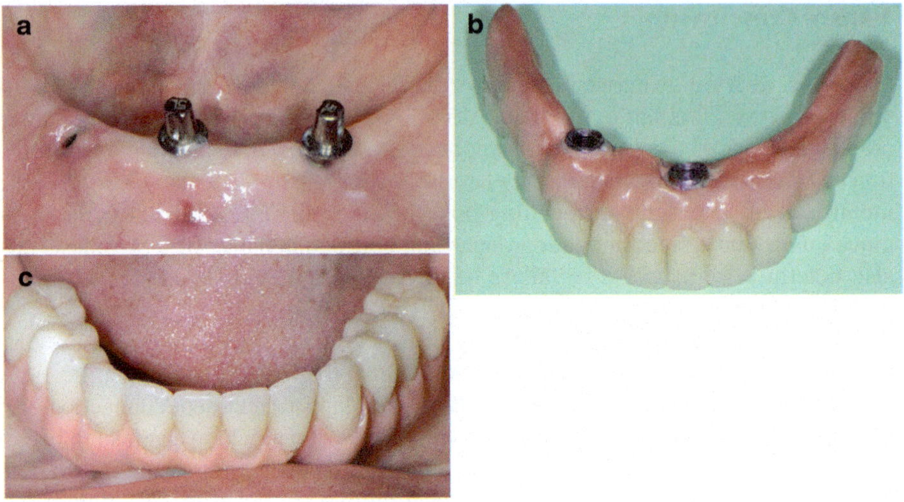

Fig. 13.247 Clinical views of a two-unit telescopic TRINIA mandibular prosthesis

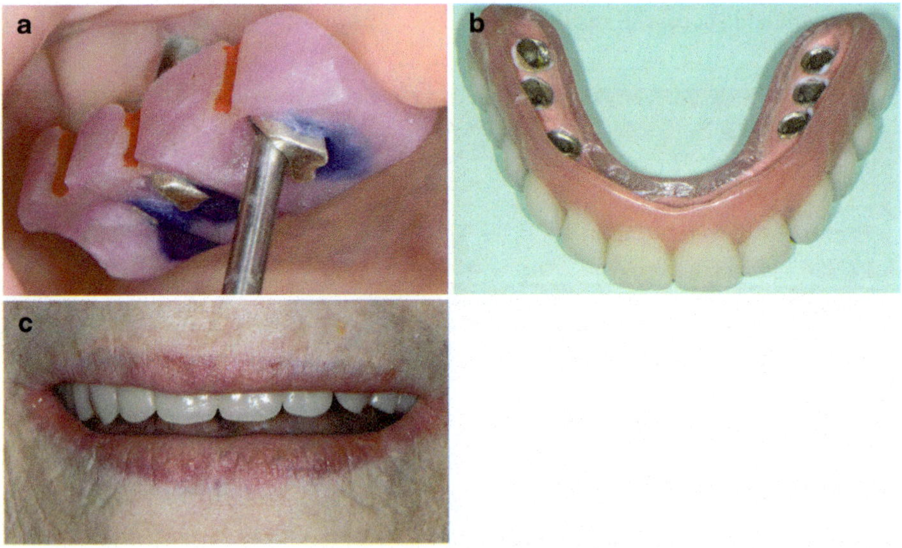

Fig. 13.248 Clinical views of six screw-retained implants with a telescopic TRINIA maxillary prosthesis

References

1. Birdi H, Schulte J, Kovacs A, Weed M, Chuang SK. Crown-to-implant ratios of short-length implants. J Oral Implantol. 2010;36:425–33.
2. Lanyon LE. Using functional loading to influence bone mass and architecture: objectives, mechanisms, and relationship with estrogen of the mechanically adaptive process in bone. Bone. 1996;18(Suppl 1):37S–43S.
3. Roberts RA. A 24-year retrospective study of bone growth after implant placement. J Oral Implantol. 2005;31:98–103.
4. Urdaneta RA, Chuang SK, Leary J, Morgan V. Factors affecting bone levels and restorations of short implants. The Bicon short implant: a thirty-year perspective. Chicago: Quintessence Publishing; 2017. p. 233–44.
5. Laurell L, Lundgren D. Marginal bone level changes at dental implants after 5 years in function: a meta-analysis. Clin Implant Dent Relat Res. 2011;13:19–28.
6. Urdaneta RA, Daher S, Leary J, Emanuel K, Chuang SK. Factors associated with crestal bone gain on single-tooth locking-taper implants: the effect of nonsteroidal anti-inflammatory drugs. Int J Oral Maxillofac Implants. 2011;26:1063–78.
7. Pilliar RM, Deporter DA, Watson PA, et al. The effect of partial coating with hydroxyapatite on bone remodeling in relation to porous-coated titanium-alloy dental implants in the dog. J Dent Res. 1991;70:1338–45.
8. Kohri M, Cooper EP, Ferracane JL, Waite DF. Comparative study of hydroxyapatite and titanium dental implants in dogs. J Oral Maxillofac Surg. 1990;48:1265–73.
9. Bell R, Beirne OR. Effect of hydroxyapatite, tricalcium phosphate, and collagen on the healing of defects in the rat mandible. J Oral Maxillofac Surg. 1988;46:589–94.
10. Geesink RG, de Groot K, Klein CP. Bonding of bone to apatite-coated implants. J Bone Joint Surg Br. 1988;70:17–22.
11. Gottlander M, Albrektsson T. Histomorphometric analyses of hydroxyapatite-coated and uncoated titanium implants. The importance of the implant design. Clin Oral Implants Res. 1992;3:71–6.
12. Oonishi H, Yamamoto M, Ishimaru H, et al. The effect of hydroxyapatite coating on bone growth into porous titanium alloy implants. J Bone Joint Surg Br. 1989;71:213–6.
13. Urdaneta RA, Seemann R, Dragan IF, Lubelski W, Leary J, Chuang SK. A retrospective study on the effect of natural tooth-implant proximity and an introduction to the concept of a bone-loading platform switch. Int J Oral Maxillofac Implants. 2014;29:1412–24.
14. Perpetuini P, Pisarik K, Morgan V, Bonfante E, Morgan K, Speratti D, Hirayama M, Murcko L, Carelli S, Hallowes D. Restorative techniques. The Bicon short implant: a thirty-year perspective. Chicago: Quintessence Publishing; 2017. p. 140.

Grow Your Practice Utilizing the Short Implant

14

Rosanna Jenkins

Contents

14.1 Internal Marketing 315
14.2 External Marketing 318
14.3 Social Media 324
References 327

Webster's dictionary defines marketing as "the process or technique of promoting, selling, and distributing a product or service". In professional practices, marketing is used to separate one's practice from the competition. In today's highly competitive arena, it is essential that the practitioner find ways to let both the public and potential referring doctors know **specifically** what you offer in your practice [1]. There are a number of ways in which one can promote a professional practice. These are inclusive of both **internal** and **external marketing** as well as the use of social media. Integrating your knowledge of short implants is essential in positioning your practice as a leader in implant technology (Fig. 14.1).

14.1 Internal Marketing

Internal marketing encompasses anything done within the confines of the practice. It begins with the first contact from the potential patient or referring doctor. Your office phone becomes THE most impactful piece of office equipment in the

R. Jenkins (✉)
Founder of "the new face of 60", CEO Rx Marketing, Denver, CO, USA
e-mail: hello@rosannajenkins.com

B. J. Tomasetti, R. Ewers (eds.), *Short Implants*,
https://doi.org/10.1007/978-3-030-44199-9_14

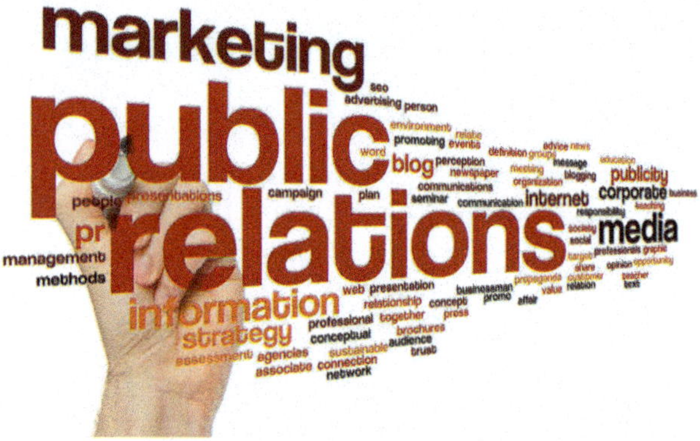

Fig. 14.1 Marketing a professional practice is a multipronged approach

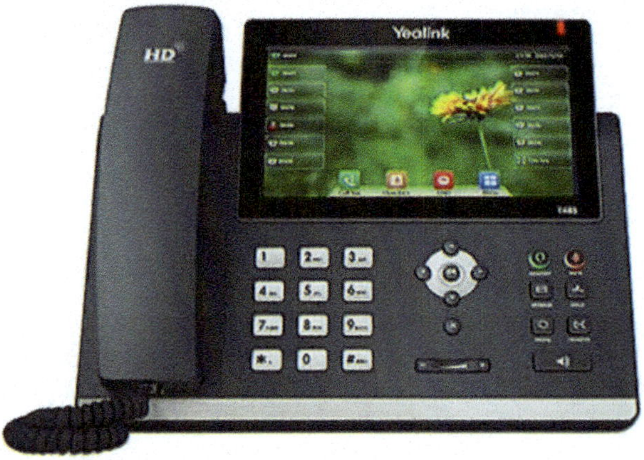

Fig. 14.2 The phone is the **most important** instrument in your office

practice. The manner in which the phone is answered can make or break your practice. Be sure that the person you have at the front desk personifies your office culture. He or she is an extension of your professionalism and your personality. **He or she has the power to help or hinder your growth** (Fig. 14.2).

Use these **simple telephone tips** to ramp up your growth:

1. **Always** answer with a smile and introduce yourself. Speak slowly and clearly.
2. Every attempt should be made to answer within the first few rings. At the very least, answer the call, and advise the caller of a short wait. Be sure to return to the call if the wait increases.
3. If you must place a patient on hold, get back to them within 30 seconds and,
4. If necessary, offer to call them back. **Do not forget to call back**!
5. Finish the call with a "thank you." Always add that patient calls are welcome should they have any questions or concerns prior to their appointment. These initial calls are full of new information that may require clarification.

Fig. 14.3 Well-branded companies are recognized simply by their logo. Make your practice stand out with a well-designed logo

Branding [2] is the first and most important part of creating and marketing your practice. It is the "identity" of your practice. Remember, branding encompasses the logo, colors, design, and personality of your business. It is what your patients and referring doctors will remember when meeting you for the first time. Be sure the overall theme transfers to your reception area, exam rooms, surgical suites, etc.

If possible, retain a professional group to assist in designing your logo, colors, stationary, etc. Once approved, it is imperative that the logo and practice name appear **on everything** involving your practice. Office signage should be consistent with respect to name, colors, and logo. Anything that leaves the office should have the practice name, logo, telephone number, and website on it (use non-serif fonts (Helvetica, Calibri) in an appropriate size for ease of reading—this includes business cards, letterhead, envelopes, billing statements, and collateral materials. Do not skimp when it comes to the quality and weight of your stationary. You can use "regular paper or copy paper" within the office or for billing statements but, anything leaving the office should be on heavy bond paper.

If you offer coffee, drinks, etc. in your reception area (and you should do this) the beverage glasses, mugs, etc. should be inscribed with the office name, telephone number, website address, and logo. If you have a tag line or quote that you use in your marketing materials, this is the place to use it (Fig. 14.3).

In order for Marketing to be at its most effective, it is essential that the doctor "buys-in" to the entire marketing plan. Unless the doctor is willing to assist in the creation, design, and promotion of his own practice exposure, Marketing will NOT succeed. Without active doctor participation all marketing efforts will fail. The doctor's participation in the Internal Marketing Plan begins by being on time for all appointments. There will be times when this is NOT possible. Completely understandable. But, be sure to keep the patient updated and offer to re-appoint if necessary.

Case in Point

An experienced surgeon, incredibly well-known for his training and surgical results loses more than half of his practice due to extreme waits and negative "word of mouth" from existing patients. Although his patients were booked every 45 min, wait times ran approximately 1–2 h.

Research indicates that patients will accept a short wait but continually being late is a sign of disrespect and the vast majority of patients will find a different provider. This is where word of mouth comes into play. These patients WILL be very open to sharing their experience not only with friends and family but, with the referring office and its staff. If the office is running late, my recommendation is that the receptionist explains it to the patient and, if a significant delay, offer to reschedule. The doctor should ***always*** apologize directly to the patient for being late. Many of my clients offer the patient a coffee gift card or two movie tickets as an apology. The doctor should always introduce themselves and thank the patient for choosing their office. When discussing proposed treatment always speak directly to the patient, using the patient's name throughout the conversation. When possible, the doctor should walk the patient to the appointment area and again thank them for choosing their office. If the doctor is unable to walk the patient to the checkout area, appoint an assistant to accompany them. Do NOT allow the patient to wander the halls.

Doctors should not be reticent in asking the patient for a referral. They may have family or friends who are looking for a new practice. Patients often assume that your office is not accepting anyone new or that they require a referral from another doctor's office. Make it clear by virtue of asking for referrals that you are indeed open to growing your practice.

Once treatment is completed, the doctor can say "we are happy to see any of your friends or family members." This can be accomplished on the way to the reception area or during the end of a follow-up visit. The receptionist should also let the patient know that all of his or her referrals are welcome. And will be treated with the utmost care and professionalism. These third-party patients are worth their weight in gold…and, because the patient is referred to you, an automatic level of "trust" is transferred at NO additional marketing cost!

Referrals, whether from patients or doctors, are the mainstay of any practice. Both the doctor and staff must ensure that these important referrals make it onto the schedule in a timely fashion. Efforts to accommodate the new patient's schedule is a great first impression. If not possible, offer the most convenient and appropriate option. It is vital to the ultimate success of your practice that **all** referrals are seen.

14.2 External Marketing

External Marketing, as the name indicates, takes place outside of your office. It includes, but is not limited to, meetings with other professionals and referral sources, attendance at CE events and meetings, presentations and office visits to referring sources by your dedicated Marketing Professional.

Today, being a physician is as much business as it is art. Long gone are the days when a doctor can get by with an occasional breakfast or lunch with a referring doctor or donut runs to their office. Most offices take a very short lunch break and/or the doctors use this time to catch up on office or personal work.

Then, you have those times when you are running late with patients and emergencies and find it necessary to cancel at the last moment. It seems much easier to schedule breakfast meetings before your day with patients begins rather than lunches.

You, the Doctor, and CEO of your practice, as well as your staff need to develop relationships with your referring offices—be certain to nurture this relationship with both referring doctor AND his or her staff. Unfortunately, this cannot be accomplished with an occasional visit to said office. Consistent interactions with current and potential referrers are mandatory in order to obtain and maintain relationships with these referrers. Relationship-building is key. The relationships must be reciprocal and mutually beneficial. A win-win. It is important to remember that more often than not, the staff in the referring office initiates the referral.

Case in Point

Mrs. Jones is checking out of her Dentist's office. She's been a patient for quite some time and now brings her children for checkups. Her oldest is in need of an implant for a congenitally missing tooth. Mary at the front desk has watched Mrs. Jones' children grow up and the two are fellow soccer moms.

Mrs. Jones asks Mary to whom she takes her own children and to whom she would take them to have implant work done. Without missing a beat a referral (valuable third-party endorsement and instant trust) is passed between the two.

This happens daily. Be sure you form a strong alliance with the entire office staff.

The referring doctor may recommend that the patient have an implant placed and may give a referral name or names to the patient. Patients, however, will invariably ask the front desk or assistants for their recommendation. Patients are going to relate to the staff far more comfortably than their doctor. Be mindful of this, doctors. The staff will refer to the office with whom they have established a relationship or, with whom they chat at soccer, pilates, yoga, camping, etc. Think of this as "extended" marketing. And, there is no monetary cost for this benefit.

The use of a Marketing Professional will help you establish the necessary relationships that will ensure that your office thrives. Regular visits by the marketing professional will allow these relationships to develop into long-lasting relationships. The doctor must be involved in order to ensure that these relationships continue. The doctor's "buy-in" to the Marketing Plan sets a precedent as to how the Staff accepts the program. Without both doctor and staff buy-in, the relationships will wither and die [3]. Consistency is KEY. Do not think that a couple of visits or events cement the relationship. These days, the business of Implantology is quite competitive. In some cities, there are several offices offering dental implants within walking distance. Your referring offices ALWAYS have a choice as to with whom they work. Make sure it's YOUR practice they want to work with every day.

As discussed, external marketing involves marketing and Public Relations done outside of your office and includes social media. It encompasses any type or promotion done to extend or expand awareness of your practice brand. Creativity and thinking "outside of the box" is crucial.

Case in Point

Dr. O has a thriving practice with lots of referring fans. But, he knows he can expand. His problem is how to reach more potential patients without expending additional marketing dollars.

Dr. O comes up with a well-designed sticker. Every patient who sees the doctor is given this sticker. It's edgy and appealing and the patients LOVE it immediately. The goal is to be given one of these stickers after a successful visit. What began to happen is that those patients who had not yet been given a sticker began to ask for them. Many of these "I've been O'd" edge stickers showed up on car bumpers, Mom's water bottles, Soccer game treat bags…you get the idea. Dr. O's relatively inexpensive concept had gone viral. The stickers were photographed online and Instagrammed out daily. The photo with the best caption was put on FaceBook. His practice grew 23% in the first 120 days.

Get creative…the Yellow Book Phone Directory days are long dead.

One of the more successful concepts in external marketing that tends to be overlooked is continuing education. As doctors start and grow their practices, it becomes much more difficult to garner time to attend these events/classes. This is a PRIME opportunity for you to facilitate a continuing education or CE event and further cement your referral relationships. Many licensing agencies now require a certain number of CE hours. Practitioners are always looking for courses that will assist them in fulfilling these requirements. With the help of an experienced Marketing Professional you can make your office a prime provider of continuing education for referring offices.

Case in Point

Dr. T's offices enjoyed a large and very loyal referral base. But, they needed to generate consistent good will and value for their referring practices. The decision to host an evening "Implant CE" event for both doctors and staff was chosen. These are rare occasions in the field as an event such as this can be a bit of an investment.

My team created an event at a local Comedy Club. The venue was a rooftop high rise and difficult to get into without a contact. Utilizing our contacts, we added a couple of top-notch comedians to perform, had a light dinner and adult beverages prior to the CE portion of the evening. Attendance topped projections and the CE space expanded. To this day, buzz exists over this creative event.

Another version of this same theme is to offer Implant Education to the public (Fig. 14.4).

Invite patients that may need this type of treatment in the future. The key is: To make the presentation or event something people WANT to attend. Choose a spot that is the new "hot" spot…. have a trendy food truck for the meeting… use your local museum and reserve it for the evening. Be creative. Make an impact. Set your practice apart. The next step is to establish yourself as "the **short implant expert**" in your community. Be sure you are up-to-date on the latest techniques and applications for your practice. Have your "A Team" staff attend and chat with staffs of

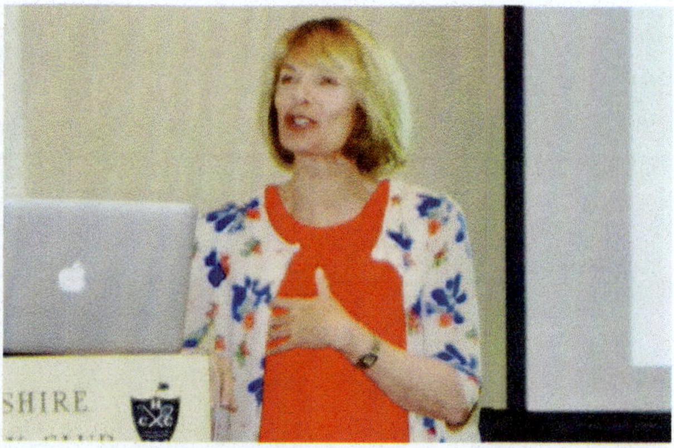

Fig. 14.4 Presentations to the public will increase your practice visibility

referring office. Establish strong relationships with your vendors. They will often assist with the cost of an event if asked (again, your marketing professional should have these contacts in place for you). Again, Short Implants can provide you with an incredible opportunity to set your practice apart from others in your community. Use this edge. While short and ultrashort implants have been around for over 40 years, many implant providers continue to offer only traditional length implants often combined with grafting thus adding unnecessary cost and potential risk. By incorporating short and ultra-short implants into your practice you have the opportunity to educate both your referring offices and your patients. Over the course of a few months and with a reasonable investment, you can become the resident expert.

The first step is to get your referring offices familiar and comfortable with short and ultrashort implants. All implant companies provide continuing education for their users and, the short implant companies are no exception. The implant companies are almost always ADA, AGD, and ACCME providers for continuing education credit. It may be possible for you to arrange a marketing partnership with the implant company thus reducing impact to your marketing budget. Often, the short implant companies are smaller operations and are more open to working with individual practitioners. This presents two great continuing education opportunities that you can use to introduce these implants to your referring offices (Fig. 14.5).

Opportunity #1 is to arrange to have a company sponsored speaker present to your referring doctors and staff. Staff should be included as they are often the people that patients will turn to with questions about recommended procedures.

When presenting these programs, it is important to obtain a venue that reflects the image that you want your practice to portray. You need to select a venue that has comfortable seating, good food/beverage offerings, and proper lighting for the presentation. The venue needs to be high end—think high quality production!

It is imperative that you provide current collateral materials containing information about short implants and your office. Be sure your staff (and ALL doctors attending the event have a good supply of their business cards). Provide good quality pens and pads (both bearing **YOUR** name, website, e-mail address and telephone number)—always with your logo imprinted. The Doctors, Marketing

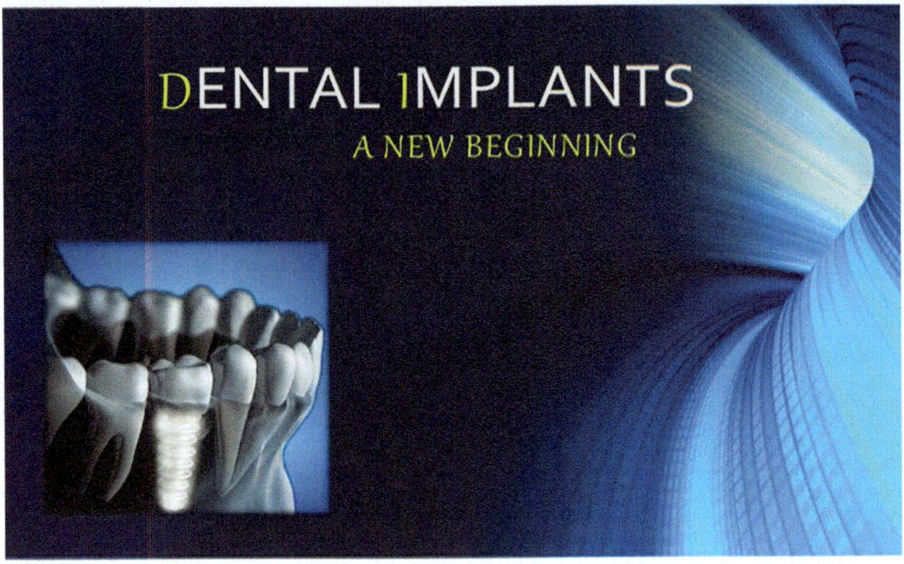

Fig. 14.5 Introductory lectures on short implants will assist in establishing you as the "resident expert" on short implants

Professional, and Staff should be in attendance throughout the presentation, greeting and talking with the guests. This is not the time for your staff to spend catching up on office gossip. Be clear with staff prior to the event that this is their practice too…when the practice grows, they reap the benefits as well. This is relationship building. Spend time getting to know your potential referral sources (and their staff). And yes, you must pay your Staff when they attend these events—they are working! There is nothing worse than having resentful staff at your event spreading malaise to your highest-value referrals sources.

The presentation should not be too lengthy. 2–3 hours tops with a scheduled break should be adequate. Depending on the timing you may want to consider providing a light dinner with the presentation starting as dessert is served.

Always provide a nice and continuing assortment of beverages. Those providers who are interested in further information about short implants will invariably want to talk with you and the speaker following the presentation. This presents you with a segue to **Opportunity #2.** If you have a large referral base, consider two or more presentations thus offering a choice of time and keeping the group to a more intimate size (under 25). It is imperative that both you and your marketing professional follow-up with attendees a short time after the presentation (I like my clients to follow up within 3 days while the experience of the meeting is still fresh).

Opportunity #2 presents itself after your initial introductory short implant presentation. Make arrangements with the implant company to invite a small group of the most interested/qualified referring or potential referral doctors to the implant company headquarters for a 2–3 day presentation.

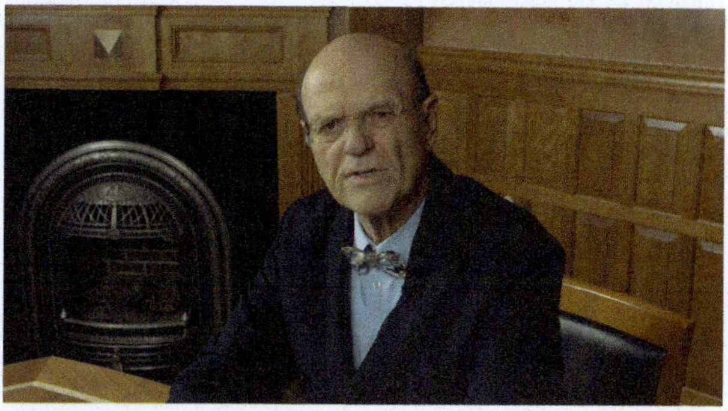

Fig. 14.6 Lectures by short implant experts will allow your referring doctors to obtain much needed CE credits

Case in Point

One of my clients, a large multilocation surgical practice chose to do this with an East Coast short implant company. The surgeons, along with my team, put together a curated a group of eight doctors who had shown great interest in short implants during a previous educational event. Some were existing referral offices, some potential offices. We went the extra mile and extended the invitation to their spouses and significant others as well. The short implant company agreed to provide flights for the doctors, hotels, breakfasts, lectures, and a couple of dinners. The surgeons paid for the spouses/SOs. Again, if you chose to promote in this fashion, do it well. Do not skimp!

The accidental added bonus to this particular trip was that a few of these doctors had never tasted Lobster. It made such a lasting impression that not only were the referral relationships cemented, but the event is STILL being talked about in the field. Again, added and FREE exposure. Do NOT underestimate the impact of these small, but important, details when setting up your event.

I cannot say this enough...reach out to your implant vendor and ask about collaborating events with them. Be clear when discussing your expectations about the financial portion of your relationship (Fig. 14.6).

Most implant companies present programs regularly at or near their headquarters and have arrangements with nearby hotels for reduced rates. You should arrange for transportation to the locale—flights, trains, etc.—and dedicated transfers to the hotel—this is critical, do not leave your referring doctors wandering around an airport looking for the taxi stand or arranging their own ride share. Do **NOT** expect these potential referring professionals to arrive late at night and awake early the following morning for presentations. Be respectful of their time and needs. They represent a large potential gain for your business. Remember, you are building a relationship**… not creating a "drive through" opportunity**.

You are the host. From the time you leave your city, to the time you arrive at the destination. Do **NOT** coordinate personal side trips and social visits…. this is a **WORKING** trip. ALL of your time and attention belong to the doctors and implant company. PERIOD. Working with the implant company, you should arrange dinners and a special event—think about a concert, sporting event, or unique tour.

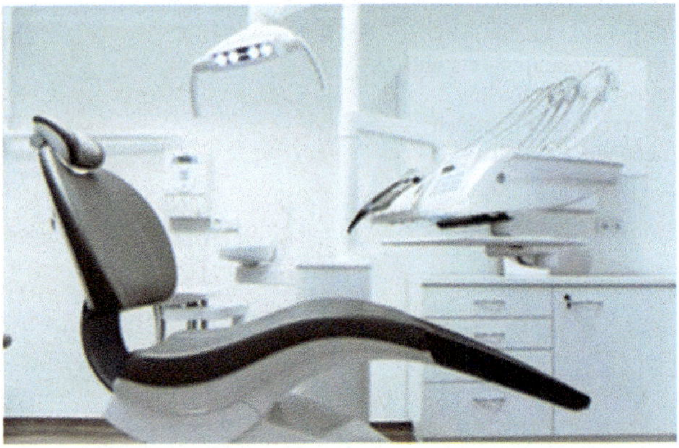

Fig. 14.7 Be aggressive in marketing your short implant practice not just when your chairs are empty. Marketing is a full-time venture. **Due to the nature of marketing and relationships in the field, your best bet for consistent patient flow is to market when your practice is at its busiest**

This is not the time to be frugal. If you plan and execute well, the return on investment will be significant as you become known as "the expert" on short and ultrashort implants. Take some time to consider what your visitors may want to do in your location. Join them and work on the relationship—not solely on business (Fig. 14.7).

14.3 Social Media

In the past decade, the integration of social media has become a **critical part of marketing** a practice [4]. It is important that your practice utilize social media platforms [5]. I would encourage you **to launch with two platforms** and expand once you have your brand established. You need to give thought to the type of platform you are going to launch. If you have **great photos and tag lines from events, patients, etc. use Instagram.** If you just want to **shoot small notes out about new technology or upcoming events, use Twitter**. Trying to get four or five different social platforms going at once may not be the most effective manner in which to promote your practice. Having a **polished and professional website is critical** but, it's not the only platform that you should be using to market your practice. This chapter is not meant to be a tutorial on social media—complete books are dedicated to this! The use of social media, however, is certainly a **place where the practitioner can showcase their expertise with short implants**.

Case in Point

Dr. M has just had his website updated and is excited about integrating Social Media. He selects ALL platforms to launch. He feels his office manager can handle updating and maintaining the platforms. She agrees…somewhat reluctantly.

Two months later, Dr. M has a free moment and decides to take a peek at his exciting new Social Media platforms. His jaw drops…only two have been done and the things that have been posted are NOT what he envisioned in promoting his practice.

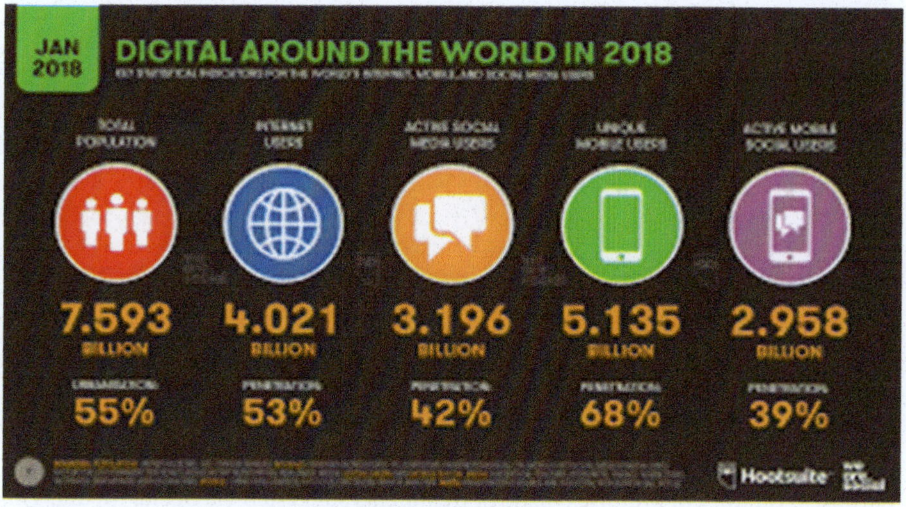

Fig. 14.8 The world is increasingly becoming digitally connected

The take-away here is that it is your practice…your license…your personality and corporate culture. Be involved…be a part of the training and setting the level of expectation when assigning someone to the task.

Needless to say, Dr. M scrapped his first attempt at Social Media and will have to begin again. He's lost both time and money. You MUST have a plan! (Fig. 14.8)

One of the biggest mistakes that professionals make with social media is inconsistency [6]. Post a mix of three or four topics that represent your personality and practice. Be sure that YOU are involved in the selection of content. You may get a shock if you leave it entirely up to a staff member. Make sure **the colors and branding are on point**—whether it is on the website, blogs or, on a platform such as Instagram. **Consistent posting** is critical to marketing your practice. Be sure it reflects your personality. People work with people they like…an old adage, but absolutely true! Appoint one person beside the doctor who will be in charge of social media posting. In an extremely busy practice, you may have to hire a specific person to be in charge of social media or have social media monitoring and posting as a part of the contract with the Marketing Professional. Be certain that **EVERY** comment is responded to**… every. single. day**. You cannot build following without engaging your viewers. If you don't respond, someone else will… (Fig. 14.9).

Your knowledge and use of short implants allow for a wealth of information to be placed on social media—for both referring offices and potential patients.

Consistent blogging—as little as once each week—that mentions short implants will help the practice establish itself as the expert on this technology. Instagram is a strong medium in which to promote your website and blog. Be sure your content supports your knowledge of short implants. Perhaps an invitation or give-away relevant to this exciting technology could be promoted. If you have a patient who has had incredible results, ask them to sign a Release and use their photos for posting

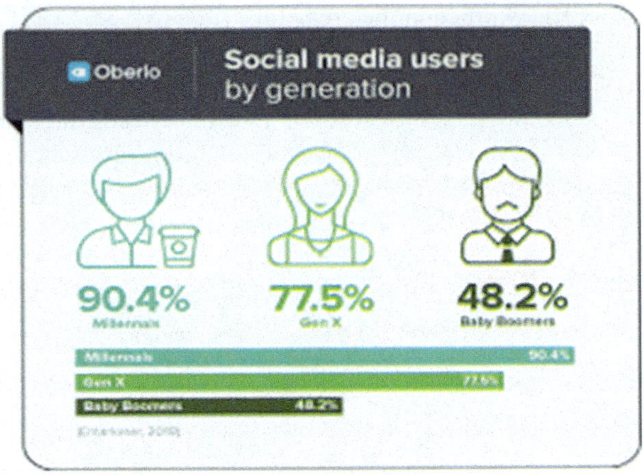

Fig. 14.9 **Know** your target demographic. Social Media usage differs dramatically between age groups and generations

purposes. Be wary of promises made or treatments suggested via Social Media. This medium is too new to know the full implication of treatment or assessment online. Social media offers an arena in which you can share educational opportunities. You can reach thousands of people with little impact to your marketing budget with Social Media. It becomes much more difficult to satisfy your continuing education requirements once you run a practice. Most states have minimums that have to be satisfied in a calendar year.

Most of all, make it easy for your referral sources to contact you. Be sure to include your contact information in a clear and concise manner. You **ARE** the expert in the field. As word spreads, your expertise in the field will widen. Elevate your practice by utilizing this cutting-edge technology.

Marketing a practice is not a sprint. Once you have developed your marketing plan/strategy, you can expect that it will take 4–6 months before you begin to see consistent results. It is important that the office track their referrals particularly with respect to short implants. You must know who is sending you patients and, more importantly, know when those referrals drop off.

Case in Point

I've seen very consistent referring offices disappear without reason. Should this occur with your practice, you, the surgeon should reach out to the referring doctor and arrange a meeting that works for both schedules.

I find that in the rush of running a practice, personal and family responsibilities and good old fashioned misunderstandings…you can lose business over absolutely nothing. Nurture these relationships. They are the life's blood of a successful and consistently growing short implant practice.

Another important consideration in marketing is to track those patients that arrive without a referral. How did they hear about you? Make sure their feedback is noted in their file.

The use of short implants is not a quick cure but, it can be a valuable tool in the growth and exposure of your practice. You may find that patients have heard about you from a new office in the area. Take time to reach out to the new doctor both by telephone and hand-written note. This kind of follow-up should take place within 3 days after the new patient has been seen. Again, cultivate these valuable relationships.

In summation, the hiring of an experienced Marketing Company is not inexpensive but, the return on your investment in terms of goodwill in the field and new relationships will make it well worthwhile. Be patient, work the Marketing Plan, and reap the benefits! Take the time to interview a variety of marketing companies. Be very clear in conveying exactly what your expectations are in terms of exposure and responsibilities. Set a budget. Empower the marketing company to implement the plan. Do not micromanage. Stay abreast of progress or concerns by having regular meetings. Most of my clients hold weekly meetings after patients to discuss findings in the field or concerns with referring offices.

Enjoy your short implant growth and prosperity.

References

1. Managing the practice American Academy of Pediatrics Newsletter 2018.
2. Hupp J. The importance of branding. J Oral Maxillofac Surg. 2019;77:1525–6.
3. Cafiero MR, et al Professional marketing strategies to staff, administrators and peers. J Wound Ostomy Continence Nurs. 2009; 30.
4. Smith A, Anderson M. Social media use in 2018. Washington, DC: Pew Research Center—Internet and Technology.
5. Social Barometer Report Hootsuite 2018.
6. Lister M. 40 Essential social media marketing strategies for 2018. The Wordstream Blog; 2018.

The manufacturer's authorised representative in the EU is Springer Nature Customer Service Centre GmbH, Europaplatz 3, 69115 Heidelberg, Germany. If you have any concerns regarding our products, please contact ProductSafety@springernature.com

Printed and bound by CPI Group (UK) Ltd, Croydon, CR0 4YY
30/09/2026
02225454-0009